AIDS and IV DRUG ABUSERS
Current Perspectives [B]

AIDS

AIDS and
IV
DRUG
ABUSERS

Current Perspectives

Edited by Robert P. Galea, PhD,
Benjamin F. Lewis, EdD, and
Lori A. Baker, MA

NHP National Health Publishing

AIDS and IV Drug Abusers: Current Perspectives is dedicated
to the clients of Spectrum House, Inc.

Contents

Contributors

Steven L. Batki, M.D.
Assistant Clinical Professor of Psychiatry, University of California at San Francisco; Medical Director, Substance Abuse Services, San Francisco General Hospital, San Francisco, California

Caroline Butkus-Small, M.D.
Department of Medicine, New York Medical College; Division of Infectious Disease, Westchester County Medical Center, Valhalla, New York

Joseph E. Caffrey, C.S.W.
Daytop Village, Inc., Parksville/Swan Lake Facilities, New York

James R. Carlson, Ph.D.
Department of Pathology, University of California, Davis, California

Kenneth G. Castro, M.D.
Medical Epidemiologist, AIDS Program, Center for Infectious Diseases, Centers for Disease Control, Public Health Service, U.S. Department of Health and Human Services, Atlanta, Georgia

Richard E. Chaisson, M.D.
Instructor in Medicine, University of California, San Francisco; AIDS Epidemiology Group, San Francisco General Hospital, San Francisco, California

Grace Christ, M.S.W.
Director, Social Work Department, Memorial Sloan-Kettering Cancer Center, New York

Mary Ann Cohen, M.D.
Director, Consultation-Liaison Psychiatry, Metropolitan Hospital Center, New York Medical College, New York

Robert L. Cohen, M.D.

Rikers Island Health Services; Department of Epidemiology and Social Medicine, Montefiore Medical Center, Bronx, New York; Albert Einstein College of Medicine, Bronx, New York

Charles P. Cox, M.A.

Department of Epidemiology and Social Medicine, Montefiore Medical Center, Bronx, New York; Albert Einstein College of Medicine, Bronx, New York

James W. Curran, M.D., M.P.H.

Director, AIDS Program, Center for Infectious Diseases, Centers for Disease Control, Public Health Service, U.S. Department of Health and Human Services, Atlanta, Georgia

William Darrow, Ph.D.

AIDS Activity Center for Infectious Diseases, Centers for Disease Control, Atlanta, Georgia

Don C. Des Jarlais, Ph.D.

Division of Substance Abuse Services and Phoenix House Research Department, New York

James W. Dilley, M.D.

Director, AIDS Health Project, San Francisco, California

Cheryl Feiner, M.P.H.

Division of Biostatistics, Montefiore Medical Center, Bronx, New York; Albert Einstein College of Medicine, Bronx, New York

Paul M. Feorino, Ph.D.

Division of Viral Diseases and Host Factors, Center for Infectious Diseases, Centers for Disease Control, Atlanta, Georgia

Donald P. Francis, M.D., D.Sc.

Division of Viral Diseases and Host Factors, Center for Infectious Disease Control, Atlanta, Georgia

John French, M.A.
New Jersey State Department of Health, Trenton, New Jersey

Gerald H. Friedland, M.D.
Associate Professor, Department of Medicine, Montefiore Medical Center, Bronx, New York

Samuel R. Friedman, Ph.D.
Narcotic and Drug Research, Inc., New York

Patricia N. Fultz, Ph.D.
Divisions of Viral Diseases and Host Factors, Center for Infectious Diseases, Centers for Disease Control, Atlanta, Georgia

Robert P. Galea, Ph.D.
President, Spectrum House, Inc., Westboro, Massachusetts

Jane P. Getchell, Ph.D.
Division of Viral Diseases and Host Factors, Center for Infectious Diseases, Centers for Disease Control, Atlanta, Georgia

Harold M. Ginzburg, M.D., J.D., M.P.H.
Chief, Epidemiology Branch, AIDS Program/NIAID/NIH, Bethesda, Maryland

Larry Gostin, J.D.
Senior Research Fellow, Faculty of Public Health, Harvard University; Counsel, Warner and Stackpole, Boston, Massachusetts

George F. Grady, M.D.
State Epidemiologist, Assistant Commissioner of the Massachusetts Department of Public Health

Ann M. Hardy, Dr.P.H.
Medical Epidemiologist, AIDS Program for Infectious Diseases, Centers for Disease Control, Public Health Service, U.S. Department of Health and Human Services, Atlanta, Georgia

Carol Harris, M.D.
Division of Infectious Diseases, Department of Medicine, Montefiore Medical Center, Bronx, New York

Peter I. Hartsock, Dr.P.H.
National Institute on Drug Abuse, Alcohol, Drug Abuse and Mental Health Administration, Rockville, Maryland

William Hopkins, M.A.
New York State Division of Substance Abuse Services and Narcotic and Drug Research, New York

Harold W. Jaffe, M.D.
Division of Viral Diseases and Host Factors, Center for Infectious Diseases, Centers for Disease Control, Atlanta, Georgia

Nancy Jainchill, M.A.
Division of Substance Abuse Services; Phoenix House Research Department, New York

Robert S. Klein, M.D.
Division of Infectious Diseases, Department of Medicine, Montefiore Medical Center, Bronx, New York

Benjamin F. Lewis, M.S.W., Ed.D.
Director of Planning and Evaluation, Spectrum House, Inc. Westboro, Massachusetts

Carl Lipshutz, M.A.
Rikers Island Health Services; Montefiore Medical Center, Bronx, New York

Mhairi Graham MacDonald, M.B.Ch.B., F.R.C.P.(E.), D.C.H.
Children's Hospital National Medical Center, George Washington University School of Medicine and Health Sciences, Washington, D.C.

J. Steven McDougall, M.D.
Divisions of Viral Diseases and Host Factors, Center for Infectious Disease, Centers for Disease Control, Atlanta, Georgia

Bernice Moll, Ph.D.
Division of Immunopathology, Department of Pathology, Montefiore Medical Center, Bronx, New York; Albert Einstein College of Medicine, Bronx, New York

W. Mead Morgan, Ph.D.
Chief, Statistics and Data Management Branch, AIDS Program, Center for Infectious Diseases, Centers for Disease Control, Atlanta, Georgia

Andrew R. Moss, Ph.D.
Department of Epidemiology and International Health, University of California, San Francisco, California

Rosemary T. Moynihan, M.S.W.
Director, AIDS Support Project; Assistant Director, Social Work Department, Memorial Sloan-Kettering Cancer Center, New York

Stuart E. Nichols, M.D.
Associate Chief, Medical and Psychiatric Services, Methadone Maintenance Treatment Program, Beth Israel Medical Center; Senior Instructor in Psychiatry, Mt. Sinai School of Medicine, City University of New York, New York

Herbet N. Ochitill, M.D.
San Francisco General Hospital, San Francisco, California

Robin Onishi, M.D.
Department of Epidemiology and International Health, University of California, San Francisco, California

Dennis Osmond, M.A.
Department of Epidemiology and International Health, University of California, San Francisco, California

Mark Perl, M.B.B.S.
San Francisco General Hospital, San Francisco, California

Ross Robak, Ph.D.
Supervising Psychologist at Parksville/Swan Lake, Daytop Village, Inc., New York

Peter A. Selwyn, M.D.
Department of Epidemiology and Social Medicine, Montefiore Medical Center; Albert Einstein College of Medicine, Bronx, New York

Earl E. Shelp, Ph.D.
Assistant Professor of Medical Ethics, Baylor College of Medicine, Waco, Texas

Daniel Shine, M.D.
Department of Social Medicine, University of California, San Francisco, California

Karolynn Siegel, M.D.
Director of Research, Department of Social Work, Memorial Sloan-Kettering Research Center, New York

Jo L. Sotheran, M.A.
Data Analyst, Narcotic and Drug Research, Inc., New York

Paul A. Volberding, M.D.
San Francisco General Hospital, San Francisco, California

Lori S. Weiner, M.S.W.
Staff Social Worker, Memorial Sloan-Kettering Cancer Center, New York

Henry Weisman, M.D.
Associate Director of Consultation-Liaison Psychiatry, Metropolitan Hospital Center, New York Medical College, New York

Foreword

Since 1981, more than 44,395 cases of Acquired Immuno-deficiency Syndrome (AIDS) have been reported in the United States. Although this fatal disease was first discovered only six years ago, it has attracted more attention and more controversy than any other illness of our time. There still is no cure for AIDS; despite on-going research, AIDS remains, for the most part, scientifically – as well as socially – frustrating. Although knowledge of AIDS virology, epidemiology, and transmission has grown, researchers estimate that an effective vaccine for this disease may not exist until well into the next decade.

Some of the most promising developments in limiting the spread of the Human Immunodeficiency Virus (HIV), the virus that causes AIDS, lie within the realm of health education. Such efforts under-taken by the homosexual and bisexual communities of San Francis-co, for example, have lead to reductions in self-reported high risk sexual behaviors among sexually active homosexual and bisexual men, as well as a reduction in the reported rates of other sexually transmitted diseases. AIDS education has become a growing con-cern among heterosexuals, as well, being incorporated more often in sex education curricula in the public schools. Despite these trends, AIDS education remains controversial; it is not yet widespread.

For intravenous drug abusers, who are the focus of this volume, AIDS education is even more complex. Many of the activities of in-travenous drug abusers are illegal, and for this reason state and federal support of measures aimed at limiting the spread of HIV among this population (such as the distribution of free, "clean" need-les to prevent needle sharing) has been limited. Because drug abusers have, stereotypically, been viewed as incapable of change, members of the general public – and even some professionals who work with intravenous drug abusers – remain skeptical of efforts to educate them regarding this syndrome. It is indeed true that there are barriers to effective AIDS education among intravenous drug abusers. Some IV drug abusers, for example, have literacy problems, making written educational materials of limited effectiveness in reaching them. The long latency period associated with HIV infec-tions makes AIDS a distant threat in comparison to the immediacy of symptoms of withdrawal, or to the other illnesses and dangers associated with drug abuse. Further, needle-sharing among intravenous drug abusers is a deeply ingrained form of social behavior which may be difficult to influence, even if free, sterile needles were made available to intravenous drug abusers on a regular basis.

Despite such difficulties, the research collected in this volume indicates that intravenous drug abusers are both aware of their high-risk for AIDS and receptive to educational interventions. Effective AIDS education for intravenous drug abusers has already begun in such key cities as New York and San Francisco. In order for these efforts to be effective, both the public and those medical and mental health practitioners who work directly with intravenous drug abusers must look beyond stereotypes and recognize that, while change may be difficult for members of this high-risk group, it is far from impossible. Presently the spread of HIV among this population also has a critical impact on the transmission of HIV to other, non-drug abusing heterosexuals.

Despite the fact that one quarter of the cases of AIDS reported in the United States occur among intravenous drug abusers, the vast majority of research published is concerned with other risk groups — sexually active homosexual/bisexual men, or hemophiliacs.

AIDS and IV Drug Abusers: Current Perspectives is the first volume devoted exclusively to addressing the various social, psychological, medical, ethical and epidemiological dimensions of HIV infection and AIDS among intravenous drug abusers. The editors of this volume are researchers and mental health professionals who have compiled these papers in recognition of the lack of information and resources available on HIV infection and AIDS in members of this risk group. For those professionals currently providing treatment to intravenous drug abusers, this book will prove an invaluable resource—the first step towards a comprehensive education on the issues surrounding AIDS in intravenous drug abusers.

Don C. Des Jarlais
Division of Substance Abuse Services

New York
November, 1987

Acknowledgements

The editors would like to thank David Mulligan, Director of Substance Abuse Services, Divisions of Alcoholism and Drug Rehabilitation, and Thomas Salmon, Assistant Commissioner, Bureau of Community Health Services, Massachusetts Department of Public Health; John Sullivan, M.D., Professor of Pediatrics, University of Massachusetts Medical School, Worcester; and Jane McCusker, M.D., Dr.P.H., Associate Professor, Epidemiology Division of Public Health, University of Massachusetts at Amherst, for their help and advice in bringing together these papers. We would also like to thank Lisa Johnson and Teresa M. Simoneau of the Northeastern University Department of Journalism for their hard work in preparing the manuscript; John Russo, M.S., computer consultant; and the Spectrum House, Inc., Board of Trustees for their support during this project.

Research for some of the articles presented in this book was supported, in whole or in part, by grants from the following: The National Institute of Allergy and Infectious Diseases, National Institutes of Health (Chapter 7); the state of California and the University of California's University-wide Task Force on AIDS (Chapter 8); The National Institute on Drug Abuse (Chapters 9 and 18); The New York State Division of Substance Abuse Services (Chapter 9); and the New York State Department of Health AIDS Institute (Chapter 19).

Introduction

Never before in this century has a disease challenged both the health and identity of western society as gravely as has acquired immunodeficiency syndrome (AIDS). There are now approximately 44,395 cases of AIDS in the United States, and researchers have estimated that as many as 2 million individuals in this country may have been exposed to the virus. As yet, there exists no cure or effective treatment to slow the course of the illness or to prolong with certainty the lives of AIDS patients. AIDS is an anomaly in a society which has come to expect miracles from medical science; because the only certain means of prevention are changes in specific behaviors (particularly sexual behaviors), AIDS exposes to question both our scientific knowledge and behavioral freedoms that have long been taken for granted.

In her book *Illness as Metaphor*, writer Susan Sontag discusses the "mythologizing" of illnesses of unknown etiology; specifically, she talks of tuberculosis and cancer as diseases which have taken on symbolic meanings because their cause or cure was unknown to medical science. Much of what Sontag says applies to AIDS, especially after the discovery of the first cases of the disease among gay men in 1981. In the beginning, AIDS (originally known as "GRID," Gay-Related Immune Disorder) was a disease of socially outcast groups: homosexual and bisexual men, intravenous (IV) drug users, and Haitian immigrants. It appeared to be a disease of retribution, a punishment for behaviors viewed as "taboo" by mainstream society. As Sontag says:

> Nothing is more punitive than to give a disease a meaning—that meaning being invariably a moralistic one. Any disease whose causality is murky, and for which treatment is ineffectual, tends to be awash in significance ... Feelings about evil are projected onto a disease. And the disease (so enriched with meanings) is projected onto the world. [1977, pp. 57-58]

When disease is viewed as punishment, inevitably the patient is blamed for his or her illness and denied the support that is typically given to the terminally ill. In the case of AIDS, societal prejudice against the groups affected by the disease resulted in a slowing of research; in fact, only in the past year, as awareness has grown that AIDS is not merely an illness of select groups, has the United States government provided funding for intensive research efforts.

Although the prejudice against AIDS sufferers has changed with increased research and media attention, there is still a stigma – a sense of deserved punishment – attached to an AIDS diagnosis or a positive test for human immunodeficiency virus (HIV) antibody. That stigma is such that patients are reluctant to seek treatment for AIDS, and some of those who might test positive for exposure to the virus avoid testing out of fear that they will be discriminated against in seeking jobs, housing, schooling, or insurance. As Sontag says, "Patients who are instructed that they have, unwittingly, caused their disease are being made to feel that they have deserved it." [1977, p. 56]

Efforts to minimize the prejudice against AIDS patients have mobilized professionals working in a variety of fields; the collaboration of medical and social scientists is a vital factor in slowing the transmission of HIV, the virus that causes AIDS. Clinicians as well as researchers, in medicine and mental health, must confront the problems of treating AIDS patients and prevent the further spread of the disease. Educators, whether in public schools or in substance abuse treatment programs, are challenged with the task of effectively spurring behavior change. Even the media has a part to play in AIDS prevention: from responsible reporting in both print and television to allowing controversial advertising geared towards AIDS prevention (e.g., condom advertisements that now air on certain television networks).

Many of the substantive challenges of AIDS prevention currently face professionals in the field of substance abuse. According to the findings of many researchers – including several of those whose work appears in *AIDS and IV Drug Abusers: Current Perspectives* – the IV drug user is the most likely link for the transmission of AIDS to nondrug-using heterosexuals. Currently, there are 5,565 cases of AIDS in IV drug users in this country; there are 1,270 cases in other heterosexuals, of which up to 73% are associated with the sexual transmission of AIDS from an IV drug user. Approximately 50% of the 444 children with AIDS have an IV drug user as a parent (Centers for Disease Control 1987). Given the fact that many IV drug users, both male and female, work as prostitutes to finance their drug habit, the potential for the further spread of HIV by members of this population exists. Therefore, educational intervention with IV drug users could profoundly influence the further course of AIDS transmission. Unfortunately, many professionals in substance abuse treatment harbor a popular prejudice about IV drug users; i.e., that they are unlikely to take the time to acquire a clean needle or to refrain from sharing needles at the time of "shooting up." The sharing of needles among IV drug users is a ritual in the IV drug-using subculture and may be difficult to discourage, since drug users may view refusal to share needles as endangering their most important friendships (Friedman, Des Jarlais, and Sotheran, 1986).

The researchers and clinicians who have contributed their work to *AIDS and IV Drug Abusers: Current Perspectives* make a number of findings about this "high-risk" population. For example, researchers have found that the majority of IV drug users "on the street" know that their needle-sharing behavior puts them at risk for AIDS; they are also able to successfully name at least one or two AIDS symptoms. Self-reported behavior change also seems common; many IV drug users are now cleaning their needles and sharing needles less. A few have stopped using drugs altogether. Some have extended their precautions to include "safe sex," such as the use of condoms. Clearly, such findings among IV drug users who are not in treatment contradict the theory that IV drug users are unable to change.

Similarly, surveys of drug addicts undergoing substance abuse treatment have found relatively high levels of knowledge about AIDS. However, one study has shown that while 80% of these clients feel that their own previous behavior may have placed them at risk for AIDS, 85% still felt that they would not have the self-control to refrain from shooting up with a dirty needle (Lewis and Galea 1986).

Because drug abuse is regarded by society as a deviant behavior – and because AIDS is widely perceived as a disease caused by excessive or deviant sexual behavior – the IV drug abuser with AIDS faces many difficulties usually spared the terminally ill. AIDS patients, in general, are often denied support by their families and friends, and many drug users are already alienated from their families. Those who are indigent have neither insurance nor resources to cover the costs of their health care. In addition, they may be reluctant to seek medical treatment because of their distrust for and alienation from the health care system. And, unlike sexually active gay and bisexual men with AIDS, IV drug users do not have a community from which they can draw support.

The epidemiology of AIDS is a pivotal aspect of the understanding of the various dimensions of the disease.

Epidemiology, which is the study of disease occurrence and patterns in groups of humans, focuses on etiology and prevention. These efforts in turn can responsibly inform and educate those who allocate fiscal resources and those involved in clinical practice.

A basic concept in epidemiology is that more than one factor contributes to the occurrence of a disease. Thus, understanding of the multiple factors that lead to HIV infection in an IV drug-abusing population, such as the tradition of needle-sharing, is critical to the activities that might be taken to reduce risk behaviors associated with risk of HIV infection.

The epidemiology of AIDS presents numerous complexities, problems, and challenges. These are in the areas of the geography of the virus, i.e., outbreaks in different areas of the world based on different modes of transmission, the prevalence of HIV infection, AIDS-related complex (ARC) and AIDS, and the implications of these considerations for intervention and consequent curtailment of the spread of HIV infection.

The epidemiology of AIDS involves both qualitative and quantitative issues. Epidemiology requires that groups of people be described and compared in a quantitative fashion. Quantitative terms, such as counts, proportions and rates, prevalence rates, and incidence and case fatality rates, are important in measuring and describing groups of people affected by AIDS. These terms are defined in the Glossary.

Clearly, accurately counting HIV-infected individuals in an IV drug-using population is problematic since: (1) there are no hard statistics that identify who, what, and where IV drug abusers are— only speculative and impressionistic appraisals are available which may under- or overestimate IV drug use; (2) testing, when available, may not be utilized by this population; (3) reporting of "counts" tends to be in discrete pockets of infection rather than for all IV drug abusers; and (4) reporting of HIV seropositivity is problematic in that it is subject to constraints involving confidentiality of cases and duplicative reporting, i.e., a positive which is retested (not an unusual situation) may be reflected as two, three, or more separate HIV-positive individuals.

Two types of quantitative measures, prevalence rates and incidence rates, are commonly used in the articles in this book.

Prevalence describes a group at a certain point in time, such as a given day or month. It is a static measure. The prevalence of HIV in a particular population may be 8%, based on blood samples drawn and analyzed in June 1987. The prevalence might be different in January 1988. For example, the prevalence of HIV antibody in a sample of IV drug abusers in New York City increased from 11% in 1977 to 27% in 1979 to 58% in 1984. *Incidence* describes the rate of development of a disease in a specific group over a time span and the continuing occurrence of new cases. Prevalence addresses all cases.

Other factors which have impact on the epidemiology of diseases like AIDS have to do with disease identification, reporting, and follow-up. Since traditionally, drug addicts are not seen as being particularly concerned about their health, and because many of the early symptoms of ARC/AIDS are similar to those experienced by individuals in various stages of withdrawal from opiates, and because of the threat of death for IV drug addicts from their often criminal lifestyle and from overdose, the identification and reporting of AIDS cases in this population are problematic. This is compounded by the fact that reported AIDS cases among IV drug abusers may go untreated and therefore are lost to reporting of treatment outcomes and perhaps ultimately to mortality statistics. Suicidal drug overdoses are becoming more common, and the inability of drug addicts to have access to health resources compounds the limitations of reporting even under the best of circumstances (Massachusetts Department of Public Health 1987).

Epidemiology also concerns itself with a study of relationships of variables to one another in its attempt to describe groups. In this regard, yet another barrier is placed in the way of uncomplicated study of the occurrence of HIV, ARC/AIDS among IV drug abusers. Information-gathering and observation often encounter a high nonresponse rate among a population which engages in illegal activities and surfaces primarily at brief encounters with the criminal justice or treatment community. Based on the consequences of their drug use, one can anticipate both inconsistent and/or otherwise unreliable data.

Finally, as with all diseases, idiosyncratic aspects of the individuals and groups affected often cannot be quantified. Anecdotal aspects of transmission and treatment are a very human and often critical dimension to the epidemiology of AIDS among IV drug abusers.

Descriptive and analytic studies of the epidemiology of this disease in the population of IV drug abusers are in their infancy. The articles in this book reflect various perspectives and problems encountered in epidemiological studies of an IV drug-abusing population. What seems to be clear, however, in spite of the methodological problems that are encountered in epidemiological studies of HIV infection in this population, is that the threat and reality of HIV infection/ARC/AIDS on a population of IV drug abusers are contributing in a critical manner to the way which addicts view their lifestyle and changes that they must make to avoid HIV infection.

With these epidemiological rules and constraints in mind, we now focus on some specific aspects of the epidemiology of AIDS as they pertain to IV drug abusers and members of their social networks.

Based on Centers for Disease Control surveillance reporting for the week of Sept. 21, 1987, individuals with only IV drug abuse as a factor in infection transmission numbered 6,147 with 1,290 or 21% female and 4,857 or 79% male. Overall, this category represents 14.8% of all reported cases of AIDS.

When one combines the risk factor of IV drug abuse with homosexual (gay and/or bisexual) activity, 2,933 or 7.1% of all reported cases, the total rises to 9,080. When all other multiple risk factor cases with IV drug use as a factor are looked at, the cumulative total of reported AIDS cases as of September 1987 with IV drug abuse is 9,982 or 24% of all reported AIDS cases.

Because of the prevalence of drug abuse in prostitutes, of cases that fall into the heterosexual transmission categories, it is likely that a significant percentage have IV drug use as one factor in transmission. Of 456 children who have been born with AIDS, it is believed that 53% have been born of mothers where IV drug abuse was the primary transmission factor (Friedman, Des Jarlais, and Sotheran, 1986).

When one looks at transmission categories by racial/ethnic group, one finds the following: total racial/ethnic distribution of reported AIDS cases is 25,452 or 61% white, not Hispanic; 10,022 or

24% black, not Hispanic; 5,733 or 14% Hispanic; and 395 or 1% other/unknown. Where the only transmission factor is IV drug abuse: 1,321 or 19% of reported AIDS cases are white, not Hispanic; 3,473 or 51% are black, not Hispanic; 2,020 or 29% are Hispanic; and 39 or .57% are other/unknown.

Prevalence of HIV in an IV drug-abusing population varies from region to region and city to city within regions, with some areas far from transmission vectors having virtually no identified cases among IV drug abusers and locations close to the New York City, northern New Jersey area, where prevalence rates among various IV drug-abusing subpopulations range from 50% to 60% (Des Jarlais, Jainchill, and Friedman, 1986). It is widely believed, based on epidemiologic studies of hepatitis B-infected parenteral drug abusers and studies of the prevalence of HIV in New York City, San Francisco, and other areas (Novick, Kreek, Des Jarlais in press), that once introduced, the virus spreads at a geometric rate among IV drug abusers in large part due to the prevalence of sharing contaminated needles, at risk sexual behaviors and prostitution, and the "incestuous" circles that addicts tend to "shoot" in. Exhibit I-1

Exhibit I-1
AIDS Cases in the United States
May 18, 1987
(N = 35,518)

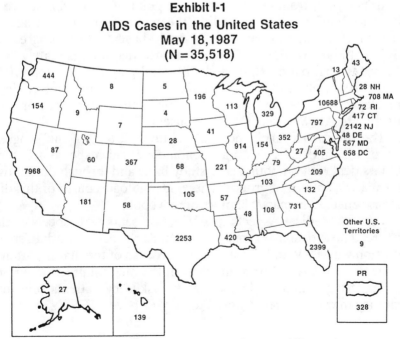

AIDS cases by state of residence at onset of illness.

presents AIDS cases by state of residence and exhibit I-2 by date of diagnosis and standard metropolitan statistical area of residence.

The number of cases of AIDS and case fatality rates by half year of diagnosis in the United States are presented in Chapter 3.

While the actual number of AIDS cases that are related to IV drug abuse cannot be specifically identified, based on the consistency of data available to date, approximately 25% can be "deemed" to involve IV drug abuse.

The projections to 1991 presented in the Morgan and Curran article (see Afterword) do not take premorbid, current and prospective education and treatment interventions into consideration, but research studies of risk reduction activities in the gay and sexually active bisexual category of transmission (Emmons et al. 1986) suggest that risk reduction interventions initiated in the past 3 to 5 years will have the result of reducing the incidence of cases in this segment of the population. Notwithstanding interventions among IV drug abusers which began later and which must overcome social traditions as well as addictive behavior, the rate at which cases among IV drug abusers will grow over the next 5 years will place this group in a disproportionately large segment of AIDS cases.

In addition, from an epidemiologic point of view, while there is no current information regarding the number and percentage of cases of HIV infection among IV drug abusers which progress to ARC or full-blown AIDS, a study indicates that approximately 34% of gay/bisexual patients infected with HIV go on to develop AIDS in 3 years (Polk 1987). The editors are currently involved in a prevalence study which includes looking at the progression of HIV infection to AIDS among IV drug abusers.

The prevalence, incidence, and natural history of the progression of HIV, ARC/AIDS is a phenomenon which the contributing authors deal with on both a case study basis and through descriptive and analytic studies of groups. The epidemiologic course of this disease is reflected in many chapters of this book.

Part I, "Medical Aspects of AIDS," presents two aspects of the disease. The article by Francis et al. details the actual mechanism of infection with HIV and the subsequent course of the illness. Grady's article discusses AIDS from the view of the medical practitioner, including the questions a doctor may be asked by patients who fear that they may have been exposed to HIV or have AIDS.

In Part II, "AIDS Epidemiology and Drug Abuse," the editors have selected contributions that examine more intensively the spread of AIDS virus among the various risk groups and, in particular, among IV drug abusers. The article by Castro, Hardy, and Curran gives a national perspective on the distribution of cases of AIDS. Ginzburg and MacDonald break down the pattern of transmission by a number of factors, including race, gender, and east- and west-coast comparisons. They also present a study comparing drug-use patterns of IV drug users with AIDS and a cohort of drug abusers participating in the Treatment Outcome Prospective Study, finding that many of the subjects who participated in the study may be at risk for developing AIDS as a result of their high-risk behaviors. Des Jarlais, Jainchill, and Friedman discuss cases of AIDS among IV drug users in New York City; their work contributes a unique perspective on AIDS epidemiology among IV drug users "on the streets," as well as those enrolled in drug treatment programs. In Chapter 7, "Intravenous Drug Abusers and the Acquired Immunodeficiency Syndrome (AIDS)," Friedland et al. compare the demographic and drug use patterns of Bronx IV drug users with and without AIDS, finding that "over half of the heterosexual IV drug abusers with AIDS or ARC were aware of sharing needles with men they thought to be homosexuals," indicating a possible link between risk groups. Chaisson et al.'s study of IV drug abusers in San Francisco finds an HIV seroprevalence rate of 10%, an indication that "the growth of the epidemic in IV drug users in San Francisco will parallel the epidemic in homosexual men."

Part III of the book, "Psychiatric and Psychosocial Aspects of AIDS," looks at mental health issues, stemming not only from the neurological complications of AIDS, but also from the reactions directed at AIDS patients by their families and society. The article by Christ, Wiener, and Moynihan looks at such issues as the psychological results of unemployment, loss of health insurance, and alienation of AIDS patients from friends and families. Dilley et al. examine the psychological reactions of the patient as a function of physical state. They also consider some of the ethical issues involved in the mental health care of the AIDS patient at each stage of the illness. Nichols describes his experience in the clinical evaluation of persons with AIDS, finding a four-stage pattern of reaction to the disease, similar in nature to reactions in other situations of "catastrophic stress."

Exhibit I-2   AIDS cases by state of residence and date of report to CDC.

State of Residence	Year Ending Sep. 21, 1986		Year Ending Sep. 21, 1987		Cumulative Total Since June 1981					
					Adult/Adolescent		Children		Total	
	No.	%	No.	%	No.	%	No.	%	No.	%
New York	3501	(29.1)	3849	(22.9)	11852	(28.5)	212	(36.6)	12064	(28.6)
California	2747	(22.8)	3867	(23.0)	9628	(23.1)	39	(6.7)	9667	(22.9)
Florida	717	(6.0)	1283	(7.6)	2827	(6.8)	67	(11.6)	2894	(6.9)
Texas	731	(6.1)	1349	(8.0)	2728	(6.6)	19	(3.3)	2747	(6.5)
New Jersey	712	(5.9)	881	(5.2)	2318	(5.6)	75	(12.9)	2393	(5.7)
Illinois	339	(2.8)	500	(3.0)	1113	(2.7)	11	(1.9)	1124	(2.7)
Pennsylvania	301	(2.5)	450	(2.7)	1010	(2.4)	11	(1.9)	1021	(2.4)
Massachusetts	253	(2.1)	395	(2.3)	891	(2.1)	16	(2.8)	907	(2.2)
Georgia	266	(2.2)	398	(2.4)	872	(2.1)	13	(2.2)	885	(2.1)
District of Columbia	209	(1.7)	324	(1.9)	756	(1.8)	8	(1.4)	764	(1.8)
Maryland	162	(1.3)	304	(1.8)	645	(1.6)	11	(1.9)	656	(1.6)
Washington	153	(1.3)	215	(1.3)	514	(1.2)	2	(0.3)	516	(1.2)
Louisiana	148	(1.2)	207	(1.2)	494	(1.2)	6	(1.0)	500	(1.2)
Virginia	154	(1.3)	195	(1.2)	479	(1.2)	8	(1.4)	487	(1.2)
Connecticut	149	(1.2)	172	(1.0)	454	(1.1)	14	(2.4)	468	(1.1)
Ohio	140	(1.2)	237	(1.4)	463	(1.1)	2	(0.3)	465	(1.1)
Colorado	115	(1.0)	218	(1.3)	439	(1.1)	2	(0.3)	441	(1.0)
Puerto Rico	113	(0.9)	123	(0.7)	371	(0.9)	23	(4.0)	394	(0.9)
Michigan	124	(1.0)	183	(1.1)	387	(0.9)	6	(1.0)	393	(0.9)
Missouri	83	(0.7)	144	(0.9)	290	(0.7)	1	(0.2)	291	(0.7)
North Carolina	71	(0.6)	152	(0.9)	285	(0.7)	4	(0.7)	289	(0.7)
Arizona	81	(0.7)	123	(0.7)	259	(0.6)	1	(0.2)	260	(0.6)
Minnesota	79	(0.7)	112	(0.7)	230	(0.6)			230	(0.5)
Oregon	58	(0.5)	116	(0.7)	216	(0.5)	1	(0.2)	217	(0.5)
Indiana	59	(0.5)	95	(0.6)	199	(0.5)	2	(0.3)	201	(0.5)
Hawaii	50	(0.4)	77	(0.5)	164	(0.4)	1	(0.2)	165	(0.4)

South Carolina	45	(0.4)	74	(0.4)	156	(0.4)	5	(0.9)	161	(0.4)
Alabama	29	(0.2)	98	(0.6)	152	(0.4)	6	(1.0)	158	(0.4)
Oklahoma	35	(0.3)	96	(0.6)	155	(0.4)	1	(0.2)	156	(0.4)
Wisconsin	34	(0.3)	82	(0.5)	146	(0.4)			146	(0.3)
Tennessee	58	(0.5)	45	(0.3)	125	(0.3)	1	(0.2)	126	(0.3)
Nevada	37	(0.3)	46	(0.3)	100	(0.2)			100	(0.2)
Rhode Island	20	(0.2)	58	(0.3)	97	(0.2)			97	(0.2)
Kentucky	29	(0.2)	31	(0.2)	87	(0.2)			87	(0.2)
Kansas	31	(0.3)	40	(0.2)	83	(0.2)	1	(0.2)	84	(0.2)
Utah	20	(0.2)	29	(0.2)	68	(0.2)	3	(0.5)	71	(0.2)
New Mexico	17	(0.1)	37	(0.2)	70	(0.2)			70	(0.2)
Arkansas	28	(0.2)	33	(0.2)	67	(0.2)			67	(0.2)
Mississippi	20	(0.2)	34	(0.2)	60	(0.1)			60	(0.1)
Delaware	20	(0.2)	19	(0.1)	54	(0.1)	1	(0.2)	55	(0.1)
Iowa	19	(0.2)	25	(0.1)	54	(0.1)	1	(0.2)	55	(0.1)
Maine	17	(0.1)	22	(0.1)	47	(0.1)	1	(0.2)	48	(0.1)
Nebraska	12	(0.1)	19	(0.1)	37	(0.1)			37	(0.1)
West Virginia	8	(0.1)	17	(0.1)	34	(0.1)	2	(0.3)	36	(0.1)
New Hampshire	12	(0.1)	18	(0.1)	33	(0.1)	2	(0.3)	35	(0.1)
Alaska	13	(0.1)	15	(0.1)	34	(0.1)			34	(0.1)
Vermont	5	(0.0)	7	(0.0)	15	(0.0)			15	(0.0)
Idaho	6	(0.0)	4	(0.0)	9	(0.0)	1	(0.2)	10	(0.0)
Montana	5	(0.0)	3	(0.0)	8	(0.0)			8	(0.0)
Wyoming	4	(0.0)	3	(0.0)	8	(0.0)			8	(0.0)
Virgin Islands	3	(0.0)			7	(0.0)			7	(0.0)
North Dakota	3	(0.0)	2	(0.0)	5	(0.0)			5	(0.0)
South Dakota	2	(0.0)	3	(0.0)	5	(0.0)			5	(0.0)
Guam	1	(0.0)			1	(0.0)			1	(0.0)
Trust Territory					1	(0.0)			1	(0.0)
Total	12048	(100.0)	16829	(100.0)	41602	(100.0)	580	(100.0)	42182	(100.0)

From Centers for Disease Control, *AIDS Weekly Surveillance Report*, Sept. 21, 1987.

The questions AIDS poses for drug treatment professionals and the potential for the development of educational programs to help IV drug abusers learn to lessen their high-risk behaviors are the focus of Part IV, "AIDS – The Therapeutic Community and Health Education." The Cohen and Weisman article considers an AIDS treatment approach for IV drug abusers in a general hospital that includes medical, psychological, and social factors. The development of therapy groups for IV drug abusers with ARC within a residential substance abuse treatment program is examined by Robak's article. Another perspective is provided by Lewis and Galea in a study of drug abusers in treatment and their perceptions and knowledge about AIDS – what it is, how it is transmitted, and whether they feel their previous lifestyle may have increased their chance of exposure to HIV. Their conclusion – that drug abusers show sufficient concern about AIDS to change their behavior – is further supported in articles by Ginzburg et al. and by Friedman, Des Jarlais, and Sotheran.

Some of the most difficult problems posed by the spread of AIDS are ethical in nature. In Part V, "Social and Ethical Implications of AIDS," the editors have selected articles that look at AIDS as a legal and ethical phenomenon. In her article, Siegel examines the prejudice that may be directed at persons with AIDS by a society that views the disease as the result of morally forbidden behaviors. Ginzburg and Gostin take this view one step further, seeing the prejudice against members of AIDS risk groups as possibly leading to difficulties in obtaining their legal rights to privacy, housing, schooling, and medical treatment. They note that the ability to maintain the confidentiality of HIV antibody status is critical because of "the potential personal, social, and economic harms that may result from disclosure of this information."

Finally, in Morgan and Curran's "Acquired Immunodeficiency Syndrome: Current and Future Trends," the authors project the pattern the AIDS epidemic may take through 1991, detailing the growth of cases among the general heterosexual population. Their conclusion is that AIDS will continue to be the major public health challenge unless a vaccine or some other means is discovered to alter its course.

The editors have also compiled an extensive Glossary and Bibliography designed to help researchers, scholars, or students who wish to obtain further information about AIDS and IV drug abuse.

References

Centers for Disease Control. 1987. AIDS Weekly Surveillance Report, March 30.

Des Jarlais, D., N. Jainchill, and S. Friedman. 1986. AIDS among IV drug users: epidemiology, natural history, and therapeutic community experiences. *Bridging Services* 69-73.

Emmons, C. et al. 1986. Psychosocial predictors of reported behavior change in homosexual men at risk for AIDS. *Health Educ. Q.* 13:331-45.

Friedman, S., D. Des Jarlais, and J. L. Sotheran. 1986. AIDS health education for intravenous drug users. *Health Educ. Q.* 13:383-93.

Lewis, B. F., and R. Galea. 1986. A survey of the perceptions of drug abusers concerning the acquired immunodeficiency syndrome (AIDS). *Health Matrix* 4:14-17.

Massachusetts Department of Public Health. 1987. Radio presentation.

Novick, D., M. Kreek, and D. Des Jarlais. Antibodies to LAV in New York City, historical and ethical considerations. In *Proceedings of the 46th Annual Scientific Meeting*, Committee on Problems of Drug Dependence, ed. L. Harris. Bethesda, Maryland: National Institute on Drug Abuse. In press.

Polk, B. F. 1987. Predictors of the acquired immunodeficiency syndrome developing in a cohort of seropositive homosexual men. *N. Engl. J. Med.* 316:61-66.

Sontag, S. 1977. *Illness as metaphor.* New York: Vintage Books.

About the Authors

Robert P. Galea, Ph.D., Benjamin F. Lewis, Ed.D., and Lori A. Baker, M.A., are researchers and administrators at Spectrum House, Inc., the largest and oldest substance abuse treatment program in Massachusetts. Recently, Spectrum House, in conjunction with the University of Massachusetts School of Public Health at Amherst, received a grant from the National Institute on Drug Abuse to study the effectiveness of cognitive versus enhanced educational modules in helping IV drug abusers alter the behaviors that place them at risk for AIDS.

About the Authors

Robert Geller, M.D., ... and Lisa ...

PART I

Medical Aspects of AIDS

Consideration of the medical aspects of acquired immunodeficiency syndrome (AIDS) must encompass two dimensions of the illness: the actual clinical course of the infection, and the issues and questions a physician may expect to hear during the course of his or her dealings with AIDS patients, those who test positive for human immunodeficiency virus (HIV), or members of high-risk groups. The articles contained in this section consider both of these aspects of AIDS. "The Natural History of Infection with the Human Immunodeficiency Virus" by Francis et al. gives an intensive examination of the physiological effects of infection with HIV. Their discussion includes all phases of illness, beginning with the carrier state and means of virus transmission, and including the progression to symptom development. They also discuss the response to infection in chimpanzees inoculated with the AIDS virus. However, Francis and colleagues note the limitation inherent in attempting to study the length of the virus' incubation in humans; the relative newness of HIV infection has as yet allowed insufficient time for an accurate assessment of how long the virus may remain dormant.

The second article in this section, "A Practitioner's Guide to AIDS" by George Grady looks at the immediate issues a physician faces when dealing with patients who may have been exposed to HIV. One of the most important issues a physician will discuss with his or her patients is HIV testing. Here, Grady discusses the accuracy and efficacy of such testing, the implications of both positive and negative results, and the possible stigma that may be attached to a positive test for exposure to HIV. He also examines policies for school attendance by children with AIDS, counseling for AIDS patients, and the possibility of occupational exposure to the virus by

1

health care workers, finding that such exposure has been rare. Both articles indicate that the "newness" of this illness leaves the physician and the patient with inevitable, and sometimes un-answerable, questions. One such question, for example, is the mean-ing of a positive test for HIV exposure in patients who are asymptomatic. The percentage of such people who will eventually develop AIDS-related complex, AIDS, or some other, lesser form of HIV-related illness is currently unknown, with studies yielding limited available results.

1
The Natural History of Infection with the Human Immunodeficiency Virus

Donald P. Francis, MD, DSc; Harold W. Jaffe, MD;
Patricia N. Fultz, PhD; Jane P. Getchell, PhD;
J. Steven McDougal, MD; and
Paul M. Feorino, PhD.

The identity of the organism that causes the acquired immunodeficiency syndrome (AIDS) was first reported in 1983, but we already possess considerable understanding of the virus, its modes of transmission, and the clinical manifestations that can occur after infection with the virus. The causative virus, the lymphadenopathy-associated virus/human T-lymphotropic virus type III, now referred to as human immunodeficiency virus (HIV) (Barre-Sinoussi, Chermann, and Rey 1983; Gallo, Salahuddin, and Popovic 1984), is capable of infecting B-cells, macrophages, and neural cells, but it preferentially infects that T4 subset of lymphocytes (Klatzmann, Barre-Sinoussi, and Nugeyre 1984). This tropism for T4 cells, with its associated cytopathic effect, is presumably responsible for the eventual loss of immunologic function that is at the root of the syndrome.

Reprinted, with changes, from "The Natural History of Infection with the Human Immunodeficiency Virus (HIV)," by Donald P. Francis et al., *Annals of Internal Medicine* 10:719-22, 1985, by permission of the authors.

Reservoir of Infection and Carrier State

How does this virus, replicating in cells that reside primarily within the vascular and lymphatic spaces, exit from one host and become available to infect the next? To answer this question, we must understand the reservoir of infection and know the length of time that a person may remain infective. For such studies, we have defined an infective person as one whose peripheral blood lymphocytes contain infectious virus as determined by cocultivation with phytohemagglutinin-stimulated normal adult lymphocytes (Barre-Sinoussi, Chermann, and Rey 1983). Virus has been isolated from a high proportion (51%) of antibody-positive (as shown by enzyme-lined immunosorbent assay [ELISA]) healthy persons and from almost all persons clinically ill with AIDS or AIDS-related conditions (table 1-1).

To study the length of the infective (carrier) state for this virus, we studied blood donors who were implicated (belonging to high-

Table 1-1

Presence of Lymphadenopathy-Associated Virus/Human Y-Lymphotropic Virus Type III in the Blood of Patients with the Acquired Immunodeficiency Syndrome (AIDS) or Lymphadenopathy and in Healthy, Antibody-Positive Persons

Group	Persons Tested	Virus Positive
	n	n (%)
Healthy, antibody-positive persons		
Blood donors*	16	16 (100)
Homosexual men	31	15 (48)
Hemophiliacs	13	1 (8)
Zairians	8	3 (38)
Total	68	35 (51)
Patients with lymphadenopathy		
Blood donors*	6	6 (100)
Homosexual men	31	20 (65)
Hemophiliacs	6	5 (83)
Total	43	31 (72)
Patients with AIDS		
Transfusion recipients	7	7 (100)
Homosexual men	13	12 (92)
Hemophiliacs	4	3 (75)
Zairians	27	23 (85)
Total	51	45 (88)

*Implicated in cases of transfusion-associated AIDS.

risk groups and having positive tests for antibody) as the source of infection for patients who developed AIDS after receiving transfusion. We assumed that these donors were infective when they donated their implicated blood, but were they still infective? We obtained blood samples from the donors to culture their lymphocytes for HIV. Blood specimens were collected from 23 antibody-positive donors 12 to 52 months after their original blood donation. All had detectable virus (exhibit 1-1) (Feorino, Jaffe, and Palmer 1985). If these donors had been infective at the time of donation (as presumed) and if they were infective at the time of specimen collection (as shown), then they were probably infective during the intervening period. Thus, we conclude that a prolonged carrier state exists for this virus.

Transmission of Infection

For HIV to be transmitted, it must exit these persistently infected carriers. One direct way for virus to gain access to the outside would be if it replicated in epithelial cells of mucous membranes, but no epithelial cell infection has been detected in vitro for HIV. Even without epithelial replication, transmission is still possible; other nonmucous-membrane-replicating, bloodborne agents, such as hepatitis B virus, do effectively exit the vascular space. This movement occurs through several mechanisms, the most obvious being a breech in the vascular bed that allows blood to exit directly. Another mechanism involves exuding plasma. Plasma itself and plasma-containing body fluids (such as saliva) could be vehicles by which infection could be transmitted. For HIV, Groopman, Salahuddin, and Sarngadharan (1984) reported isolating virus from the saliva of 8 to 18 patients studied, and Levy, Kaminsky, and Morrow (1985) have expanded these numbers by reporting isolates from saliva of 3 of 4 patients. Another mechanism of virus transmission is unique for lymphotropic viruses, such as HIV, in that any fluid or exudate that contains lymphocytes can be expected to contain some infected cells. For example, Ho, Schooley, and Rota (1984) and Zagury, Bernard, and Leibowitch (1984) successfully cultured virus from cell-containing semen from a few men, and Levy, Kaminsky, and Morrow (1985) report the isolation of virus from semen of 4 of 19 patients.

Early epidemiologic observations of AIDS implied – and more recent experiments with chimpanzees have proved – that virus can

Exhibit 1-1

Time (mos.) from Donation to Specimen Collection

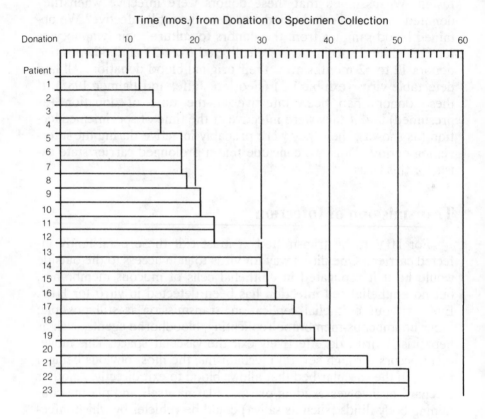

infect hosts after either direct intravascular exposure, as occurs with blood transfusion, exchange of blood in shared needles and syringes, or after mucous membrane exposure, as occurs during sexual intercourse. For such an exposure to transmit infection, virus from the index person would have to contact susceptible target cells in the next person. With what we know now, lymphocytes and macrophages would appear to be the most likely target cells, although as mentioned above, the susceptibility of other cell types has not been eliminated. Direct intravascular exposure would certainly allow virus adequate access to susceptible lymphocytes. Mucous membrane exposure might be less likely to result in virus-lymphocyte contact, but our recent success in infecting a chimpanzee via vaginal exposure

Exhibit 1-1, continued.

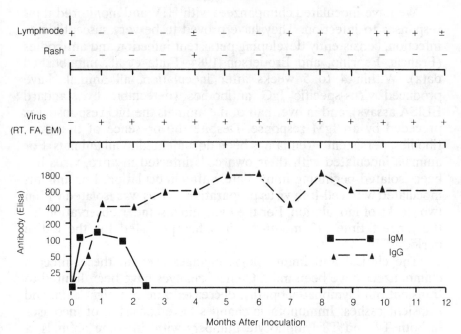

Interval between implicated blood donation and virus isolation from 23 antibody-positive blood donors. Data from Feorino and colleagues. Clinical, virologic, and serologic response of a chimpanzee to infection with lymphadenopathy-associated virus/human T-lymphotropic virus type III. A culture was considered virus-positive if it showed reverse transcriptase *(RT)* activity, antigen on direct immunofluorescence testing *(FA)*, and virus particles on electron microscopy *(EM)*. ELISA = enzyme-linked immunosorbent assay.

without trauma or coexisting infection shows that transmission can occur readily (Fultz et al., unpublished data). Virus entry via mucous membranes would presumably be facilitated in inflamed or traumatized tissues where, because of increased concentrations of reactive cells, transmitted virus would have a better chance of contacting susceptible target cells. The high prevalence of both traumatic and inflammatory anorectal lesions in homosexual men could, at least theoretically, increase their susceptibility to infection by this route.

Early Responses to Infection

We have inoculated chimpanzees with HIV and monitored their responses to infection. They have proved to be very susceptible to infection, consistently developing persistent infection and antibodies (Francis, Feorino, and Broderson 1984; Fultz et al., unpublished data). Within 4 to 5 weeks after inoculation, all animals have produced virus-specific IgG antibodies (detectable by standard ELISA assays), and in over half of the animals the IgG response was preceded by an IgM response. Despite the presence of these antibodies, persistent viremia has been documented in all animals. For animals inoculated with their own cells infected in vitro, virus has been isolated beginning immediately after inoculation. For animals inoculated with cell-free virus preparations, virus was isolated within two weeks of inoculation. For the two animals under observation for the longest time (12 months), virus has persisted for the entire period.

The clinical and immunologic changes seen in these infected chimpanzees have been mild. Clinical changes have been limited to transient mild lymphadenopathy, decreased rate of weight gain, and transient rashes. Immunologic changes have consisted of increases in both T4 and T8 lymphocyte numbers with, in some animals, a lower T4/T8 ratio. Functional assays using mitogen or antigen stimulation of lymphocytes from infected animals have shown no changes.

An acute clinical syndrome may be associated with infection with lymphadenopathy-associated/human T-lymphotropic virus type III. Recent reports have described a 3- to 14-day mononucleosis-like illness during the first few weeks after infection (Cooper, Gold, and Maclean 1984; Tucker, Ludlam, and Craig 1984). We have not seen a similar condition in chimpanzees, but because many of the acute symptoms described by human patients are constitutional, they could have escaped detection in chimpanzees. Constitutional symptoms in chimpanzees may have been reflected in the decreased rate of weight gain that was prominent in all animals during the first 6 months after infection.

Incubation Period

To discuss the clinical manifestations of AIDS that occur at times late after infection, we must first deal with possible biases resulting from the shortness of our observation times. How long must we follow a group of infected humans for all of those who are going to develop disease to do so? One estimate of the average incubation period can be gleaned from studying patients with transfusion-associated AIDS; for them, infection coincides with the receipt of blood. In these patients, the average time from transfusion to diagnosis of AIDS has been estimated to be 19.4 months for children and 29.6 months for adults.

Another estimate of the incubation period can be gleaned by testing stored serum from patients with AIDS and measuring the time from seroconversion to the diagnosis of AIDS. In collaboration with the San Francisco City/County Health Departments, we have tested serum obtained as part of previous hepatitis B virus studies on homosexual men. Multiple serum specimens taken since 1978 were available for six study participants who developed AIDS. The time from the midpoint between last negative serologic test and first positive serologic test to the diagnosis of AIDS in these men has ranged from 16 to 65 months, with a mean of 38 months.

Thus, the incubation period for AIDS is long. It may be even longer than our current estimates because this infection has only recently been introduced into the United States, and we may not have observed infected persons for enough time in order for the longest incubating cases to have developed. As a result, our estimates of average incubation period may be short, and our estimates of outcome may be low.

Late Clinical Manifestations

Realizing these potential biases, we can now examine cohorts of infected persons to determine what proportion have developed AIDS or AIDS-related conditions. Members of three well-studied cohorts have been followed for more than 12 months. One cohort was reported by Goedert, Sarngadharan and Biggar (1984), and two have been followed by the Centers for Disease Control (Feorino, Jaffe, and Palmer 1985; Jaffe, Darros, and Echenberg 1985). Two of these cohorts consist of homosexual men whose stored serum specimens showed that they had been infected in years past. Of 35 patients from private physician's offices who have been followed for a mean of 21 months, 8 (23%) have developed AIDS-related conditions and 5 (14%) have developed AIDS (Goedert, Sarngadharan, and Biggar 1984). Of 31 patients from a sexually transmitted disease clinic who have been followed for 48 to 72 months, 8 (26%) have developed AIDS-related conditions and 2 (7%) have developed AIDS (Jaffe, Darros, and Echenberg 1985). The other cohort consists of blood donors, mostly homosexual men, who were presumed to have been already infected when they donated blood that was later implicated as the source of infection for patients developing transfusion-associated AIDS. Of 26 blood donors followed for 12 to 52 months, 6 (23%) have developed AIDS-related conditions and 4 (15%) have developed AIDS (Feorino, Jaffe, and Palmer 1985).

The consistency of outcomes for the three cohorts is striking. During follow-up, between 23% and 26% of infected members have developed AIDS-related conditions and between 7% and 15% have developed AIDS. It should be stressed that the cohort members in these studies were almost all homosexual men. Whether such high rates of clinical disease can be expected for other infected persons who are not homosexual men who are infected with this virus, the projected morbidity and mortality in this group alone are going to be huge.

Major questions remain about persons who are infected but who have not developed AIDS. Will they remain healthy, or will they develop AIDS or some equally serious condition? The recent reports of replication of this virus in the central nervous system and the development of dementia and myelopathy in patients with AIDS (Petito et al. 1985) suggest that infected persons may be susceptible to other disease. Certainly, a large proportion of HIV-infected persons have abnormal immunologic features, even in the absence of disease. For example, many infected persons without AIDS (9%) have low numbers of T4 cells, the hallmark of AIDS. One can presume that if this deficit is not corrected, it will be associated with various other infectious and neoplastic diseases.

We do not understand what determines who will and who will not develop serious disease after infection. It appears from studies of humans and chimpanzees that elevations in both T4 and T8 lymphocyte counts may be early host responses to infection with HIV. In contrast, the late disease, especially those categorized as AIDS, almost invariably occur in persons whose T4 cells are depleted. But there is a gap in our knowledge about the pathogenic process that occurs between these two periods. Are the early elevations of lymphocyte subsets part of a continuum that will eventually result in the loss of T4 cells and an adverse outcome, or are these elevations an early sign of infection from which some patients will recover and return to normal? To date, no prognostic marker has been identified to differentiate those whose infection will progress to AIDS from those who will remain healthy.

References

Barre-Sinoussi, F., J. C. Chermann, and F. Rey. 1983. Isolation of a T-lymphotropic retrovirus from a patient at risk for acquired immune deficiency syndrome (AIDS). *Science* 220:868-71.

Cooper, D. A., J. Gold, and P. Maclean. 1984. Acute AIDS retrovirus infection: definition of a clinical illness associated with seroconversion. *Lancet* 1:537-40.

Feorino, P. M., H. Jaffe, and E. Palmer. 1985. Transfusion-associated acquired immunodeficiency syndrome: evidence for persistent infection in blood donors. *N. Engl. J. Med.* 312:1293-96.

Francis, D. P., P. Feorino, and J. Broderson. 1984. Infection of chimpanzees with lymphadenopathy-associated virus (letter). *Lancet* 2:1276-77.

Gallo, R. C., S. Salahuddin, and M. Popovic. 1984. Frequent detection and isolation of cytopathic retroviruses (HTLV-III) from patients with AIDS and at risk for AIDS. *Science* 224:500-503.

Goedert, J. J., M. Sarnagharan, and R. Biggar. 1984. Determinants of retrovirus (HTLV-III) antibody and immunodeficiency conditions in homosexual men. *Lancet* 2:711-15.

Groopman, J. E., S. Salahuddin, and M. Sarngadharan. 1984. HTLV-III in saliva of people with AIDS-related complex and healthy homosexual men at risk for AIDS. *Science* 226:447-49.

Ho, D. D., R. Schooley, and T. Rota. 1984.

HTLV-III in the semen and blood of a healthy homosexual man. *Science* 226:451-53.

Jaffe, H. W., W. Darros, and D. Echenberg. 1985. The acquired immunodeficiency syndrome in a cohort of homosexual men: a 6-year follow-up study. *Ann. Intern. Med.* 103:210-14.

Klatzmann, D., F. Barre-Sinoussi, and M. Nugeyre. 1984. Selective tropism of lymphadenopathy associated virus (LAV) for helper inducer T lymphocytes. *Science* 225:59-63.

Levy, J. A., L. Kaminsky, and W. Morrow. 1985. Infection by the retrovirus associated with the acquired imunodeficiency syndrome: clinical, biological, and molecular features. *Ann. Intern. Med* 103:604-9.

Petito, C. K., B. Navja, E. Cho, B. Jordan, D. George, and R. Prince. 1985. Vacuolar myelopathy pathologically resembling subacute combined degeneration in patients with the acquired immunodeficiency syndrome. *N. Engl. J. Med.* 312:874-78.

Tucker, J., C. Ludlam, and A. Craig. 1984. HTLV-III infection associated with glandular-fever-like illness in a haemophili ac (letter). *Lancet* 1:585.

Zagury, D., J. Bernard, and J. Leibowitch. 1984. HTLV-III in cells cultured from semen of two patients with AIDS. *Science* 226:451-53.

2
A Practitioner's Guide to AIDS

George F. Grady, MD.

It is a rare practitioner, social worker, or psychologist who has not been asked to interpret some media announcement about the acquired immunodeficiency syndrome (AIDS). In addition to quelling anxieties, physicians may need to assess patients' specific exposures to AIDS. Less often, it may be necessary to consider AIDS or the clinically milder AIDS-related complex (ARC) in a differential diagnosis. In still other situations, practitioners may be called upon to provide the primary clinical judgment and to argue against unnecessary isolation or restricted mobility of patients infected with the AIDS-associated virus. Dealing with these concerns requires a careful case-by-case assessment and knowledge of public health policies that have been developed recently; in addition, there must be an awareness of the rationale for caution and confidentiality in serologic testing, a caution that should extend beyond the usual prudence.

Our knowledge of how AIDS is transmitted has developed not only from direct observation of AIDS, but also by longer study of the close parallels seen in hepatitis B. The public cannot be blamed

Excerpted with permission from "A Practitioner's Guide to AIDS," by George F. Grady, *Massachusetts Medicine*, January/February, 1986.

for mistakenly believing that AIDS's transmission pattern includes airborne spread (as in influenza or measles) or enteric spread (as in polio or hepatitis A). Although physicians can rebut these misconceptions, pointing out that virus transmission patterns are predictable, that casual transmission of AIDS has not been seen, and that the similarities to hepatitis B are also reassuring, there are some unspoken fears that must also be appreciated. For example, parents may fear that they will have to choose between their deeply ingrained protective instincts and their desire to appear as progressive, rational, and calm role models for their children. The acceptance of policies on school attendance (described later) have succeeded in part because of sensitivity to that conflict; this has enabled parents to suspend judgment long enough to learn that AIDS is not transmissible in the normal interactions of school children.

Another anxiety relates to the ignorance and fear of mainstream society regarding such "forbidden behaviors" as drug addiction and homosexuality. When it was initially recognized that AIDS was concentrated among drug addicts and homosexual men, there was a feeling that the disease might not get the same attention and funding that otherwise would be given. The rare but more randomly distributed risk of infection via blood transfusions and blood products heightened public consciousness and helped overcome inertia in federal support. Now, somewhat paradoxically, the belated strong support for research and education risks being misinterpreted as an indication that AIDS is a universal threat destined to work its way inexorably through all segments of society. The swings between underappreciation and overreaction should now give way to dispassionate description of the requirements necessary to reduce needle and sexual transmissions, whether homosexual or heterosexual.

It has become clear that everyone must have a social, humanitarian, and economic concern about AIDS. However, we can also conclude by analogy to hepatitis B that at least 95% of the population at large are unlikely to become infected, even while the prevalence in subgroups at high risk reaches saturation. For example, whereas serologic markers of previous or continuing hepatitis B infection are found in 80% or more of parenteral drug users who share contaminated needles and gay males with multiple partners, the nationwide seroprevalence among blood donors has not exceeded 5%. Because the AIDS-associated virus is neither more hardy nor more abundant in the circulation than hepatitis B virus, projections based on the hepatitis B model would seem to identify the limits of the worst-case scenario for AIDS.

The approximately 700 cases of AIDS in Massachusetts include 576 residents and 116 treated in Massachusetts hospitals who were nonresidents when symptoms first appeared. The Massachusetts data resemble national statistics, in that slightly less than three-quarters of adult cases are in homosexuals. All such cases are in males, thus skewing state and national figures toward 93% males overall, and incidentally indicating by the absence of females in the homosexual category that certain sexual practices rather than sexual preference per se dictate risk.

Because Massachusetts has ongoing outbreaks of hepatitis B and delta hepatitis attributable to parenteral drug abusers and their sexual partners, this is an area that is attracting concern. Presumed heterosexual transmission continues to account for 7% of cases in the state and 4% nationally. There is no theoretical reason why heterosexual transmission could not occur, but the impact overall is difficult to evaluate. The numbers could underestimate future trends or could be overestimates if the category includes persons with concealed histories of other risk factors, such as intravenous drug use. Although there are slightly fewer cases among nonwhites here than nationally, there are slightly more cases in immigrants from countries where AIDS may be endemic.

Pediatric AIDS cases have accounted for between 1% and 2% nationally and currently account for 2% in Massachusetts. Typically, most of these would occur through infection in utero or at birth to mothers who had contracted AIDS from contaminated intravenous drug injections. Other cases would follow blood transfusion or use of contaminated antihemophilic-factor concentrates. (Fortunately, the latter causes should become increasingly rare now that blood donations are screened serologically and blood products undergo appropriate virus inactivation processes.)

The clinical profiles of cases in Massachusetts are similar to those seen nationally, except that the preponderance of *Pneumocystis carinii* pneumonia and other opportunistic infections is not quite as great.

With regard to the geographic distribution of cases within Massachusetts, approximately half the resident cases are in Suffolk County (Boston), and there is a small cluster in Provincetown (Barnstable County).

Patients who consult you to evaluate specific exposures will first have decided to risk embarrassment about the confidential nature of their concerns and the uncertainty of whether definitive reassurance can be given. These inquiries may be resolved quickly and satisfactorily if the feared contact is incompatible with transmission (e.g., by food or water, donating blood, or sitting near a patient with AIDS) or falsely assumed to have taken place by superficial exposure to individuals belonging to groups at risk for AIDS. In the latter situation, the source of anxiety may be obscured by additional uncertainty about the physician's reaction to any homophobic or homosexual feelings the patient has. Members of the Massachusetts Governor's Task Force on AIDS have suggested that the following reassuring approach would be useful.

"It may not seem obvious to you why I need to ask about your sexuality, but there are some diseases that are contracted through bodily fluids. To help me in treating you, I need to ask you a few questions."

"Are you sexually active?"

(If sexually active:)

"Are you sexually active with men, women, or both?"

"Is this information socially known?"

"Are you an IV drug user?"

(If so:)

"Do you share needles?"

(If so:)

"Do you sterilize or disinfect your needles?"

Some patients may be worried about exposures that carry only statistically remote risks of causing AIDS, e.g., having received a blood transfusion before serologic screening became available. Although the likelihood of infection from such a transfusion appears to be less than one in 100,000, many patients will want reassurance that they are not destined to become victims.

What most patients may be seeking is the "blood test" that they have heard is available and in use primarily to screen blood donors. Indeed, because some people fear loss of confidentiality, or may be uncomfortable about consulting their physician, they have posed as blood donors in order to obtain the test anonymously. Blood transfusion centers have worried that if persons in risk groups for AIDS were to ignore admonitions not to donate, the value of implementing the screening test might be more than offset by the influx of potentially infective donors, some of whom could be missed owing to the test's technical limitations. To reduce these risks, various Departments of Public Health throughout the country have initiated "alternative sites" for anonymous testing, a service that became available at the same time that routine blood-donor screening began. These sites, established in collaboration with the American Red Cross Blood Services and various groups representing addicts and gay men, appear to have been successful in diverting many AIDS-prone individuals who indicated that they would have donated blood had not the alternative sites been available.

Physicians should know how to obtain serologic testing and integrate the test into practice. Assimilation of these services into good general medicine is the most hopeful and logical means of meeting the growing demand.

The limits of sensitivity of HIV antibody testing can only be inferred from prospective studies of high-risk populations, such as intravenous drug users or homosexual males with multiple exposures. In such settings, an occasional individual has been detected in the process of seroconversion such that a period of viremia may be detected before seroconversion. Still rarer are those believed to have immune systems so deranged by HIV infection that antibody is not produced. The proportion of antibody-negative infective persons has been estimated at 1% to 5%. This proportion should not necessarily be extrapolated to blood donors, however, because high-risk donors would have to ignore admonitions, be well enough to donate, and pass the limited physical exam that could detect significant lymphadenopathy. Apart from the biologic limitations of the antibody test, there may be technical limitations to its sensitivity. Nevertheless, except for the possibility of frank technical error, the enzyme-linked immunoassay (ELISA) and the more accurate Western blot test (which is the federally licensed national standard) are extremely sensitive and should detect any significant antibody response to current or past HIV infection.

Because the antibody test was devised as a screening test for blood donors, and because the proportion of presumptively positive units of blood to be diverted was assumed to be acceptably small, there was an inherent design bias toward sensitivity and possible "overdiagnosis." However, recognition that informing a donor of HIV antibody positivity carries a substantial psychological impact has created the need for confirmatory tests with maximum specificity and with sensitivity not significantly less than that of the screening test. A research technique called Western blot analysis, which examines the reactivity of antibody against electrophoretically separated HIV components, is the working standard.

In summary, a negative screening test means that there is a probability on the order of 95% to 99% that the individual has not been sufficiently exposed to HIV recently enough to develop antibody. An antibody response has been described within 4 to 5 weeks of exposure in a nurse sustaining an accidental inoculation; in studies of nonhuman primates, antibody has also appeared within 4 to 12 weeks after experimental challenge. Incubation periods of several years between transfusion and the onset of clinical disease have been reported, but this should not necessarily imply an equally long latency for seroconversion. Clearly, one cannot use a negative antibody test to absolve a potential exposure within the previous month, much less for the "morning after." However, a negative test might have some value in easing the mind of someone focusing on a single potential exposure that occurred in the past few months.

The national average for the prevalence of HIV antibody repeatably positive by ELISA screening of blood donors is 0.25% and is 0.05% for Western blot confirmable donors (1/5 of 0.25%). The comparable figure in Massachusetts is 0.03%.

In the differential diagnosis of AIDS, it is important to remember that congenital forms of immune deficiency have been well described in the pediatric literature, and that acquired immunodeficiency of unknown origin has occurred at all ages long before the intrusion of HIV upon Western cultures. Thus, not every patient with these clinically similar syndromes should be automatically assumed to have AIDS or ARC. *Pneumocystis carinii* pneumonia and other opportunistic infections are not unique to AIDS. However, the diagnosis is highly likely when one observes the purple raised skin lesions of Kaposi's sarcoma, a malignancy rare in all populations except elderly men of Mediterranean origin. Lymphopenia is to be expected; a finding that the "helper" T cells (T4 lymphocytes) are differentially depressed is also highly consistent. However, especially when other diagnoses such as Hodgkin's disease, sarcoid, and tuberculosis are entertained, and when one wants to minimize invasive diagnostic procedures, testing for HIV antibody is indicated.

Access to HIV antibody tests for medical management was intentionally restricted initially because there had been isolated instances of mishandling of test results. There was fear of widespread abuse that could be psychologically damaging and cause discrimination in insurance, housing, and employment. Restricted access policies were initiated in mid-1985 by various emergency regulations throughout the country by legislators and public health officials.

The policy for school attendance by children with AIDS flows from the right and legal obligation of every child to be in grades kindergarten through 12 unless there is a medical exemption. Exemptions should include only those children with AIDS who are too sick to attend school, are at unacceptable risk of contracting an infection from classmates, or who have inappropriate behavior, such as biting. The primary personal physician judges the child by these criteria and arranges school attendance through communication with the limited number of school personnel who have a need to know (e.g., the superintendent, teacher, and school nurse).

Policy for attendance of younger children in group settings, such as day care, has received additional review by the Governor's Task Force. Although day care is recognized as potentially important to child development and has economic implications, it lacks the legal mandate for education in grades K-12 as described previously. In addition, although there have been no examples of horizontal transmission of AIDS among young children in group settings or households, a theoretical risk is recognized when an HIV-infected child is not yet toilet-trained or may drool and occasionally bite. Therefore, children under four years of age who have AIDS or HIV antibody are thought to be inappropriate candidates for formal group settings outside the household. Children aged four, or five year olds not yet in kindergarten, should be considered on an individual basis with regard to a given facility's ability to provide the necessary degree of supervision. Older individuals with developmental disabilities producing a mental age equivalent to that of pre-schoolers should be considered accordingly.

Routine screening for HIV antibody is not recommended. However, we recognize that there may be situations where the clinician will be presented with such data or may believe it to be in the interest of the child's medical management to obtain the test. In the case of the very young child, where some theoretical risk of transmission to contacts may exist, no distinction is made between symptomatic and asymptomatic (seropositive only) individuals. The reason that no similar comment is made regarding older schoolchildren is because the question seems moot in the absence of a significant risk of transmission in that age group.

Advocacy regarding continued employment depends upon concepts that are similar to those described for older schoolchildren. There is no public health reason, in the absence of open weeping lesions, for an individual to stop working, and there may be many positive effects if he or she is well enough to continue. The employer should be expected to treat the employee's illness as a disability with regard to health benefits and tenure. There may be, however, circumstances in which the employer will invoke additional concerns, such as in food handling.

Because AIDS is not a foodborne disease, and because any employee with open lesions on his or her hands is already prohibited from handling food, no sanctions are required.

Counseling is made difficult by many factors, including uncertainty about the prognostic meaning of positive serologic findings and their relation to mild clinical syndromes (ARC) or full-blown AIDS. In a study conducted in San Francisco, there has been progressive evolution toward symptomatic disease in a consistently enlarging proportion of homosexual men identified initially by serologic tests. Other studies with drug addicts and gay men have shown variable rates of progression, with long, relatively static periods in each phase. Some individuals, especially hemophiliacs, may have HIV antibody as an indication of an immunization-like response analogous to that in early studies of recipients of blood products containing noninfective hepatitis B virus components, such as hepatitis B surface antigen. Viral cultures, especially in HIV antibody-positive hemophiliacs, may be worthwhile for estimating infectivity. However, potential limitations of sensitivity and availability will always raise the question of whether an antibody-positive individual should have to consider his blood and semen, and possibly saliva, infectious until proven otherwise.

The antibody-positive individual who is a drug addict or gay would like a choice other than abstinence from needle-sharing or sexual activity needs help in learning how to communicate fairly with prospective sex partners. A substantial amount of literature describing sterilizing needles and "safe sex" techniques is available and can be obtained through various AIDS action groups. Initiation of discussion about these issues has been suggested as a means of conveying the message without being frighteningly abrupt. Advice regarding expected outcomes of pregnancy in antibody-positive women is even more difficult. At the moment there are no recognizable markers of virulence analogous to the e antigen in hepatitis B, so all antibody-positive pregnancies must be viewed with equal concern.

Several hundred needle-stick or accidental surgical exposures to blood from patients with clinical AIDS or HIV antibody have been recorded in a prospective study coordinated by the Centers for Disease Control. To date there has been no evidence of AIDS or ARC except in one subject. The incidence of seroconversion is estimated at less than 1%, a much lower figure than found in comparable studies of hepatitis B.

There is no official recommendation for postexposure prophylaxis. Some lots of hepatitis B immune globulin are known to contain HIV antibody. There has been no clinical evidence that the globulin is infective, and virus has not been recovered from it experimentally. However, it is also unknown whether passively administered HIV antibody would be protective or even present in adequate quantity.

Unlike infectious diseases reportable through local boards of health, AIDS is reportable directly to the State Department of Public Health, which makes reports to the Centers for Disease Control.

The importance of reporting has never been so important as now, while we try to monitor the early natural history of AIDS. The data do suggest that the rate of increase of new cases is slowing. For example, the annual number of new cases increased fourfold between October 1983 and October 1984 but increased only twofold through October 1985. We must strive for continued consistent reporting in order to know whether we are indeed on our way toward containment, relying entirely on education in the absence of a vaccine.

PART II

AIDS Epidemiology
and Drug Abuse

Since the first cases of acquired immunodeficiency syndrome (AIDS) appeared in homosexual/bisexual men in 1981, researchers have been puzzled by the epidemiology of the disease, which appeared to exclusively infect members of certain high-risk groups: sexually active homosexual/bisexual men, intravenous (IV) drug users, and even recent Haitian immigrants. Today, research has clarified the means of transmission of the human immunodeficiency virus (HIV), finding that it parallels the transmission of hepatitis B, another illness found among homosexuals and IV drug users. Epidemiological studies have determined that HIV is transmitted through blood to blood or semen to blood contact; ongoing studies still seek to discover the role played by various demographic characteristics, specific high-risk behaviors, and the role of the frequency of exposures to the virus in the development of AIDS-related complex or full-blown AIDS. One of the most important discoveries of the past several years, however, is that AIDS is a disease of specific behaviors rather than of specific groups.

The authors whose papers are presented in Part II consider AIDS epidemiology primarily among IV drug users, although general epidemiology and risk factors among all "high-risk" groups are also considered. One of the most interesting comparisons drawn for the reader by this group of articles is that between east- and west-coast patterns of AIDS transmission. As authors Ginzburg, Des Jarlais, and Friedland note, a large number of AIDS cases in metropolitan New York and New Jersey are among IV drug users; in those states, studies of the rates of HIV seroprevalence among IV drug users are as high as 56%. In Chapter 8, on the other hand, Chaisson et al. discuss rates of HIV exposure among IV drug users

23

in treatment in San Francisco. There, they note, seroprevalence rates are relatively low, and the vast majority of cases of AIDS are among homosexual/bisexual men. However, the results of testing in San Francisco indicate that HIV exposure in drug users now mirrors similar rates of exposure found among homosexual men at the beginning of the AIDS "epidemic," indicating that a similar pattern may emerge in San Francisco's IV drug-using population.

3

The Acquired Immuno-deficiency Syndrome: Epidemiology and Risk Factors for Transmission

Kenneth G. Castro, MD; Ann M. Hardy, DrPH; and James W. Curran, MD, MPH.

Epidemiology of AIDS

Acquired immunodeficiency syndrome (AIDS) was first recognized in the spring of 1981, when the Centers for Disease Control (CDC) received reports of multiple cases of two rare diseases – *Pneumocystis carinii* pneumonia and Kaposi's sarcoma – occurring in young, previously healthy, homosexual men from New York City and California (CDC 1981, 1982a). All of these patients had similar patterns of underlying immunosuppression without any apparent cause. Because of the unusual and severe nature of these diseases, the CDC established a task force to study this apparently new syndrome.

An early observation was that patients with AIDS had a specific impairment in the cell-mediated component of the immune system and that they developed diseases predictive of this impairment

Reprinted, with changes, from "The Acquired Immunodeficiency Syndrome: Epidemiology and Risk Factors for Transmission," by Kenneth G. Castro, Ann M. Hardy, and James W. Curran, *Medical Clinics of North America* 70:635-49, 1986, by permission of W. B. Saunders Co. (Philadelphia, Pa.). Copyright 1986.

(Gottlieb, Schroff, and Schanker 1981; Siegal, Lopez, and Hammer 1982; Masur, Michelis, and Green 1984). This observation was used to formulate the case definition that the CDC use for surveillance purposes. The CDC define AIDS as a reliably diagnosed disease at least moderately predictive of underlying cellular immune deficiency occurring in a person with no known underlying cause of immune deficiency or other cause of reduced resistance associated with that disease (CDC 1982; Selik, Haverkos, and Curran 1984). Eleven opportunistic infections and diseases are considered specific enough to be indicative of AIDS (exhibit 3-1). Because the surveillance case definition was designed with more emphasis on specificity than sensitivity, the cases of AIDS represent only the "tip of the iceberg" of the disease spectrum (exhibit 3-2). Other disease entities, such as non-Hodgkin's lymphoma, generalized unexplained lymphadenopathy, thrombocytopenia, and oral candidiasis, are part of the AIDS disease spectrum, as well as infection with the virus without signs of symptoms (CDC 1982b; Morris, Distenfeld, and Amorosi 1982; Klein, Harris, and Small 1984).

Recent laboratory and epidemiologic evidence demonstrates that a retrovirus is the cause of AIDS (Barre-Sinoussi, Cherman, and Rey 1983; CDC 1984b; Gallo, Salahuddin, and Popovic 1984; Laurence, Brun-Vezinet, and Schutzer 1984; Levy, Hossman, and Kramer 1984; Weiss, Goedert, and Sarngadharan 1985a; Weiss, Saxinger, and Rechtman 1985b). Three morphologically similar protype isolates, termed lymphadenopathy-associated virus, human T cell lymphotropic virus type III and AIDS-associated retrovirus,

Exhibit 3-1

Opportunistic Diseases Considered to Be Indicative of AIDS

PROTOZOAL INFECTIONS	FUNGAL INFECTIONS
Pneumocystis carinii pneumonia	*Candida* esophagitis
Toxoplasma gondii encephalitis or disseminated infection (excluding congenital infection)	Cryptococcal meningitis or disseminated infection
Chronic (>1 month) *Cryptosporidium* enteritis	Bacterial infection
Noncongenital Viral Infections	Disseminated (not just pulmonary or lymphatic)
Chronic (>1 month) mucocutaneous herpes simplex	*Mycobacterium avium-intracellulare*
Histologically evident cytomegalovirus infection of an organ other than liver or lymph node	Cancers
Kaposi's sarcoma (in a person under age 60)	
Progressive multifocal leukoencephalopathy	Primary brain lymphoma (limited to the brain)

Exhibit 3-2

"Iceberg"

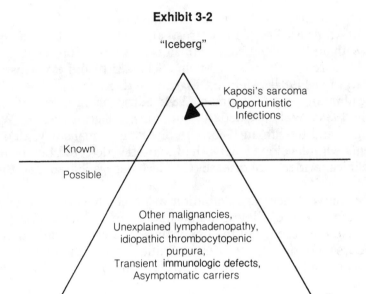

Clinical spectrum of AIDS.

later designated human immunodeficiency virus (HIV), have been described (Barre-Sinoussi, Chermann, and Rey 1983; Gallo, Salahuddin, and Popovic 1984; Levy, Hossman, and Kramer 1984) and represent independent isolates of the same virus group. These retroviruses have been isolated from patients with AIDS, AIDS-related conditions, such as generalized lymphadenopathy, and asymptomatic members of groups with an increased incidence of AIDS (Barre-Sinoussi, Chermann, and Rey 1983; Gallo, Salahuddin, and Popovic 1984; Groopman, Salahuddin, and Sarngadharan 1984; Levy, Hossman, and Kramer 1984; Zagury, Bernard, and Leibowitch 1984; Feorino, Jaffe, and Palmer 1985). Antibodies to HIV have been found in 68% to 100% of AIDS patients and in patients with AIDS-related conditions (Laurence, Brun-Vezinet, and Schutzer 1984; Levy, Hossman, and Kramer 1984; Safai, Sarngadharan, and Groopman 1984; Sarngadharan, Popovic, and Bruch 1984) and in 22% to 87% of high-risk-group members (CDC 1984b; Goedert, Sarngadharan, and Biggar 1984; Melbye, Biggar, and Ebbesen 1984;

Ramsey, Palmer, and McDougal 1984; Spira, Des Jarlais, and Marmor 1984; Weiss 1985). In contrast, antibodies have been detected in less than 1% of persons with no known risk for AIDS (CDC 1985d; Laurence, Brun-Vezinet, and Schutzer 1984; Levy, Hossman, and Kramer 1984; Melbye, Biggar, and Ebbesen 1984; Safai, Sarngadharan, and Groopman 1984; Sarngadharan, Popovic, and Bruch 1984; Weiss, Goedert, and Sarngadharan 1985a; Weiss, Saxinger, and Rechtman 1985b). In one longitudinal study, all of the patients who developed AIDS had anti-HIV detected before there was clinical evidence of disease (Goedert, Sarngadharan, and Biggar 1984).

The surveillance case definition was recently revised to include other, more severe, clinical manifestations of HIV infection (CDC 1985c). In the absence of the opportunistic diseases required by the previous AIDS surveillance case definition, any of the following diseases is considered indicative of AIDS if the patient has a positive serologic or virologic test for HIV:

1. Disseminated histoplasmosis, diagnosed by culture, histology, or antigen detection.

2. Isosporiasis, causing chronic diarrhea (> month), diagnosed by histology or stool microscopy.

3. Bronchial or pulmonary candidiasis, diagnosed by microscopy or by the presence of characteristic white plaques on the bronchial mucosa.

4. Non-Hodgkin's lymphoma of high-grade pathologic type and of B-cell or unknown immunologic phenotype, diagnosed by biopsy.

5. Histologically confirmed Kaposi's sarcoma in patients who are 60 year of age or younger (when diagnosed).

6. Histologically confirmed diagnosis of chronic interstitial pneumonitis in a child under 13 year of age.

Revision of the AIDS case definition resulted in the reclassification of less than 1% of cases previously reported to the CDC. The number of AIDS cases reported to the CDC is steadily increasing (exhibit 3-3). The first cases of AIDS in the United States were diagnosed in 1978. Statistical analysis of the trends indicates that cases

Exhibit 3-3

Reported Cases of AIDS by Half Year of Diagnosis United States, May 18,1987

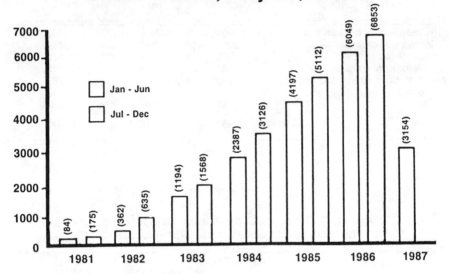

will continue to increase substantially through 1991 (Morgan and Curran 1984). Thirty-four percent of AIDS cases have been reported from New York (see Introduction); most of these are New York City residents. California (primarily San Francisco and Los Angeles) reported 23% of the cases. Other states with numerous cases include Florida, New Jersey, and Texas.

Cases of AIDS in adults can be divided into six patient categories that suggest a possible means of disease acquisition (table 3-1). These categories are arranged hierarchically, so that each patient falls into only the first appropriate category. Seventy-three percent of the cases are reported in homosexual or bisexual men. Past or present abusers of intravenous (IV) drugs compose 17% of the total; another 8% are both homosexual/bisexual and IV drug abusers, and more than half the women with AIDS are IV drug abusers. One percent of the patients are hemophiliacs, and another

Table 3-1

Reported Cases of AIDS in Adults, by Patient Characteristic and Gender, United States, June 1981 — January 21, 1986

PATIENT GROUP	MEN		WOMEN		TOTAL	
	No.	%	No.	%	No.	%
Homosexual or bisexual man	11,998	79	—	—	11,998	73
Intravenous drug user	2206	14	572	53	2778	17
Hemophiliac	128	1	4	<1	132	1
Heterosexual contact	27	<1	158	15	165	1
Transfusions with blood/blood products	162	1	101	9	263	2
Other	747	5	240	22	987	6
Total	15,268		1075		16,343	

Table 3-2

Reported Cases of AIDS, by Disease Category and Case: Fatality Ratio, United States, June 1981 — January 21, 1986

PRIMARY DISEASE	AIDS CASES		NO. OF DEATHS	CASE FATALITY RATIO (%)
	No.	%		
KS without PCP	3056	18	1167	38
Both KS and PCP	920	6	598	65
PCP without KS	9539	58	4986	52
OI without KS or PCP	3059	18	1672	55
Total	16,574		8423	51

KS = Kaposi's sarcoma. PCP = *Pneumocystis carinii* pneumonia. OI = Other opportunistic infection.

1% were heterosexual partners of persons in one of the first three groups. Approximately 2% were recipients of single-donor blood transfusions in the 7 year before diagnosis of AIDS.

More than half the patients with AIDS were reported with *P. carinii* pneumonia, 18% with Kaposi's sarcoma, 6% with both *P. carinii* pneumonia and Kaposi's sarcoma, and 18% with another opportunistic disease only (table 3-2). The distribution of diseases varies by patient category. *P. carinii* pneumonia is more common in

IV drug users and hemophiliacs. Homosexual or bisexual men are more likely to have Kaposi's sarcoma than the other groups.

Fifty-one percent of patients are reported to have died. Mortality varies both by disease group and by time from diagnosis of AIDS. Patients with Kaposi's sarcoma alone appear to have a lower mortality than those in other disease groups (table 3-2). The reported mortality increases as time from diagnosis of AIDS increases. For patients diagnosed prior to 1983, the mortality is 77%. Patients diagnosed in 1983 have a 73% mortality, those diagnosed in 1984 have a 61% mortality, and 31% of those diagnosed in 1984 have died. No patients with definite AIDS have been reported to have recovery of immune function, although a very small percentage survive.

The age distribution of AIDS patients has remained relatively constant: about 90% are between the ages of 20 and 49. Forty-seven percent are between 30 and 39 year old. The racial/ethnic distribution of AIDS patients is as follows: 60% are white, 24% are black, and 14% are Hispanic. Fewer than 1% of patients are Asian, even though the United States, especially New York City and San Francisco, has a large Asian population.

The CDC has received reports of 416 children (229 boys, 187 girls) under the age of 13 who meet a provisional case definition for pediatric AIDS (CDC 1983c). Three percent of these children were diagnosed with Kaposi's sarcoma, 58% have *P. carinii* pneumonia, and 40% had another opportunistic disease. Fifty-nine percent of these children are known to have died.

Cases of AIDS have also been reported from over 47 countries other than the United States.

Risk Factors for HIV Transmission

Homosexuality

Because more than 70% of those with AIDS in the United States are homosexual men, much attention has been focused on the transmission of HIV in this group. A national case-control study performed by the CDC compared 50 homosexual men with AIDS with 120 healthy homosexual men selected from outpatient clinics and private physician practices (Jaffe, Choi, and Thomas 1983). The most important variables in differentiating AIDS cases from controls were measures of homosexual activity. AIDS cases had a larger number of male sex partners per year, began having sex at an earlier age, and were more likely to have had syphilis and non-B hepatitis during their lifetime than did controls. Although AIDS cases used a greater variety of "street" drugs over their lifetime than did controls, no one drug was associated with AIDS. AIDS cases were also more likely than controls to have inserted their tongue ("rimming") or hand ("fisting") into a partner's rectum within the last year; however, a substantial proportion of cases never engaged in either of these activities.

Another case-control study, carried out in New York City, compared 20 men with Kaposi's sarcoma with 40 homosexual controls from a private physician's practice (Marmor, Friedman-Kien, and Zolla-Pazner 1984). This study also found that the number of male sex partners in the year prior to diagnosis was significantly higher in AIDS cases. Other important variables identified included anal-receptive intercourse and "fisting."

The sexual transmission hypothesis generated by the two case-control studies was further strengthened by the discovery of a cluster of AIDS cases linked by sexual contact (Auerbach, Darrow, and Jaffe 1984). When 13 of the first 19 AIDS patients reported from southern California were interviewed, nine were found to have had sexual contact with one or more AIDS patients within the 5 year of onset of symptoms. An AIDS patient who did not live in California was found to have had sex with four of these nine California patients and also with AIDS patients in New York City. Ultimately, the investigators were able to link 40 AIDS patients in 10 different cities by sexual contact, accounting for over 16% of the first 248 cases of AIDS reported in homosexual men in the United States.

Serologic studies for antibodies to the implicated retrovirus in asymptomatic homosexual men have yielded seropositivity rates ranging from 22% to 65% (CDC 1984b; Goedert, Sarngadharan, and Biggar 1984; Melbye, Biggar, and Ebbesen 1984; Weiss, Goedert, and Sarngadharan 1985a; Weiss, Saxinger, and Rechtman 1985b). In a cohort of homosexual men attending a city clinic in San Francisco, the seroprevalence of anti-HIV has increased from 4.5% (13 of 290) in 1978 to 24.1% (7 of 29) in 1980 and 67.4% (293 of 435) in 1984 (Hirsch, Wormser, and Schooley 1985; Jaffe, Darrow and Echenberg 1985). This increasing seroprevalence is similar to the epidemic curve for AIDS in San Francisco. Factors associated with anti-HIV seropositivity in homosexual men were found to be similar to those associated with AIDS in the two case-control studies: seropositive persons reported a larger number of homosexual partners and more frequent anal-receptive intercourse than did seronegative persons (Goedert, Sarngadharan, and Biggar 1984). A statistical association has also been seen between AIDS and seropositivity and "fisting"; however, a proportion of subjects in all studies never engaged in this practice, making its role less clear. Longitudinal studies show that antibody prevalence is rising in groups of homosexual men; infection with the implicated retrovirus is much more common than is AIDS itself, and most of those exposed have not developed overt AIDS.

IV Drug Use

Coincident with the first published reports of AIDS in homosexual men were reports of the same syndrome in IV drug abusers (Small, Klein, and Friedland 1983; Masur, Michelis, and Greene 1984). These patients were first diagnosed in early 1984, about 2 year after the first male homosexual patients (Selik, Haverkos, and Curran 1984). By 21 January 1986, 77% of these patients had been reported from New York or neighboring northern New Jersey. About 11% of homosexual patients give a history of IV drug use, providing a potential mechanism of transmission between the two populations (exhibit 3-4). The route of transmission is presumed to be by parenteral exposure to contaminated equipment used for injection. Needle-sharing has been reported to be a risk factor in these patients (Harris, Cabradilla, and Klein 1983b), but the significance of this practice as a risk factor has not been examined in controlled studies. Seroepidemiologic studies have demonstrated that 87% of recent IV drug users enrolled in a detoxification program in New York City had anti-HIV (Spira, Des Jarlais, and Marmor 1984). In contrast, much lower rates (10%) of antibody prevalence have been reported in IV drug users in San Francisco, where very few AIDS cases are in IV drug users (Spira, 1985, personal communication).

Exhibit 3-4

Cases of AIDS in Adults by Risk Group United States, May 11, 1987
N = 35,020

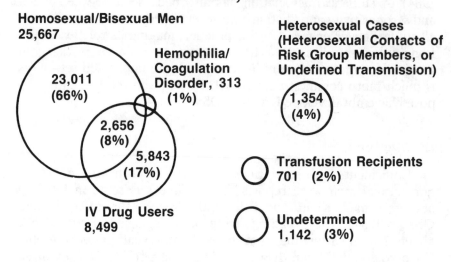

Homosexual/Bisexual Men
25,667

23,011
(66%)

Hemophilia/
Coagulation
Disorder, 313
(1%)

2,656
(8%)

5,843
(17%)

IV Drug Users
8,499

Heterosexual Cases
(Heterosexual Contacts of
Risk Group Members, or
Undefined Transmission)

1,354
(4%)

Transfusion Recipients
701   (2%)

Undetermined
1,142   (3%)

Blood Transfusions

Additional evidence for blood-borne transmission of AIDS came with the reporting of probable transfusion-associated cases to the CDC (CDC 1982f; Ammann, Wara, and Dritz 1983; Jett, Kuritsky, and Katzmann 1983). Transfusion-associated cases were defined for surveillance purposes as AIDS patients meeting the criteria for adult or pediatric AIDS, having a history of blood transfusion within 7 year prior to diagnosis, having abnormal immunologic studies, and having no evidence to suggest that the patient was a member of a group at risk for AIDS. As of January 1987, 588 such cases had been reported, of whom 537 were adults and 51 were children.

In investigations of the donors to these transfusion-associated cases, a "high-risk" donor has been identified in nearly every case (Curran, Lawrence, and Jaffe 1984; Peterman, Jaffe, and Feorino 1985). A "high-risk" donor was defined as a person in an AIDS risk group and/or with persistently abnormal T-helper:T-suppressor cell ratios. Of the 53 "high-risk" donors found in 48 completed investigations, only 9 developed AIDS; an additional 9 developed diffuse generalized lymphadenopathy (part of the broader spectrum of AIDS-associated disease), and the rest have been asymptomatic. Implicated blood components included packed red cells, fresh frozen plasma, platelets, and whole blood, but no single blood component was found to be associated with a markedly higher risk of AIDS virus transmission than the others. (For further information about transfusion-related AIDS, please see the introduction.)

The discovery of HIV and the development of tests for detecting both the presence of virus and antibodies to this agent have permitted the identification of asymptomatic carriers (Feorino, Jaffe, and Palmer 1985). Lymphocyte cultures were evaluated for HIV in 22 of the 25 completed investigations: specimens obtained an average of 28 month (range of 12 to 52 mo) after blood donation were virus-positive for 91% (20 of 22) of the completed evaluations. At the time of examination, 68% (15 of 22) of the virus-positive donors remained healthy, 2 had been diagnosed with AIDS, and 5 had generalized lymphadenopathy. In addition, the isolation of HIV from both donors and recipients in six of the investigations has further strengthened the etiologic role of HIV in AIDS. The study of these transfusion-associated cases has provided important information regarding the natural history of AIDS. Besides confirming that blood can transmit AIDS, we have learned that the disease has a long incubation period and that asymptomatic persons may transmit the disease.

Recommendations for preventing transmission of the disease were issued by the U.S. Public Health Service in March 1983 (CDC 1983b), with subsequent specific guidelines being issued by the Food and Drug Administration (1983, unpublished data). These recommendations have been implemented by the major blood service organizations and are aimed at discouraging blood and plasma donation by persons at an increased risk for AIDS. Donated blood will be tested for anti-HIV to supplement these prevention measures.

Heterosexual Transmission

Reports of AIDS from Zaire and Rwanda also implicate heterosexual transmission as an important mode of spread of this disease in those countries (Piot, Tailman, and Minlangu 1984;

Vande Perre, Le Page, and Kestlyn 1984). In the United States, AIDS has been reported among heterosexual partners of IV drug abusers, bisexual men, Haitians, hemophiliacs, and partners of other persons at risk for developing AIDS (CDC 1983a; Harris, Small, and Klein 1983a). Eighty-six percent of these patients have been residents of New York, New Jersey, California, and Florida. Twenty-six percent of the men who reported to the CDC with no risk factors for AIDS gave a history of sexual contact with female prostitutes (CDC 1984d). Most lived in New York City, where the largest number of cases in female IV drug users have been reported. Further evidence of HIV transmission through heterosexual contact comes from a study of 25 heterosexual partners of 21 patients with AIDS and four patients with AIDS-related conditions (Harris, Cabradilla, and Klein 1984). Forty-one percent of these sex partners (9 of 22) had anti-HIV. One of these heterosexual partners developed AIDS and four patients with AIDS-related conditions had detectable anti-HIV. Specific risk factors for heterosexual transmission of AIDS have not been conclusively identified. Controlled studies are in progress to explore the potential role of multiple sex partners and exposure to prostitutes in heterosexual AIDS transmission.

Other Factors

Approximately 6% of AIDS diagnosed in adults occurs in persons who cannot be classified into one of the previously described groups. This includes persons born in Haiti or central Africa, for whom risk factors for HIV infection were not identified. The first cases of AIDS in Haitian-born immigrants without other risk factors were diagnosed in 1980 (CDC 1982d). This characterized a distinct group with increased incidence of AIDS (Hardy, Allen, and Morgan 1985). Most had entered this country after 1977. Ninety-seven percent of these patients are residents of Florida, New Jersey, and New York. Eighty-four percent are male and 16% are female. *P. carinii* pneumonia and other opportunistic infections are more prevalent than Kaposi's sarcoma in these patients.

AIDS has been well documented in Haiti (Pape, Liautaud, and Thomas 1983). Reports from an epidemiologic study of AIDS in Haiti indicate that, of 93 male patients, 36% gave a history of bisexuality, 5% had received blood transfusions, and 58% had no identified risk factors (Pape, Liautaud, and Thomas 1985). Of 35 Haitian women with AIDS, 40% gave a history of blood transfusions, 6% were heterosexual partners of persons at risk for AIDS, and 54% had no identified risk factors. In a case-control study of the AIDS patients without known risks, significant differences were reported: AIDS patients were more likely to have received injections from nonmedical personnel than were controls; and both male and female patients were more likely to have had multiple sex partners (Pape, Liautaud, and Thomas 1985). Factors underlying the occurrence of AIDS in Haitians living in the United States have recently been described in a case-control study conducted in New York and Miami (Castro, Fischl, and Landesman 1985). Haitian men with AIDS differed significantly from controls in that they were more likely to report a history of previous gonorrhea and sexual contact with prostitutes. Among women, the variable most significantly associated with disease was having been offered money for sexual favors.

In conclusion, risk factors for Haitians may well be the same as in other groups, and heterosexual transmission is likely to be more important because of a higher prevalence of AIDS in predominantly heterosexual men and women. The much higher incidence of AIDS in recent Haitian entrants (post-1977) is consistent with the hypothesis that AIDS and HIV infection are relatively new as important public health problems in Haiti as well as the United States.

An epidemiologic analysis of the first 136 noncharacteristic AIDS cases reported in the United States revealed that information regarding risk factors was incomplete for most (65%) of these patients. However, because many of these patients were similar with regard to age, race, and area of residence to populations recognized to be at increased risk of AIDS (e.g., IV drug users and heterosexual partners of persons at risk for AIDS), some may belong to previously recognized risk groups (Chamberland, Castro, and Haverkos 1984).

Surveillance for AIDS and HIV infection in health-care workers has been undertaken. To date, none of the reported cases of AIDS in health-care workers can be linked to a specific occupational exposure. In the United States, prospective evaluations of health workers with documented parenteral exposure to blood and body fluids of patients with AIDS have only identified four persons with anti-HIV (CDC 1984a, 1985b, 1985e; Weiss, Goedert, and Sarngadharan 1985a). In none of these persons was a preexposure serum sample available to date the onset of the infection. However, one nurse in London reportedly developed anti-HIV 49 days after an accidental needle-stick injury while she drew blood from an AIDS patient (Anonymous, 1984). Available data suggest that occupational transmission of AIDS and HIV infection will remain uncommon.

References

Ammann, A. J., D. Wara, and S. Dritz. 1983. Acquired immunodeficiency in an infant: possible transmission by means of blood products. *Lancet* 1:956-58.

Anonymous. 1984. Needlestick transmission of HTLV-III from a patient infected in Africa. *Lancet* 1:1376-77.

Auerbach, D. M., W. Darrow, and H. Jaffe. 1984. Cluster of cases of the acquired immune deficiency syndrome: patients linked by sexual contact. *Am. J. Med.* 76:487-92.

Barre-Sinoussi, F., J. Chermann, and F. Rey. 1983. Isolation of a T-lymphotropic retrovirus from a patient at risk for acquired immune deficiency syndrome (AIDS). *Science* 220:868-71.

Castro, K. G., M. Fischl, and S. Landesman. 1985. Risk factors for AIDS among Haitians in the United States. Paper presented at the International Conference on the Acquired Immunodeficiency Syndrome (AIDS), 14-17 April, session 11, Atlanta, Georgia.

Centers for Disease Control. 1981a. *Pneumocystis pneumonia*—Los Angeles. *M.M.W.R.* 30:250-52.

———. 1981b. Kaposi's sarcoma and *Pneumocystis pneumonia* among homosexual men—New York City and California. *M.M.W.R.* 30:305-8.

———. 1982a. Diffuse, undifferentiated non-Hodgkin's lymphoma among homosexual males. *M.M.W.R.* 31:277-79.

———. 1982b. *Pneumocystis carinii* pneumonia among persons with hemophilia A. *M.M.W.R.* 31:315-67.

———. 1982c. Update on acquired immune deficiency syndrome (AIDS)—United States. *M.M.W.R.* 31:507-14.

———. 1982d. Opportunistic infections and Kaposi's sarcoma among Haitians in the United States. *M.M.W.R.* 31:353-54.

———. 1982e. Acquired immunodeficiency syndrome (AIDS): precautions for clinical and laboratory staffs. *M.M.W.R.* 31:577-80.

———. 1982f. Possible transfusion-associated acquired immune deficiency syndrome (AIDS)—California. *M.M. W.R.* 31:652-54.

———. 1983a. Prevention of acquired immunodeficiency syndrome (AIDS): report of inter-agency recommendations. *M.M.W.R.* 32:101-3.

———. 1983b. Update: acquired immunodeficiency syndrome (AIDS)—United States. *M.M.W.R.* 32:688-91.

———. 1983c. Immunodeficiency among female sexual partners of males with acquired immunodeficiency syndrome (AIDS)—New York. *M.M.W.R.* 31:697-98.

———. 1984a. Prospective evaluation of health-care workers exposed via parenteral or mucous-membrane routes to blood and body fluids of patients with acquired immunodeficiency syndrome. *M.M.W.R.* 33:181-82.

———. 1984b. Antibodies to a retrovirus etiologically associated with acquired immunodeficiency syndrome. *M.M.W.R.* 33:377-79.

———. 1984d. Acquired immunodeficiency syndrome (AIDS)—United States. *M.M.W.R.* 33:661-64.

———. 1985b. Update: prospective evaluation of health-care workers exposed via the parenteral or mucous-membrane route to blood or body fluids of patients with acquired immunodeficiency syndrome—United States. *M.M.W.R.* 34:101-3.

———. 1985c. Revision of the case definition of acquired immunodeficiency syndrome for national reporting—United States. *M.M.W.R.* 34:373-75.

———. 1985d. Results of human T-lymphotropic virus type III test kits reported from blood collection centers—United States, April 22-May 19, 1985. *M.M.W.R.* 34:375-76.

———. 1985e. Update: evaluation of human T-lymphotropic virus type III/lymphadenopathy-associated virus infection in health-care personnel—United States. *M.M.W.R.* 34:575-78.

Curran, J. W., D. Lawrence, and H. Jaffe. 1984. Immunodeficiency syndrome (AIDS) associated with transfusions. *N. Engl. J. Med.* 310:69-75.

Feorino, P. M., H. Jaffe, and E. Palmer. 1985. Transfusion-associated acquired immunodeficiency syndrome: evidence for persistent infection in blood donors. *N. Engl. J. Med.* 312:1293-96.

Gallo, R. C., S. Salahuddin, and M. Popovic. 1984. Frequent detection and isolation of cytopathic retroviruses (HTLV-III) from patients with AIDS and at risk for AIDS. *Science* 224:500-3.

Goedert, J. J., M. Sarngadharan, and R. Biggar. 1984. Determinants of retrovirus (HTLV-III) antibody and immunodeficiency conditions in homosexual men. *Lancet* 2:711-16.

Gottlieb, M. S., R. Schroff, and H. Schanker. 1981. *Pneumocystis carinii* pneumonia and mucosal candidiases in previously healthy homosexual men. *N. Engl. J. Med.* 305:1425-31.

Groopman, J. E., S. Salahuddin, and M. Sarngadharan. 1984. HTLV-III in saliva of people with AIDS-related complex and healthy homosexual men at risk for AIDS. *Science* 226:447-49.

Hardy, A. M., J. Allen, and W. Morgan. 1985. The incidence rate of acquired immunodeficiency syndrome in selected populations. *J.A.M.A.* 253:215-20.

Harris, C., C. Small, and R. Klein. 1983a. Needle sharing as a route of transmission of the acquired immune deficiency syndrome (abstract 632A). Paper presented at the Twenty-Third Interscience Conference on Antimicrobial Agents and Chemotherapy, American

Society for Microbiology, Las Vegas, Nevada.

Harris, C. A., C. Cabradilla, and R. Klein. 1983b. Immunodeficiency in female sexual partners of men with acquired immune deficiency syndrome. *N. Engl. J. Med.* 308:1181-84.

Harris, C. A., C. Cabradilla, and R. Klein. 1984. Antibodies to a core protein of lymphadenopathy-associated virus and immunodeficiency in heterosexual partners of AIDS patients (abstract 64). Paper presented at the Twenty-Fourth Interscience Conference on Antimicrobial Agents and Chemotherapy, American Society for Microbiology, Washington, D.C.

Hirsch, M. S., G. Wormser, and R. Schooley. 1985. Risk of nosocomial infection with human T-cell lymphotropic virus III (HTLV-III). *N. Engl. J. Med.* 312:1-4.

Jaffe, H. W., K. Choi, and P. Thomas. 1983. National case-control study of Kaposi's sarcoma and *Pneumocystis carinii* pneumonia in homosexual men. Part 1. Epidemiologic results. *Ann. Intern. Med.* 99:145-51.

Jaffe, H. W., W. Darrow, and D. Echenberg. 1985. The acquired immunodeficiency syndrome in a cohort of homosexual men: a six-year follow-up study. *Ann. Intern. Med.* 103:210-14.

Jett, J. R., J. Kuritsky, and A. Katzmann. 1983. Acquired immunodeficiency syndrome associated with blood-product transfusions. *Ann. Intern. Med.* 99:621-24.

Klein, R. S., C. Harris, and C. Small. 1984. Oral candidiasis in high-risk patients as the initial manifestation of the acquired immunodeficiency syndrome. *N. Engl. J. Med.* 311:354-58.

Laurence, J., F. Brun-Vezinet, and S. Schutzer. 1984. Lymphadenopathy associated viral antibody in AIDS: immune correlations and definition of a carrier state. *N. Engl. J. Med.* 311:1269-73.

Levy, J. A., A. Hossman, and S. Kramer. 1984. Isolation of lymphocytopathic retroviruses from San Francisco patients with AIDS. *Science* 225:840-42.

Marmor, M., A. Friedman-Kien, and S. Zolla-Pazner. 1984. Kaposi's sarcoma in homosexual men: a seroepidemiologic case-control study. *Ann. Intern. Med.* 100:809-15.

Masur, H., M. Michelis, and J. Greene. 1984. An outbreak of community-acquired *Pneumocystis carinii* pneumonia: initial manifestation of cellular immune dysfunction. *N. Engl. J. Med.* 305:1431-38.

Melbye, M., R. Biggar, and P. Ebbesen. 1984. Seroepidemiology of HTLV-III antibody in Danish homosexual men: prevalence, transmission, and disease outcome. *Br. Med. J.* 289:573-75.

Morgan, W. M., and J. Curran. 1984. Acquired immunodeficiency syndrome: current and future trends. *Public Health Reports* 101:459-64.

Morris, L., A. Distenfeld, and E. Amorosi. 1982. Autoimmune thrombocytopenic purpua in homosexual men. *Ann. Intern. Med.* 96(pt. 1):714-17.

Pape, J. W., B. Liautaud, and F. Thomas. 1983. Characteristics of the acquired immunodeficiency syndrome in (AIDS) in Haiti. *N. Engl. J. Med.* 309:945-50.

———. 1985. The acquired immunodeficiency syndrome in Haiti. *Ann. Intern. Med.* 103:674-78.

Peterman, T. A., H. Jaffe, and P. Feorino. 1985. Transfusion-associated acquired immunodeficiency syndrome in the United States. *J.A.M.A.* 254:2913-17.

Piot, P., H. Tailman, and K. Minlangu. 1984. Acquired immunodeficiency syndrome in a heterosexual population in Zaire. *Lancet* 2:65-69.

Ramsey, R. B., E. Palmer, and J. McDougal. 1984. Antibody to lymphadenopathy-associated virus in hemophiliacs with and without AIDS. *Lancet* 2:397-98.

Safai, B., M. Sarngadharan, and J. Groopman. 1984. Seroepidemiological studies of human T-lymphotropic retrovirus type III in acquired immunodeficiency syndrome. *Lancet* 1:1438-40.

Sarngadharan, M. G., M. Popovic, and L. Bruch. 1984. Antibodies reactive with human T-lymphotropic retroviruses (HTLV-III) in the serum of patients with AIDS. *Science* 224:506-8.

Selik, R. M., H. Haverkos, and J. Curran. 1984. Acquired immune deficiency syndrome (AIDS) trends in the United States, 1978-1982. *Am. J. Med.* 76:493-500.

Siegal, F. P., C. Lopez, and G. Hammer. 1982. Severe acquired immunodeficiency in male homosexuals, manifested by chronic perianal ulcerative herpes simplex lesions. *N. Engl. J. Med.* 305:1439-44.

Small, C. B., R. Klein, and G. Friedland. 1983. Community acquired opportunistic infections and defective cellular immunity in heterosexual drug abusers and homosexual men. *Am. J. Med.* 74:433-34.

Spira, T. J., D. Des Jarlais, and M. Marmor. 1984. Prevalence of antibody to lymphadenopathy-associated virus among drug-detoxification patients in New York. *N. Engl. J. Med.* 311:467-68.

Van de Perre, P., P. Le Page, and P. Kestlyn. 1984. Acquired immunodeficiency syndrome in Rwanda. *Lancet* 2:62-65.

Weiss, S. H., J. Goedert, and M. Sarngadharan. 1985a. Screening test for HTLV-III (AIDS agent) antibodies: specificity, sensitivity, and applications. *J.A.M.A.* 253:221-25.

Weiss, S. H., W. Saxinger, and D. Rechtman. 1985b. HTLV-III infection among health-care workers. *J.A.M.A.* 254:2089-93.

Zagury, D., J. Bernard, and J. Leibowitch. 1984. HTLV-III in cells cultured from semen of two patients with AIDS. *Science* 226:449-51.

4
The Epidemiology of the Human Immunodeficiency Virus

Harold M. Ginzburg, MD, JD, MPH; and
Mhairi Graham MacDonald, MBChB,
FRCP(E), DCH.

The first recognized cases of the acquired immunodeficiency syndrome (AIDS) were described in mid-1981 (Gottlieb, Schroff, and Shanker 1981; Siegal, Lopez, and Hammer 1981). By the end of 1986, 29,000 cases of AIDS had been reported to the Centers for Disease Control (CDC).

Case Identification

The initial cases of AIDS were reported before a causative agent had been identified (Gottlieb, Schroff, and Shanker 1981). Almost two years of intense scientific exploration were required before the probable cause of AIDS, a retrovirus known as human T-cell leukemia (lymphotropic) type III (Gallo, Salahuddin, and Popovic 1984), or the lymphadenopathy-associated virus (Barre-Sinoussi, Chermann, and Rey 1984) now known as human immunodeficiency

Reprinted with permission and updated figures from "The Epidemiology of Human T-Cell Lymphotrophic Virus, Type III (HTLV-III Disease)" by Harold M. Ginzburg and Mhairi Graham MacDonald, *Psychiatric Annals* 16:153-57, 1986.

virus (HIV), was isolated and identified in 1983. The following year, an enzyme-linked immunosorbent assay was developed to detect the presence of antibodies to HIV (Weiss, Saxinger, and Rechtman 1985c). This enzyme-linked immunosorbent assay test indicates whether or not an individual has been infected with the virus. The Western blot technique provides a more specific, but less sensitive, confirmatory test for the presence of HIV antibodies (Weiss, Saxinger, and Rechtman 1985c). However, unlike antigen tests, antibody tests indicate only that an individual has been infected with the virus and has mounted an immune response. Either a viral culture or an antigen test (presently under development) is required to confirm that an individual is infectious.

There appears to be a spectrum of clinical illnesses associated with infection with the HIV virus and loss of the integrity of the T-helper cell population (Landesman, Ginzburg, and Weiss 1985). The symptom complex for early case identification includes weight loss, chronic unexplained fever or diarrhea, oral candidiasis (thrush), generalized lymphadenopathy, thrombocytopenia, and T-helper cell count below 400 cells/mm (CDC 1984; Landesman, Ginzburg, and Weiss 1985).

Patients with chronic unexplained lymphadenopathy and persistent depletion of T-helper cells are given the diagnosis "AIDS-related complex" (CDC 1985). The number of HIV seropositive persons in whom full-blown AIDS has developed during follow-up periods of one to five years has ranged from 4% to 19% (Landesman, Ginzburg, and Weiss 1985). In these studies, nonspecific symptoms suggesting early stages of HIV-related illnesses have occurred in an additional 25% of individuals who have demonstrated antibodies to HIV.

Basic Epidemiology

HIV diseases are not uniformly distributed across this country (exhibit 4-1). New York State, California, and Florida have reported the greatest number of cases of AIDS. Within these states, the vast majority of the cases are in four cities—New York City, Los Angeles, San Francisco, and Miami. Approximately 30% of the AIDS cases have occurred within the New York City metropolitan area (this includes northern New Jersey). In these cities, there is a non-

Exhibit 4-1

Cases of AIDS by State
Cases as of March 31, 1987

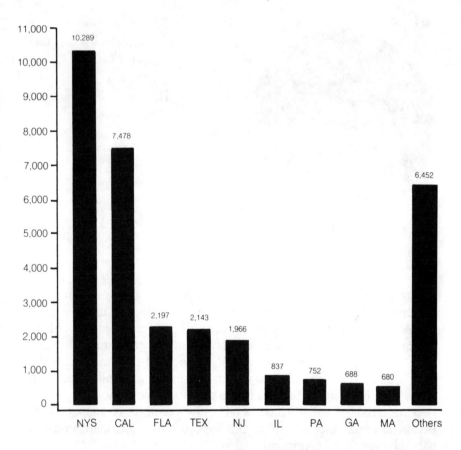

random distribution of patients with AIDS among the high-risk groups.

Exhibit 4-2 illustrates the current high-risk groups, as identified by the CDC. Sexually active homosexual and bisexual men, regardless of whether they admit to a history of intravenous drug use, account for more than 70% of the cases of AIDS. More than one-fourth of all patients with AIDS, independent of sexual preference, give a history of intravenous drug use. There is an overlap among

Exhibit 4-2

33,482 Cases of AIDS in the Country
by Risk Group (As of March 30, 1987)

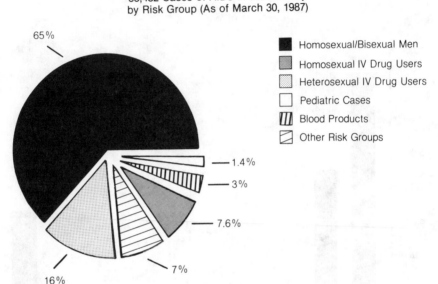

■ Homosexual/Bisexual Men
▨ Homosexual IV Drug Users
▨ Heterosexual IV Drug Users
☐ Pediatric Cases
▥ Blood Products
▨ Other Risk Groups

the two principal risk groups; nationally, 11% of the homosexual patients with AIDS have a history of intravenous drug use.

Although attracting a great deal of media attention, hemophiliacs (1% of the AIDS cases), recipients of contaminated blood transfusions (2%), the heterosexual contacts of persons with AIDS (2%), and children (1%) together represent a small number of cases. The incidence of AIDS in the pediatric population may be underestimated, since it has been only recently recognized that pediatric cases may not meet the formal diagnostic criteria established by the CDC (Ammann 1985).

CDC removed Haitian immigrants from the list of high-risk categories in April 1985. Haitians presently represent more than half of those patients with AIDS who are placed in the "other" category. The majority of the remaining cases in the "other" category are individuals for whom only partial data are available. However, at the present time, it appears that essentially all patients with AIDS have been exposed to HIV either through contaminated blood products, needles and syringes, or by intimate sexual contact with an individual infected with the virus.

Less than 2,000 cases of AIDS have occurred among women (CDC 1985). More than half (53%) of the women with AIDS have a history of intravenous drug use. These women represent 20% of all heterosexual intravenous drug users with AIDS. The National Institute on Drug Abuse estimates that approximately 1 in 4 intravenous drug users is a woman; however, their relative rate of self-injection is less than men. Therefore, intravenous drug-using women appear to be at similar risk for developing AIDS as their male counterparts, when frequency of intravenous drug use is taken into consideration.

Table 4-1 presents the two principal risk groups by their racial composition. More than 74% of all homosexuals with AIDS are white; the homosexual/bisexual men who provide a history of intravenous drug use are also predominantly white. However, approximately 80% of all heterosexual intravenous drug users with AIDS are nonwhite (blacks, 50%; Hispanics, 30%). Many of this latter group are economically disadvantaged (Maayan, Wormser, and Hewlett 1985).

Exhibits 4-3 and 4-4 present a unique view of the different distribution patterns among the high-risk groups in the eastern and western cities with the largest number of reported cases of AIDS. Sexually active homosexual and bisexual men, independent of their history of intravenous drug use, account for approximately 96% of

Table 4-1

Racial Distribution Among Major Risk Groups

	White Not Hispanic	Black Not Hispanic	Hispanic	Other	Total
Homosexual/ Bisexual Men (n = 21,707)	74%	15%	10%	1%	100%
Homosexual IV Drug Users (n = 2535)	65%	21.7%	12.7%	.6%	100%
Heterosexual IV Drug Users (n = 5540)	19%	50%	30%	1%	100%
Other (n = 3700)	37.3%	47%	14.5%	1.2%	100%
Total (n = 33,482)	20,122 60%	8,271 25%	4,766 14%	323 1%	33,482

Exhibit 4-3

2,963 Cases of AIDS in San Francisco
As of February 1987

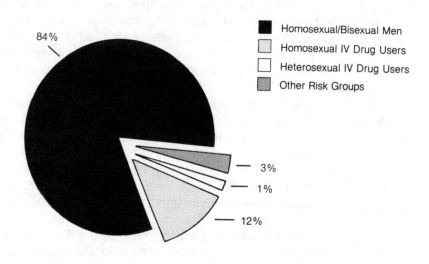

Exhibit 4-4

9,188 Cases of AIDS in New York City
As of February, 1987

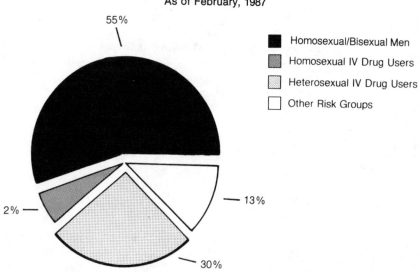

the cases of AIDS in San Francisco; in New York City, they account for only 55%. Intravenous drug use independent of sexual preference is reported by approximately 15% of the patients with AIDS in San Francisco and 32% of the patients with AIDS in New York City.

Because the majority of the patients with AIDS are men (93%), the importance of this disease among women has often been overlooked. Yet, 20% of all heterosexual patients with AIDS who give a history of intravenous drug use are women. At the present time, the majority of the female intravenous drug users diagnosed with AIDS are in the New York City metropolitan area. In addition, heterosexual acquisition of HIV and the development of AIDS have been reported among female sexual partners of male members of high-risk groups (Harris, Small, and Klein 1984), prostitutes (Redfield, Markham, and Salahuddin 1985b), and wives of patients with AIDS-related complex and AIDS (Redfield, Markham, and Salahuddin 1985a).

The National Institute on Drug Abuse, the National Cancer Institute, and the New Jersey State Department of Health (1984) conducted a seroprevalence study among intravenous drug users in drug abuse treatment programs during the autumn of 1984 (Weiss, Goedert, and Sarngadharan 1985b). The results of that seroprevalence study indicated that the relative rate of infection with HIV is the same for male and female intravenous drug users. One-third of all of the intravenous drug users sampled were infected with HIV. Seropositivity rates varied by geographic proximity to New York City. A city within 5 miles of downtown New York had a seropositivity rate of 56% among its clients in a methadone maintenance treatment program. A city approximately 100 miles from downtown New York had a seroprevalence rate of 2% among its clients in a methadone maintenance treatment program. Two intermediate cities had intermediate rates. Needle-sharing behavior was common among the intravenous drug users in all four cities. Overall, more than 95% of these intravenous drug users reported some needle-sharing behavior in the year prior to admission to drug abuse treatment programs.

The State of New Jersey estimates that there were 40,000 intravenous drug users, in New Jersey, at the time of the National Institute on Drug Abuse/National Cancer Institute/New Jersey State Department of Health seroprevalence study (J. French, 1985, personal communication). This would seem to indicate that, overall, approximately 13,200 intravenous drug users (one-third of all intravenous drug users in New Jersey appear to be seropositive) had been infected with HIV. At the time the seroprevalence study was conducted in New Jersey, 455 cases of AIDS had been reported to the New Jersey Department of Health; 55% of these individuals gave a history of intravenous drug use (New Jersey State Department of Health 1984). It is thus possible to estimate crudely that for every case of clinically diagnosed AIDS in New Jersey, among intravenous drug users there were 53 individuals who have been infected with the virus. These findings are similar to the estimates developed for the male homosexual community in San Francisco (Curran, Morgan, and Hardy 1985).

In Zaire, the male-to female ratio for AIDS is 1.1:1 (Plot, Taelman, and Minlangu 1984), supporting the hypothesis that recurrent heterosexual exposure results in male-to-female transmission of HIV. Thus, active public health campaigns directed to women are necessary. This is especially true for women of child-bearing age because intrauterine transmission of HIV to the fetus has been documented (Rubinstein, Sickick, and Gupta 1983; Scott, Buck, and Letterman 1984; Ammann 1985).

Social, Psychological, and Ethical Considerations

Current estimates are that between 500,000 and 1,000,000 residents of this country have already been infected with HIV (Curran, Morgan, and Hardy 1985). As noted previously, this is based on an infection-to-AIDS ratio of 50:1 to 100:1. Thus, an estimated annual attack rate (rate of being diagnosed as having AIDS), once an individual is HIV antibody-positive, is between 1% and 2%. The incubation period has been reported to be as long as 5 years (Curran, Laurence, and Jaffe 1984). More than half of the patients with AIDS are diagnosed during their 30s (CDC 1985).

Parental concern regarding the spread of the virus in schools has not abated, despite the publication of school attendance guidelines by the CDC (Current Trends 1985). Occupational exposure has been a concern among health care workers, again despite CDC guidelines indicting the efficacy of certain precautionary procedures (Current Trends 1983). That HIV virus infection can result from an accidental needle-stick is not surprising (Weiss, Ginzburg, and

Goedert 1985a). Hepatitis B has been known to be spread in this manner for many years. However, there is a fundamental difference between AIDS and hepatitis: hepatitis is only infrequently fatal.

Those individuals who are either HIV antibody-positive or who are closely associated with someone who is, are fearful. Responsible counseling for those who are concerned about AIDS is crucial. It is also important not to label those who are requesting such counseling as psychiatrically ill or psychologically disturbed. A phobia is an irrational fear; those who are concerned about HIV diseases feel that their attitudes and behaviors are rational, based on the available scientific data as presented by the media.

Conclusions

The mass media attention given to AIDS reflects our society's growing concern. At the present time, neither a cure nor a vaccine is on the horizon. Many members of our society who are low risk for contracting AIDS may develop increasing fears about the spread and transmission of the disease. An active public health prevention and education program should help to relieve HIV and AIDS-associated anxieties. Mental health professionals must become more knowledgeable about HIV-related diseases and their neuropsychiatric and psychosocial consequences, in order that they may effectively participate in the education of other health care workers and the lay public.

HIV diseases, including AIDS, will not be eradicated in the foreseeable future. We can minimize the associated physical morbidity through the implementation of effective prevention initiatives in our communities; we can also minimize the associated psychic morbidity through the dissemination of accurate information.

References

Ammann, A. J. 1985. The acquired immunodeficiency syndrome in infants and children. *Ann. Intern. Med.* 103:734-37.

Barre-Sinoussi, F., J. Chermann, and F. Rey. 1984. Isolation of a T-lymphotropic retrovirus from a patient at risk for acquired immune deficiency syndrome (AIDS). *Science* 220:868-71.

Centers for Disease Control. 1984. Acquired immunodeficiency syndrome (AIDS). Weekly surveillance report, 31 December.

——. 1985. Acquired immunodeficiency syndrome (AIDS). Weekly surveillance report, 25 November.

Curran, J. W., D. Laurence, and H. Jaffe. 1984. Acquired immunodeficiency syndrome associated with transfusions. *N. Engl. J. Med.* 310:69-75.

Curran, J. W., W. Morgan, and M. Hardy. 1985. The epidemiology of AIDS: current status and future prospects. *Science* 229:1352-57.

Current Trends. 1983. Acquired immune deficiency syndrome (AIDS): precautions for clinical and laboratory staff. *M.M.W.R.* 31:577-80.

Current Trends. 1985. Education and foster care of children infected with human T-lymphotropic virus type III/lymphadenopathy-associated virus. *M.M. W.R.* 34:517-21.

Gallo, R. C., S. Salahuddin, and M. Popovic. 1984. Frequent detection and isolation of cytopathic retroviruses (HTLV-III) from patients with AIDS and at risk for AIDS. *Science* 224:500-3.

Gottlieb, M. S., R. Schroff, and H. Shanker. 1981. *Pneumocystis carinii* pneumonia and mucosal candidiasis in previously healthy men. *N. Engl. J. Med.* 305:1425-31.

Harris, C., C. Small, and R. Klein. 1984. Immunodeficiency in female sexual partners of men with the acquired immunodeficiency syndrome. *N. Engl. J. Med.* 310:69-75.

Landesman, S. H., H. Ginzburg, and S. Weiss. 1985. Special report: the AIDS epidemic. *N. Engl. J. Med.* 312:521-25.

Maayan, S., G. Wormser, and D. Hewlett. 1985. Acquired immunodeficiency syndrome (AIDS) in an economically disadvantaged population. *Arch. Intern. Med.* 145:1607-12.

New Jersey State Department of Health. 1984. Monthly AIDS data.

Plot, P., H. Taelman, and K. Minlangu. 1984. Acquired immunodeficiency syndrome in a heterosexual population in Zaire.

Lancet 2:65-69.

Redfield, R. R., P. Markham, and S. Salahuddin. 1985a. Frequent transmission of HTLV-III among spouses of patients with AIDS-related complex (ARC) and the acquired immunodeficiency syndrome (AIDS): a family study. *J.A.M.A.* 253:1571-73.

———. 1985b. Heterosexually acquired HTLV-III/LAV disease (AIDS-related complex and AIDS): epidemiologic evidence for female-to-female transmission. *J.A.M.A.* 254:2094-96.

Rubinstein, A., M. Sickick, and A. Gupta. 1983. Acquired immunodeficiency with reverse T4/T8 ratios in infants born to promiscuous and drug-addicted mothers. *J.A.M.A.* 249:2350-56.

Scott, G. B., B. Buck, and J. Letterman. 1984. Acquired immunodeficiency syndrome in infants. *N. Engl. J. Med.* 310:76-81.

Siegal, F. P., C. Lopez, and G. Hammer. 1981. Severe acquired immunodeficiency in homosexual males manifested by chronic perianal and herpes simplex lesions. *N. Engl. J. Med.* 305:1439-44.

Weiss, S. H., H. Ginzburg, and J. Goedert. 1985a. Risk for HTLV-III exposure and AIDS among parenteral drug users. Paper presented at the International Conference on the Acquired Immune Deficiency Syndrome (AIDS), Atlanta, Georgia.

Weiss, S. H., J. Goedert, and M. Sarngadharan. 1985b. Screening test for HTLV-III (AIDS agent) antibodies: specificity, sensitivity, and applications. *J.A.M.A.* 253:221-25.

Weiss, S. H., W. Saxinger, and D. Rechtman. 1985c. HTLV-III infection among health care workers: association with needle-stick injuries. *J.A.M.A.* 254:2089-93.

5

AIDS among IV Drug Users: Epidemiology, Natural History, and Therapeutic Community Experiences

Don C. Des Jarlais, PhD; Nancy Jainchill, MA; and Samuel R. Friedman, PhD.

Introduction

The number of cases of acquired immunodeficiency syndrome (AIDS) represents only a small fraction of the persons who have been exposed to human immunodeficiency virus (HIV), the virus that is the primary cause of AIDS. Estimates of the number of persons who already have been exposed range up from 1 to 2 million. At present, the number of exposed persons who will develop the full syndrome is unknown, with most estimates around 10% to 40%.

Currently, there are no effective treatments for AIDS, and the disease is fatal. Approximately three-quarters of diagnosed cases die within 2 years of initial diagnosis (Curran, Morgan, and Hardy 1985). There is also no effective vaccine for the prevention of the syndrome. While there is intensive research in developing a vaccine, the rate of genetic change in the virus makes development of a vaccine much more difficult (Wong-Stall, Shaw, and Hahn 1985).

Reprinted from "AIDS among IV Drug Users: Epidemiology, Natural History, and Therapeutic Community Experience," by Don C. Des Jarlais, Nancy Jainchill, and Samuel R. Friedman, *Bridging Services* 69-73, 1986, by permission of Alfonso P. Acampora (Editor) and the authors.

In this paper, we will summarize data on the epidemiology of AIDS among intravenous (IV) drug users, the natural history of HIV infection, and the experiences of therapeutic communities with AIDS.

Epidemiology

The development of antibody tests for exposure to HIV has greatly improved our ability to conduct epidemiologic studies of AIDS among IV drug users for several reasons. Previously, epidemiologic research had to use actual cases of surveillance definition AIDS as a dependent variable. The long and variable time period between viral exposure and development of the disease (Lawrence, Lui, and Bregman 1985) and the high ratio of exposed persons to AIDS cases at any single point in time both make numbers of exposed persons a much more powerful variable for analysis than numbers of AIDS cases.

It is clear that the sharing of needles for injecting drugs is the primary method of transmitting HIV virus among IV drug users (Cohen, Marmor, and Des Jarlais 1985; Weiss, Ginzburg, and Goedert 1985). In terms of viral transmission, "needle-sharing" should be defined to include the sharing of the syringes used for injection and possibly even the "cookers" used for preparation of the drugs. Heroin and cocaine are by far the most commonly injected drugs among IV drug users who have been exposed to the HIV virus, but the particular drug being injected does not appear to play an important part in the spread of the virus (Cohen, Marmor, and Des Jarlais 1985).

In the United States, the AIDS epidemic in IV drug users is centered in the New York City metropolitan area. Our 1984 studies of HIV seropositivity among IV drug users in New York City showed approximately 60% of the IV drug users tested had been exposed to the virus. This did not vary significantly among subjects recruited from methadone maintenance, detoxification, or therapeutic communities (Cohen, Marmor, and Des Jarlais 1985). Studies conducted by Weiss, Ginzburg, and Goedert (1985) in New Jersey show a range from 50% seropositive in the northern part of the state, near New York City, to only 2% in the southern part of the state. Studies of seroprevalence in San Francisco and Chicago found approximately 10% of those tested positive in both cities (Spira, Des

Jarlais, and Bokos 1985). Clearly, the AIDS epidemic among IV drug users is most advanced in the New York City area, but it has also started in other cities with large numbers of IV drug users. Prevention efforts are needed throughout the country, but particularly in areas like San Francisco and Chicago, where the great majority of IV drug users have not yet been exposed to the virus.

We have also conducted historical studies of the epidemic in New York City, using serum samples that were originally collected for other purposes. We have sera from IV drug users that go back to the middle 1960s. HIV virus appears to have been introduced among IV drug users in the late 1970s in New York City, and the seroprevalence rate has increased by about 5% per year since then. The first indication of HIV antibody presence is 1 of 11 samples from 1978. Seroprevalence then increases greatly: 29% of 40 samples in 1979 were positive, 44% of samples from 1980 were positive, and 52% of samples from 1982 were positive (Novick, Kreek, and Des Jarlais 1985).

Data on HIV seroprevalence among IV drug users outside of the United States is somewhat limited, but does indicate that the virus is well-established among IV drug users in continental Europe. There are published reports showing 35% seropositivity among IV drug users tested in Zurich (Schupbach, Haller, and Vogt 1985) and 34% among IV drug users tested in Germany (Hunsmann, Schneider, and Bayer 1985). There are preliminary data showing approximately 20% among IV drug users in Holland, 30% among IV drug users in Milan, and 20% among IV drug users in Stockholm. In contrast to the continent, a report from London showed only 1.5% seropositivity among IV drug users (Cheingsong-Popov, Weiss, and Dalgleish 1984). At present, there is no comprehensive explanation for the variation in HIV seropositivity rates among IV drug users in different parts of the world. Hypotheses are being tested to see if differences in needle-sharing between male homosexual and heterosexual IV drug users, or in male homosexual prostitution among IV drug users, may account for the variation. Regardless of the exact reasons for these geographical differences, it is clear that the AIDS problem among IV drug users must be considered a truly international one and not confined to the United States.

In the United States, IV drug users form a link to two other groups at increased risk for AIDS: heterosexual partners and children. Of the 423 cases of AIDS among children reported through January 1987, 53% had an IV drug-using parent. Of the 1,111 cases reported where heterosexual transmission appears to be the route of exposure, 73% involved transmission from an IV drug user. In the United States, heterosexual transmission appears to be almost exclusively male to female. Reasons for the great preponderance of females are currently under investigation.

Risk Reduction

There is a common stereotype that IV drug users are not at all concerned about health and are not likely to change their behavior in order to avoid exposure to human T-lymphotropic virus type III/lymphadenopathy-associated virus. Much of the stereotype appears to be based on observations of very unsanitary "shooting galleries" (Califano 1982; Des Jarlais, Friedman, and Strug 1985). Despite this stereotype, there is consistent evidence from a variety of sources to show that IV drug users in New York City have changed their behavior in order to reduce the chances of exposure to the AIDS virus.

We have conducted studies using interviews of IV drug users in treatment (Friedman, unpublished data), those not in treatment (Des Jarlais, Friedman, and Hopkins 1985b), and persons selling needles for drug injection (Des Jarlais, Friedman, and Spira 1985a). All of these studies showed that IV drug users in New York City knew of AIDS, and the great majority (approximately 90%) knew that it was spread through sharing needles. Approximately 60% of the subjects reported efforts to reduce the chances of exposure to the AIDS virus, primarily through increased use of sterile needles. This self-reported increase in sterile needles was confirmed in our interviews of persons selling needles, who reported an increase in demand for sterile needles as a direct result of the AIDS epidemic. Limited availability of sterile needles was also noted as a major constraint on risk reduction in our studies of IV drug users not in treatment.

It is not yet possible to quantify precisely the amount of reduced needle-sharing that has occurred among IV drug users in New York City. Drawing a truly random sample of IV drug users, and then monitoring their behavior over time, would be an enormously complex research undertaking. All of our present evidence, however, does indicate that efforts to reduce transmission of HIV are occurring as a result of knowledge of AIDS. IV drug users should not be considered unresponsive to the threat of AIDS.

Natural History

The course of HIV infection after a diagnosis of AIDS has been well studied, but there is comparatively little knowledge of the early "natural history" of HIV infection among IV drug users. Important aspects of the natural history yet to be determined include significant events in the early course of the infection, the different possible outcomes for IV drug users exposed to the HIV virus, and the distribution of exposed persons across the different outcomes.

We are currently following a group of over 300 IV drug users, approximately 60% of whom have been exposed to HIV. This will permit us to monitor the early course of HIV infection as well as to determine the various possible outcomes. The decline of T4 (helper) cells to an abnormally low level appears to be an important marker in the infection process. This event is associated with a variety of changes in immunologic status, including increases in serum immunoglobulins and serum (beta)$_2$-microglobulin, and increases in AIDS-related complex symptoms (Des Jarlais, Friedman, and Hopkins 1985b). It may mark a point where serious impairment of the immune system begins, and, after which, treatment may need to include reconstitution of the immune system as well as halting HIV viral replication.

Surveillance definition AIDS and AIDS-related complex are the two best-known outcomes of HIV infection, but certainly not the only possible ones. Most IV drug users exposed to HIV will probably not develop AIDS or any other significant health problems as a result. There is, however, increasing evidence of direct HIV effects upon the central nervous system, leading to a syndrome that resembles Alzheimer's disease (Holland 1985). There have also been epidemics of non-AIDS pneumonia and tuberculosis among IV drug users in New York City that coincide with the AIDS epidemic (Stoneburner and Kristal 1985), and preliminary indications in our data of increased rates of endocarditis among IV drug users exposed to HIV. It is important to determine if exposure to HIV does increase susceptibility to these other serious illnesses that are not normally associated with AIDS. Given the large number of persons who have already been exposed to HIV, we need knowledge of the full range of possible outcomes from exposure.

One of the most frequently asked questions regarding the natural history of HIV infection is the likelihood of developing AIDS. The most common estimates center on 20% to 40% of those exposed developing surveillance definition AIDS. In light of the other possible outcomes noted previously, many of which are disabling or fatal in themselves, the percentage of persons who develop severe health problems as a result of HIV exposure will very likely be much greater.

Cofactors

Our follow-up of HIV-exposed IV drug users is also being used to examine possible cofactors that might influence the progression of HIV infection. Given the absence of effective treatment and the large numbers of persons who have already been exposed to the virus, identification of cofactors may have great potential for reducing the adverse consequences of viral exposure. If cofactors involve modifiable behavior, then it may be possible for many persons who have already been exposed to take actions that would reduce the chances of adverse outcomes.

The potential cofactors that we are examining include continued drug injection/repeated exposure to the virus, exposure through multiple routes, use of noninjected drugs (particularly alcohol and marijuana), stress, and other illnesses. Our preliminary findings indicate that multiple exposure to the virus may have deleterious effects, and recommendations to persons who have already been exposed should advise against activities that may lead to additional exposures.

Therapeutic Communities and AIDS

The most knowledgeable individual at each of 15 therapeutic communities in different parts of the United States was interviewed by telephone in order to assess the prevalence, treatment, and particular concerns about AIDS in therapeutic communities. Results of the interviews are briefly summarized below.

Five of the therapeutic communities reported having residents with AIDS in treatment. In an additional therapeutic community, there were clients who tested positive for HIV, but who were otherwise asymptomatic. All of the therapeutic communities with active cases made the existence of the cases known to residents, but only one community disclosed the client's identity. Five of the 15 therapeutic communities reported that residents had been diagnosed as having AIDS after leaving treatment.

Programs were also asked if clients who had already been diagnosed with AIDS or AIDS-related illness had been accepted into treatment. Four programs had accepted individuals who were asymptomatic, one program had refused admission to such an individual, and the other 10 had not yet been asked to admit anyone diagnosed with the disease. Of these 10, 3 said they would admit based on the individual's medical condition, 3 said they would refuse admission, and 4 stated they had no policy or established guidelines on which to base an admission decision.

The therapeutic communities were also asked what forms of AIDS education had been conducted at the program. All but two of the programs had provided some form of AIDS education to staff and/or residents. Of these programs, most (Cohen, Marmor, and Des Jarlais 1985) involved both staff and residents in the educational effort (e.g., seminars, counseling, or literature distribution), while four involved only their staff.

From the phone interviews, it became apparent that a minority of programs had not begun facing either the moral or the practical issues involved in AIDS among IV drug users, particularly regarding therapeutic community treatment for persons with AIDS-related illness. For some of these programs, the interview process appeared to spur consideration of the issues. The majority of the programs had begun to address the issues, but lacked necessary information and had not resolved the potential value/philosophical conflicts.

Finally, the therapeutic communities were asked about what information and services they needed to deal with AIDS. The predominant issues and needs expressed by the 15 therapeutic communities included: the availability and dissemination of comprehensive and reliable information concerning the disease (Curran, Morgan, and Hardy 1985), the delineation of a rational admissions policy based on facts (Wong-Stall, Shaw, and Hahn 1985), the availability of resources for testing of individuals prior to admission into treatment (Lawrence, Lui, and Bregman 1985), the elucidation of issues specific to the treatment of the terminally ill (Cohen, Marmor, and Des Jarlais 1985), and the establishment of a therapeutic community for the care of substance abusers with AIDS or AIDS-related illnesses.

Summary

Over the last 4 years, AIDS has emerged as a major health problem for IV drug users, with great impact on persons involved in drug abuse treatment. AIDS is creating many new relationships between IV drug use and death. First, it is increasing the death rate among IV drug users. Second, the long latency period means that an individual may now successfully cease drug use, only to die a few years later. Formerly, one could be essentially certain that the health risks from IV drug use could be immediately controlled simply by ceasing to inject. Third, heterosexual and in utero transmission of the virus place the spouses and newborn children of IV drug users at risk of a fatal disease, even though they do not inject drugs themselves. Fourth, it is creating demands for types of services, centered around issues of death and dying, that were not previously required in drug abuse treatment. Finally, even though there is no evidence for casual contact or shared living arrangement transmission, AIDS does provoke fears of death among persons associating with IV drug users.

Specific policy questions for therapeutic communities related to the emergence of AIDS are discussed in an accompanying paper. Our review of the epidemiology and therapeutic community experiences with AIDS indicates that spread of the virus is generally well ahead of the development of strategies for coping with the difficult problems that AIDS presents for therapeutic communities. It is apparent that therapeutic communities need to consolidate efforts and resources for coping with the philosophical/value and practical issues related to the epidemic.

References

Califano, J. A. 1982. *Report on drug abuse and alcoholism*. New York: Warner Books.

Cheingsong-Popov, R., R. Weiss, and A. Dalgleish. 1984. Prevalence of antibody to human T-lymphotropic virus type III in AIDS and AIDS-risk patients in Britain. *Lancet* 2:477-80.

Cohen, H. W., M. Marmor, and D. Des Jarlais. 1985. Behavioral risk factors for HTLV-III/LAV seropositivity among intravenous drug abusers. Paper presented at the International Conference on Acquired Immune Deficiency Syndrome (AIDS), 14-17 April, Atlanta, Georgia.

Curran, J. W., W. Morgan, and A. Hardy. 1985. The epidemiology of AIDS: current status and future prospects. *Science* 229:1352-57.

Des Jarlais, D. C., S. Friedman, and T. Spira. 1985a. A stage model of HTLV-III/LAV infection in intravenous drug users. In *Problems of drug dependence*, ed. L. Harris. Bethesda, Maryland: National Institute on Drug Abuse.

Des Jarlais, D. C., S. Friedman, and W. Hopkins. 1985b. Epidemiology and risk reduction for AIDS among intravenous drug users. *Ann. Intern. Med.*

Des Jarlais, D. C., S. Friedman, and D. Strug. 1985. AIDS and needle sharing within the intravenous drug use subculture. In *The social dimensions of AIDS: methods and theory*, eds. D. Feldman and T. Johnson. New York: Praeger.

Holland, J. C. B. 1985. Psychosocial and neuropsychiatric sequelae of AIDS and AIDS-associated disorders: an overview. Paper presented at the International Conference on Acquired Immune Deficiency Syndrome (AIDS), 14-17, April, Atlanta, Georgia.

Hunsmann, G., J. Schneider, and H. Bayer. 1985. Seroepidemiology of HTLV-III/LAV in the Federal Republic of Germany. *Klin. Wochen.* 63:233-35.

Lawrence, D. N., K. Lui, and D. Bregman. 1985. A model-based estimate of the average incubation and laboratory period for transfusion-associated AIDS. Paper presented at the International Conference on Acquired Immune Deficiency Syndrome (AIDS), 14-17 April, Atlanta, Georgia.

Novick, D. M., M. Kreek, and D. Des Jarlais. 1985. Antibody to LAV, the putative agent of AIDS, in parenteral drug abusers and methadone maintenance patients: therapeutic, historical, and ethical aspects. In *Problems of drug dependence*, ed. L. Harris. Bethesda, Maryland: National Institute on Drug Abuse.

Schupbach, J., O. Haller, and M. Vogt. 1985. Antibodies to HTLV-III in Swiss patients with AIDS and pre-AIDS and in groups at risk for AIDS. *N. Engl. J. Med.* 312:265-70.

Spira, T. J., D. Des Jarlais, and D. Bokos. 1985. HTLV-III/LAV antibodies in intravenous drug (IV) abusers—comparison of high and low risk areas for AIDS. Paper presented at the International Conference on Acquired Immune Deficiency Syndrome (AIDS), 14-17 April, Atlanta, Georgia.

Stoneburner, R. L., and A. Kristal. 1985. Increasing tuberculosis incidence and its relationship to acquired immunodeficiency syndrome in New York City. Paper presented at the International Conference on Acquired Immune Deficiency Syndrome (AIDS), 14-17 April, Atlanta, Georgia.

Weiss, S. H., G. Ginzburg, and J. Goedert. 1985. Risk for HTLV-III exposure to AIDS among parenteral drug abusers in New Jersey. Paper presented at the International Conference on Acquired Immune Deficiency Syndrome (AIDS), 14-17 April, Atlanta, Georgia.

Wong-Stall, F., G. Shaw, and B. Hahn. Genetic diversity of human T-lymphotropic virus type III (HTLV-III). *Science* 229:759-65.

6
Acquired Immune Deficiency Syndrome (AIDS) and Drug Abuse

Harold M. Ginzburg, MD, JD, MPH.

No single disease or medical condition seems to have evoked as much interest and concern from the health care community and the information media as acquired immune deficiency syndrome (AIDS), a new epidemic disease characterized by dysfunction of cellular immunity.

Despite widespread alarm, this immunodeficiency syndrome does not uniformly attack the general population. Initial reports (Centers for Disease Control [CDC] 1981a, 1981b; Masur 1981) indicated that homosexual and bisexual males with multiple sexual partners and the users of illicit intravenous drugs were particularly at risk. More recently, additional risk groups have been identified and defined: recent Haitian immigrants to the United States (Vieira 1983), hemophiliacs receiving factor VIII concentrate (Davis 1983), and "others," including recipients of multiple blood transfusions (CDC 1982) and steady sexual partners of persons with AIDS (Harris 1983). There has been much controversy over reports that AIDS has appeared at higher than expected rates among prison inmates (Womser 1983) and infants in households where other high-risk individuals reside (Oleske 1983).

Reprinted with permission and updated figures from "Acquired Immune Deficiency Syndrome (AIDS) and Drug Abuse," by Harold M. Ginzburg, *Public Health Reports* 99:206-12, 1984.

This paper focuses on drug users who may be most at risk for AIDS, the concerns of drug users about AIDS, and the concerns of their treatment service providers. Techniques are described that can be utilized to educate both drug users and their health care providers.

The term "drug user" or "drug abuser" refers to any person who uses psychoactive substances in a manner that does not constitute an approved medical intervention prescribed by a health professional. This definition applies to misadventure with legally prescribed medications as well as to the use of illicit substances. The term "intravenous drug user" refers to a person who voluntarily injects psychoactive substances directly into his or her blood circulation.

Although intravenous drug users have been recognized as a unique "at-risk" group, they have not attracted as much media attention as the homosexual, Haitian, or hemophiliac groups. Each of these groups has constituencies that can direct attention to their plight.

Drug abusers in general, and intravenous drug users in particular, have no organized advocacy. On the contrary, these groups have been identified as reservoirs of medical problems (such as serum hepatitis) and social ills. Drug abusers are traditionally associated with self-destructive activities; high rates of unemployment and criminality among abusers are frequently reported. Despite these apparent similarities, drug abusers are an extremely heterogeneous group. They display no common type of social, economic, or political behavior that distinguishes them from the general population.

Although they prefer to remain anonymous, drug abusers are generally identified in one of two circumstances: as they seek treatment or when they are arrested. Thus, the drug abuse treatment community and the criminal justice system have traditionally been the primary sources of information on persons with serious drug abuse problems (National Institute on Drug Abuse 1982a, 1982b; Chaiken and Chaiken 1982).

Many drug abusers are not regular abusers (Miller 1983) nor are they readily identified by either of these systems. Treatment for drug-related problems may be provided by the general medical care delivery system without the patient ever being labeled a drug abuser. Drug abusers frequently present with clinical signs of depression or other psychiatric illnesses (Weissman 1976) and these, rather than the substance abuse behavior, may be the reported clinical diagnoses. Most importantly, many persons abuse and misuse drugs and never receive any therapeutic intervention.

As a rule, the general medical community has preferred not to treat either the social or medical ills of drug abusers. Instead, society relies upon the substance abuse treatment community, predominantly a nonmedically oriented treatment system, to provide services for drug users.

Because the drug-abusing community is poorly defined and services to it are typically provided by a potpourri of resources, containment of AIDS among this group becomes a serious public health issue.

Epidemiology of AIDS among Drug Users

The hierarchical presentation of AIDS data by CDC places a person with more than a single risk factor in the most prevalent risk group. For example, according to the CDC method, a drug-abusing homosexual is classified solely as a homosexual. Assignment of cases to risk groups in this manner has limitations; notably, the size differences between risk groups are exaggerated. Not only are the data misleading because they force each case into one category without regard to the separate risks of, say, homosexual intercourse or intravenous drug use, but this is also compounded by using absolute prevalence rather than relative prevalence. That is, if denominator data were developed for homosexuals and intravenous drug users in the geographic areas where AIDS is prevalent, it would probably show that intravenous drug abusers are at substantially higher risk for AIDS than are homosexuals.

When sexual preference is disregarded, intravenous drug a-busers represent more than one-fourth of all AIDS cases. One-third of persons with a history of intravenous drug use are homosexual or bisexual, but only 12% of homosexuals or bisexuals have a history of intravenous drug use. This subgroup of homosexuals or bisexuals who abuse drugs may be an "ultra high-risk" category, and further study may be required to determine if the other risk factors are more likely to predispose this group to AIDS than they are to affect homosexuals or bisexuals who do not self-administer drugs intravenously.

Patterns of illicit drug use among intravenous and nonintravenous drug users who enter treatment programs have been well documented (Sells 1974; Bray 1982; National Institute on Drug Abuse 1982a, 1982b). There are much more limited data on intravenous drug users who do not seek treatment (Levengood, Lowinger, and Schoof 1973; O'Donnell 1976). Data from the Treatment Outcome Prospective Study (TOPS), a large-scale longitudinal study supported by the National Institute on Drug Abuse, are presented here as representative of the subpopulation of drug users who enter treatment. This data base has been determined to be representative of the national census of admissions to all drug abuse treatment programs in the United States (Craddock 1983). The demographic characteristics of TOPS clients and AIDS patients with a history of illicit intravenous drug use, however, are not identical. Slightly more than one-fourth of the TOPS clients reporting intravenous drug use are women, while only 7% of all AIDS victims are women. Ninety percent of AIDS victims are between the ages of 20 and 49 years, with half being between the ages of 30 and 39; approximately one-fourth of the TOPS clients reporting intravenous drug use are between the ages of 30 and 39 (table 6-1).

TOPS is based on three annual cohorts (1979, 1980, and 1981) of clients admitted to more than 40 drug abuse treatment programs throughout the country (Sells 1974; Bray 1982). These clients were interviewed on admission to treatment and reinterviewed periodically while they remained in treatment. A stratified random sample of all clients was interviewed at 90 days, 1 year, and 2 year posttreatment to determine the relative effectiveness of their treatment experiences.

The demographic characteristics of TOPS clients entering drug abuse treatment programs during calendar years 1979, 1980, and 1981 are presented in table 6-1. The most striking observation is that a minimum of three-fourths (8,809) of the 11,623 clients participating in the TOPS study self-administered intravenous drugs in the year before they entered treatment. The median age of these clients was 28 year, and approximately three-fourths were men. Although Caucasians constitute about 74% of the total population of the United States, they constituted only 45% of the intravenous drug users among TOPS clients. Blacks, who make up approximately 13% of the nation's population, constituted nearly 40% of the intravenous drug users. Hispanics, who form approximately 13% of

Table 6-1

Demographic characteristics of TOPS clients who self-
administered their drugs intravenously in the year before
they entered treatment

Characteristic	Number	Percent
Age		
Under 16	14	0.2
16 - 18	140	1.6
19 - 21	641	7.3
22 - 25	1,840	20.9
26 - 30	3,065	34.8
31 - 35	1,719	19.5
36 - 40	681	7.7
41 - 45	351	4.0
Over 45	344	3.9
Total	[1]8,795	[2]99.9
Sex		
Male	6,397	72.6
Female	2,411	27.4
Total	[1]8,808	100.0
Race		
Caucasian	3,956	44.9
Black	3,512	39.9
Hispanic	1,256	14.3
Other	83	0.9
Total	[1]8,807	100.0
Treatment modality		
Methadone detoxification	1,017	11.5
Methadone maintenance	3,907	44.4
Outpatient drug free	1,299	14.7
Therapeutic communities	2,176	24.7
Unassigned or never entered treatment ..	410	4.7
Total	[1]8,809	100.0

[1] Sample size may vary slightly because of incomplete data collection forms.

[2] Does not add to 100.0 because of rounding.

the nation's population, constituted approximately 14%. The racial distribution among AIDS victims reporting illicit intravenous drug use is similar.

TOPS examined drug use patterns in a hierarchical manner. The classification presented in table 6-2 is the result of a cluster analysis. In order to be classified within a given group, a client had to indicate that he or she had used the drug or group of drugs in question at least weekly during the entire year before entering treatment.

Periods of incarceration were considered "no opportunity periods" and were discounted despite frequent reports of the relative accessibility of drugs within detention facilities.

Heroin and narcotics, together and separately, were the drugs used by 70% of all who reported using intravenous drugs during the year before beginning treatment. However, persons who had a minimal drug use pattern (those who did not use even alcohol or marijuana at least weekly), or persons who acknowledged using only alcohol or marijuana and/or a single nonnarcotic, accounted for nearly one-fourth of the clients with a history of intravenous drug use. By the standard CDC definition, these persons would seem to be at added risk for AIDS, despite the fact that they did not have a history of regular opioid abuse.

It is not surprising that the majority of heroin users among TOPS clients reported administering the drug intravenously (table 6-3). However, more than half of all cocaine users reported that their principal route of administration was intravenous, and one-third of those who abused amphetamines preferred the intravenous route. (Thirty-eight percent of all clients did not use any amphetamines.)

TOPS clients were asked to report the manner in which they most commonly self-administered drugs. If a client reported snorting cocaine most of the time and using it intravenously only occasionally, his intravenous use would not be recorded. Thus, the data presented here are conservative estimates of the prevalence of

Table 6-2

Characteristics of TOPS clients self-administering their drugs intravenously—drug use pattern in the year before entry into treatment

Pattern	Number	Percent
Both heroin and narcotics	1,406	16.0
Heroin	3,727	42.3
Narcotics except heroin	1,068	12.1
Multiple nonnarcotics	455	5.2
Single nonnarcotic	762	8.7
Alcohol or marijuana	949	10.7
Minimal drug use	442	5.0
Total	8,809	100.0

Table 6-3

Route of administration of heroin, cocaine, and amphetamines for 11,623 TOPS clients during the year before their admission to a drug abuse treatment program

Route	Heroin		Cocaine		Amphetamines	
	Number	Percent	Number	Percent	Number	Percent
Oral	39	0.3	69	0.6	4,570	39.6
Smoke	48	0.4	55	0.5	2	0.0
Snort	725	6.2	4,475	38.8	163	1.4
Inject:						
Intravenous	7,902	68.0	5,236	45.4	2,391	20.7
Intramuscular	120	1.0	46	0.4	47	0.4
Other	1	0.0	2	0.0	1	0.0
Never used	2,788	24.0	1,657	14.4	4,362	37.8
Total	[1]11,623	[2]99.9	[1]11,540	[2]100.1	[1]11,536	[2]99.9

[1]Sample size may vary slightly because of incomplete data collection forms.
[2]Percentages do not add to 100.0 because of rounding.

intravenous drug use. No comparable data are available for AIDS patients.

Table 6-3 demonstrates the relatively high percentage of clients, irrespective of the specific substance they use, who might be at risk for AIDS, especially if the disease is associated with frequency of the use of needles and the sharing of those needles. Preliminary unpublished estimates from both New York City and New Jersey have indicated that it is a very common practice for intravenous drug users to share needles. In fact, intravenous drug users who do not share needles appear to be the exceptions. In both New York City and New Jersey, several clusters of intravenous drug users who share needles have been identified because all or nearly all of the members of these isolated clusters have developed either AIDS or its prodrome.

If frequency of drug use and frequency of needle-sharing are related to an increased risk of contracting AIDS, then which drug-abusing populations are at greatest risk? Table 6-4 provides a view of the patterns of intravenous drug use among persons reporting either heroin or cocaine use. Nearly half of the heroin abusers and one-fifth of the cocaine abusers use their drugs at least daily. While there may be some overlap between these two groups, the numbers

Table 6-4

Patterns of intravenous drug use among TOPS clients using
heroin or cocaine in the year before their entry into treatment

Pattern	Number	Percent
Heroin		
Less than monthly.................	2,005	25.1
At least monthly..................	1,249	15.6
At least weekly...................	1,156	14.5
At least daily....................	3,574	44.8
Total.....................	7,984	100.0
Cocaine		
Less than monthly.................	1,309	24.9
At least monthly..................	1,767	33.6
At least weekly...................	1,177	22.4
At least daily....................	1,000	19.0
Total.....................	5,253	[1]99.9

[1]Does not add to 100.0 because of rounding.

who are at risk of being exposed to a contaminated needle are very
great.

Until now, questions about the route of self-administration of
cocaine have not been a regular part of national household or high
school survey data, yet more than half of all cocaine users seeking
treatment report some intravenous drug use (Allison, et al. 1983). It
is estimated that 19% of young adults (age 18 to 25 years) and 4%
of older persons have used cocaine at least once, and 11.6% of all
young adults and 2.8% of all older persons have estimated that they
have used cocaine no fewer than 10 times (Miller 1983). Through
this "casual" drug abuse behavior, a significant portion of the
general population may be exposed to the risk of AIDS via contaminated syringes. If this is the case, the dangers associated with
cocaine use require an additional serious public health dimension.

The National Institute on Drug Abuse estimates that there are
at least 350,000 to 400,000 active intravenous heroin users. No
precise estimate of the number of periodic "chippers," or casual
users, of heroin is available, but it is thought to be well over 1 million. No estimates of the numbers of intravenous cocaine and am-

phetamine abusers are available, but these numbers would appear to be reasonably large.

Considered together, these data suggest that the population at risk of contracting AIDS through intravenous self-administration of drugs may be at least several million people.

Concerns of Drug Abusers about AIDS

It might be asked whether drug abuse clients are aware of AIDS occurring within their communities. A small survey was conducted in August 1983 in New York City by a research group directed by Dr. George DeLeon and his Colleagues, Yasser Hijazi and Dr. Harrison Trigg (Ginzburg 1984). One hundred thirty-two clients in four different treatment programs participated. Eighty (61 percent) of the clients were in residential treatment programs; the remainder were in either a methadone maintenance or a methadone detoxification treatment program. Only two of those interviewed (1.5%) had not heard of AIDS. Six additional clients indicated that, although they had heard of the disease, they could not recall any specific details about it. Half of these eight persons were less than 17 years of age. The remainder of all clients interviewed (94%) were able to identify one or more facts about the disease. Only four of the clients (3%) had first learned about AIDS from the treatment program that they were attending.

Almost all of the clients who learned about AIDS while in treatment programs were living in therapeutic communities. Staff of residential treatment programs have more extensive contact with intravenous drug users than staff of either methadone maintenance or methadone detoxification programs. Staff of residential programs appear more interested in gathering additional information on any condition that might affect the residents of their programs and ultimately themselves.

One-third of all of the clients in this special study indicated that they were personally "very concerned" about AIDS, and an additional one-third indicated that they were personally "somewhat concerned about it." Nearly 30% indicated that drug abusers were "very concerned" about AIDS, and an additional 29% indicated that drug users on the street were "somewhat concerned" about it. Clients in residential treatment programs indicated that AIDS had a significant impact on drug users seeking treatment for their drug-related problems. Nearly 20% indicated that they perceived a great increase in clinic attendance, while an additional 58% indicated that they perceived some increase in clinic attendance. No client felt that fears concerning AIDS infectivity were causing any substantial decrease in clinic attendance.

Only 19% of the clients in the methadone programs indicated that the existence of AIDS had influenced many people to stop "shooting up" drugs; however, 59% indicated that the existence of AIDS had influenced some people to stop sharing needles. One in six indicated that AIDS had had no effect on the sharing of needles.

Sixteen percent of all clients interviewed indicated that AIDS had influenced "many" people who had never used drugs to stay away from drugs. An additional 32% felt that AIDS had influenced "some" (but not many) people who had never used drugs to stay away from drugs.

Treatment Program Staff Concerns

AIDS cases among intravenous drug users are currently estimated at 1 per 1,000; approximately 50 AIDS victims have been identified among about 35,000 drug abuse treatment slots in New York City in 1983 (New York State Office of Substance Abuse Services 1983). (The treatment slot concept is similar to that of the hospital bed—more than a single person will occupy a slot during the course of 1 year, but only one person occupies a slot at any point in time.)

Drug abuse treatment staff have expressed concerns about the dangers of handling specimens from a population that might be at great risk of developing AIDS. Although the cause of AIDS is not yet known, these treatment personnel must be reminded that they have been handling specimens with a high prevalence of hepatitis B for many years without contracting hepatitis. Historically, the standards of protection have been adequate when they have been maintained as recommended by State and Federal (CDC) authorities.

A task force at the University of California at San Francisco has developed infection control guidelines for AIDS patients (Conte 1983). These recommendations are more descriptive than the CDC guidelines, but are generally directed to inpatient care settings. The University of California at San Francisco group, like many other research groups, is operating under the basic assumption that AIDS is transmitted through blood products and body fluids.

There are nearly 200,000 clients in drug abuse treatment programs at any point in time, nearly all of them outpatients or in residential environments; during the course of 1 year, more than 400,000 distinct treatment episodes occur (National Institute on Drug Abuse 1982b). If exposure of drug abuse program staff to drug abusers were a significant risk, several cases of AIDS should already have occurred among drug treatment personnel. To date, there has not been a case reported.

Educational Programs for Treatment Providers

The vast majority of treatment services provided in drug abuse programs are not provided by physicians or nurses. While program directors may be medically trained personnel who will understand journal articles and scientific presentations on AIDS, the social workers, counselors, and vocational rehabilitation experts who provide the bulk of direct patient care may not. Therefore, presentations on AIDS need to be specifically tailored for these service providers. Adequate time for the presentation and for question-and-answer sessions is vital. Private consultation time with the presenters should be provided, since some persons are sensitive about displaying their ignorance in wording a "dumb" question, and others may have a question about a personal matter that might be too sensitive for public airing.

Educational programs on AIDS for treatment providers have been organized and administered in New York City by the New York State Office of Drug Abuse Services (1983). Treatment program staff have been uniformly appreciative of these presentations. After the initial sessions, follow-up programs are held. Small group workshops help staff verbalize their concerns about the possibility of contracting AIDS and spreading it to their families and friends. After the staff has participated in these education and ventilation sessions, joint staff-patient discussions are often very useful.

Summary

AIDS appears to be spread through exposure to infected blood products and body fluids. Sharing of needles ("works") appears to be the most significant factor in transmission of AIDS among intravenous drug users, rather than the type of drug administered through that needle.

There is no evidence that close, nonintimate contact with an AIDS victim results in transmission of the disease. No health care worker has developed AIDS as a result of caring for AIDS patients.

Targeted educational programs and research activities are required for intravenous drug users and the health professionals who care for them. The fears and anxieties of treatment program clients, their families, and treatment staff need to be addressed directly. Specific recommendations that meet the needs of outpatient and residential treatment staff should be developed.

Drug abuse treatment program staff are known to share foods, beverages, and cigarettes with their clients. While these practices have not been associated with the development of AIDS, they should be discouraged for general health reasons and not for the possibility of casual transmission of the AIDS virus. Those treatment staff who handle blood or other body fluids should continue to use the CDC infectious disease precautions that have been in use for years. The original precautions were established (and have proved adequate) to protect clinical staff from hepatitis.

Education of drug users with regard to general preventive measures is important. Special attention needs to be directed to those intravenous drug users who do not own their own "works" or who share their works with other drug users. Needle-sharing should be actively discouraged.

Although drug abusers and personnel who provide direct services to them have received little media attention and, until very recently, no significant amount of research interest, this trend is changing. As public information campaigns directed to changing the sexual practices of very sexually active homosexuals become more effective, it is quite possible that an increasing proportion of new cases of AIDS will emanate from the drug-using community. Education measures are required immediately. Drug users, their families, their friends, and those who provide treatment services need to know more about AIDS, its etiology, the mode(s) by which it is spread, and methods for limiting exposure.

References

Allison, M., R. Hubbard, E. Cavanaugh, and J. Rachal. 1983. *Drug abuse treatment process: descriptions of TOPS methadone, residential, and outpatient drug free programs.* Research Triangle Park, North Carolina: Research Triangle Institute.

Bray, R. M. 1982. *Approaches to the assessment of drug use in the Treatment Outcome Prospective Study.* Research Triangle Park, North Carolina: Research Triangle Institute.

Centers for Disease Control. 1981a. *Pneumocystis* pneumonia—Los Angeles. *M.M.W.R.* 30:250-52.

Centers for Disease Control. 1981b. Kaposi's sarcoma and *Pneumocystis* pneumonia among homosexual men—New York City and California. *M.M.W.R.* 30:305-8.

Centers for Disease Control. 1982. Possible transfusion-associated acquired immune deficiency syndrome (AIDS)—California. *M.M.W.R.* 31:652-54.

Chaiken, J. M., and M. Chaiken. 1982. *Varieties of criminal behavior.* Santa Monica, California: Rand Corporation.

Conte, J. E., Jr. 1983. Infection-control guidelines for patients with acquired immunodeficiency syndrome (AIDS). *N. Engl. J. Med.* 309:740-44.

Craddock, S. G. 1983. *Drug use before and during drug abuse treatment: 1979-81 TOPS admission cohorts. Research Triangle Park, North Carolina: Research Triangle Institute.*

Davis, K. C. 1983. Acquired immune deficiency syndrome in a patient with hemophilia. *Ann. Intern. Med.* 98:284-86.

Ginzburg, H. M. 1984. *A survey of attitudes concerning AIDS among clients in treatment. Clinical research notes.* Rockville, Maryland: National Institute on Drug Abuse.

Harris, C. 1983. Immunodeficiency in female sexual partners of men with the acquired immunodeficiency syndrome. *N. Engl. J. Med.* 308:1181-84.

Levengood, R., P. Lowinger, and K. Schoof. 1973. Heroin addiction in the suburbs—An epidemiologic study. *Am J. Public Health* 63:209-14.

Masur, H. 1981. An outbreak of community acquired *Pneumocystis carinii* pneumonia: initial manifestation of cellular immune dysfunction. *N. Engl. J. Med.* 305:1431-38.

Miller, J. D. 1983. *National Survey on Drug Abuse: main findings, 1982.* Rockville, Maryland: National Institute on Drug Abuse.

National Institute on Drug Abuse. 1982a. *Client oriented data acquisition process (CODAP), annual data 1981.* Statistical Series, series E, no. 25. Rockville, Maryland.

National Institute on Drug Abuse. 1982b. *National drug and alcoholism treatment utilization survey.* Summary report on drug abuse treatment units. Rockville, Maryland.

New York State Office of Substance Abuse Services. 1983. *AIDS newsletter.*

O'Donnell, J. A. 1976. *Young men and drugs A nationwide survey.* National Institute on Drug Abuse. Research Monograph Series 5. DHEW publication no. (ADM) 76-311. Washington, D.C.: U.S. Government Printing Office.

Oleske, J. 1983. Immune deficiency syndrome in children. *J.A.M.A.* 249:2345-49.

Sells, S. B., ed. 1974. *The effectiveness of drug abuse treatment: evaluation of treatment,* vol. 1. Cambridge, Massachusetts: Ballinger Publishing Company.

Vieira, J., E. Frank, T. Spira, and S. H. Landesman. 1983. Acquired immune deficiency in Haitians; opportunistic infections in previously healthy Haitian immigrants. *N. Engl. J. Med.* 308:125-29.

Weissman, M. W. 1976. Clinical depression among addicts maintained on methadone in the community. *Am J. Psychiat.* 13:1434-38.

Womser, G. P. 1983. Acquired immunodeficiency syndrome in male prisoners: new insights into an emerging syndrome. *Ann. Intern. Med.* 98:297-303.

7

Intravenous Drug Abusers and the Acquired Immunodeficiency Syndrome (AIDS)

Gerald H. Friedland, MD; Carol Harris, MD; Catherine Butkus-Small, MD; Daniel Shine, MD; Bernice Moll, PhD; William Darrow, PhD; and Robert S. Klein, MD.

The second largest group of cases of the acquired immunodeficiency syndrome (AIDS) has appeared in persons who use illegal drugs intravenously (IV drug abusers). This risk group constitutes 17% of all cases (1). Together, with sexually active gay/bisexual men who are also IV drug abusers, this group accounts for almost 25% of all reported cases of AIDS. Approximately half of all cases of AIDS have been reported from New York City, and the New York metropolitan area accounts for over 85% of all cases in IV drug abusers (Jaffe, Bregman, and Selik 1983a; Jaffe, Choi, and Thomas 1983b). The hospitals associated with the Albert Einstein College of Medicine provide care for a large number of IV drug abusers in the Bronx, New York City. The majority of our patients with AIDS belong to this risk group (Small, Klein, and Friedland 1983).

Reprinted with permission from "Intravenous Drug Abusers and the Acquired Immunodeficiency Syndrome (AIDS)," by Gerald H. Friedland, Carol Harris, Catherine Butkus-Small, Daniel Shine, Bernice Moll, William Darrow, and Robert S. Klein, *Archives of Internal Medicine* 145:1413-17, 1985.

The population affected by AIDS are also those with high rates of hepatitis B (Sherlock 1981). Transmission of AIDS via a blood-borne route through the infusion of contaminated blood products is suggested by the appearance of AIDS in hemophiliacs (Centers for Disease Control 1982) and multiply transfused patients without other risk factors (Curran, Lawrence, and Jaffe 1983). Blood-borne transmission of the virus among IV drug abusers takes place through the sharing of needles and syringes; such needle-sharing behavior has also been implicated as the most likely epidemiological connection between IV drug abusers and sexually active gay and bisexual men who use IV drugs (Des Jarlais, Jainchill, and Friedman 1986).

To clarify these issues related to the transmission of AIDS, we studied the demographic characteristics, drug use, and sexual practices of IV drug abusers with AIDS and AIDS-related complex (ARC) and then compared them with those of a group of IV drug abusers without evidence of AIDS.

Subjects and Methods

Subjects

The study population consisted of all IV drug abuser patients with AIDS or ARC who were identified by the investigators during hospitalization at Montefiore Medical Center, North Central Bronx Hospital, of Bronx Municipal Hospital Center, from July 1981 to March 1983. These patients were referred to the investigators by house officers, infectious disease fellows, and infection control nurses. A comparison control group of IV drug abusers with no evidence of AIDS or ARC was identified from two sources: hospitalized IV drug abusers admitted with illnesses unrelated to AIDS who were brought to the attention of the investigators by house officers and infectious disease fellows (Jaffe, Bregman, and Selik 1983a; Jaffe, Choi, and Thomas 1983b) and healthy IV drug abusers who were sequentially enrolled into the Montefiore Medical Center Drug Abuse Treatment Program (Small, Klein, and Friedland). Subjects from both sources were excluded from the control group if they had generalized lymphadenopathy and/or oral candidiasis, abnormal T-cell ratios, or opportunistic infections.

Definitions

Patients were defined as having AIDS according to the Centers for Disease Control criteria (Centers for Disease Control 1983). Patients with AIDS were previously healthy adults below the age of 60 years who had biopsy or culture-proven opportunistic infection suggestive of immune dysfunction and/or disseminated Kaposi's sarcoma. Patients with ARC were previously healthy adults below the age of 60 years who manifested generalized lymphadenopathy (hyperplastic, if biopsied), without known cause, in association with an inverted T4/T8 ratio and other parameters of immune dysfunction characteristic of that seen in AIDS (lymphopenia and cutaneous anergy), and/or unexplained oral candidiasis. Generalized lymphadenopathy was defined as the presence of palpable lymph nodes larger than 1 cm at two or more extrainguinal sites, excluding draining sites of IV injection.

Subject Evaluations

After informed consent was obtained, AIDS, ARC, and control subjects underwent a detailed, standardized interview conducted by one of the investigators. The interview focused on demographic characteristics and sexual and drug use practices. All subjects were examined by one of the investigators and underwent an immunologic laboratory screening evaluation. This included lymphocyte count, immunoglobulin levels, testing for cutaneous hypersensitivity, and quantitation of T-cell subsets. Standard techniques were used to determine absolute lymphocyte counts and immunoglobulin levels. Intradermal injections of *Candida*, mumps, Trichophyton, and tuberculin-purified protein derivative antigens were used to test for cutaneous anergy. In vitro studies included identification of all peripheral T-cells, helper/inducer T-cells (T4), and suppressor/cytotoxic T-cells (T8), with the use of monoclonal antibodies OKT3, OKT4, and OKT8, respectively, in an indirect immunofluorescence assay or on the fluorescent-activated cell sorter as previously described (Moll, Emeson, and Small 1983; Rubinstein, Siclick, and Gupta 1983).

The Fisher's exact test was used to assess statistical independence.

Results

Seventy-nine adult patients with AIDS or ARC were seen at our institutions between July 1981 and March 1983. Sixty (76%) gave a history of IV drug abuse. Of these, 20 were not available for study. Fifteen patients died and five were unavailable for follow-up before complete evaluation could be performed. The remaining 40 drug abuse patients (16 patients with AIDS and 24 with ARC) were completely studied. These 40 were similar in age, sex, and sexual preference to the total population of 60 drug abusers. The mean T helper/suppressor ratio among AIDS patients was 0.23, and among ARC patients, 0.45. Twenty of 24 ARC patients had T-cell ratios determined; these ranged from 0 to 0.98. The remaining four had unexplained lymphadenopathy and oral candidiasis. Three of these had cutaneous anergy and two had lymphopenia. In the "healthy" IV drug abuser control population, 24 IV drug abusers without clinical evidence of AIDS or ARC were initially identified. Ten were eliminated because of inverted T-cell ratios. The remaining 14 were included for study (six hospitalized patients and eight drug abuse treatment program enrollees). Their mean T-cell ratio was 1.77 (range: 1.4 to 3.40).

The demographic characteristics of the 40 patients and the 14 "healthy" IV drug abusers are shown in table 7-1. There were no demographic differences between the AIDS and ARC patients, and we therefore grouped them together for comparison with the "healthy" IV drug user control population. Patients and controls were young, of lower socioeconomic status, and predominantly from the geographic area immediately surrounding our hospitals. Foreign travel and even travel outside of New York City was rare. The majority were men of Hispanic (predominantly Puerto Rican) background. None were Haitian or had known close contact with Haitians. Eighty-three percent of the AIDS and ARC patients were heterosexuals, as were 79% of the control IV drug abusers; 17% of the patients and 21% of the controls were homosexual males. There were no significant differences between the homosexual and heterosexual populations with respect to age, residence, ethnic background, or income status. Twenty percent of AIDS and ARC patients were women, as were 14% of the "healthy" IV drug abuser controls. The women were similar to the men in age, income, and ethnic and geographic backgrounds. The median number of total

Table 7-1

Demographic Features and Sexual Practice of Intravenous (IV) Drug Abusers

	No. (%)			
	AIDS* Patients (n = 16)	ARC* Patients (n = 24)	Total Patients (n = 40)	"Healthy" IV Drug Abuser Controls (n = 14)
Age, yr				
Mean	32.5	32.6	32.6	32.8
Range	22-51	23-41	22-51	23-50
Sex				
M	13 (81)	19 (79)	32 (80)	12 (86)
F	3 (19)	5 (21)	8 (20)	2 (14)
Residence				
Bronx	13 (81)	23 (96)	36 (90)	12 (86)
Other areas of New York City	3 (19)	1 (4)	4 (10)	2 (14)
Background				
Hispanic	12 (75)	15 (62)	27 (68)	8 (57)
Black	3 (19)	9 (38)	12 (30)	4 (29)
White	1 (6)	0 (0)	1 (2)	2 (14)
Income, dollars/yr				
<10,000	10 (63)	19 (82)	29 (73)	9 (64)
10,000-20,000	5 (31)	2 (8)	7 (18)	3 (21)
>20,000	0 (0)	1 (4)	1 (2)	2 (14)
Unknown	1 (6)	2 (8)	3 (7)	0 (0)
Sexual orientation				
Heterosexual	12 (75)	21 (88)	33 (83)	11 (79)
Male homosexual or bisexual	4 (25)	3 (12)	7 (17)	3 (21)
No. of lifetime sexual partners				
Heterosexuals				
Median	6	15	15	12
Range	1-250	1-200	1-250	1-150
Homosexuals				
Median	50	15	25	17
Range	2-500	3-25	2-500	10-150

*AIDS indicates acquired immunodeficiency syndrome; and ARC, AIDS-related complex.

lifetime sexual partners is recorded for each group in table 7-1. There were no significant differences in median numbers of sexual partners or in sexual practices between the heterosexual patients and heterosexual controls or between the homosexual patients and homosexual controls. The heterosexual patients all denied male prostitution.

Table 7-2

Drug Use in Intravenous (IV) Drug Abusers

	No. (%)			
	AIDS* Patients (n = 16)	ARC* Patients (n = 24)	Total Patients (n = 40)	"Healthy" IV Drug Abuser Controls (n = 14)
Type				
Heroin	16 (100)	23 (96)	39 (98)	14 (100)
Cocaine	14 (88)	20 (83)	34 (85)	14 (100)
Mixed	12 (75)	15 (63)	27 (68)	14 (100)
Frequency				
Daily	10 (63)	16 (67)	26 (65)	12 (86)
2-5/wk	1 (6)	1 (4)	2 (5)	0 (0)
≤ 1/wk	3 (21)	1 (4)	4 (10)	1 (7)
Unknown	2 (13)	6 (25)	8 (20)	1 (7)
Duration, yr				
>5	15 (94)	19 (79)	34 (85)	12 (86)
1-5	0 (0)	4 (17)	4 (10)	1 (7)
<1	1 (6)	1 (4)	2 (5)	1 (7)
Current use	12 (75)	24 (100)	36 (90)	12 (86)
Nitrite use (inhaled)				
Total	5 (31)	1 (4)	6 (15)	3 (21)
Heterosexual	2/12 (17)	0/21 (0)	2/33 (6)†	1/10 (10)
Homosexual	3/4 (75)	1/3 (33)	4/7 (57)	2/3 (67)
Alcohol use				
Moderate/heavy	9 (56)	13 (54)	22 (55)	8 (57)
Occasional	4 (25)	10 (42)	14 (35)	5 (36)
None	3 (19)	1 (4)	4 (10)	1 (7)
Marijuana use				
Moderate/heavy	10 (63)	17 (71)	27 (68)	13 (93)
Occasional	1 (6)	1 (4)	2 (5)	0 (0)
None	5 (31)	0 (0)	5 (13)	1 (7)
Unknown	0 (0)	6 (25)	6 (19)	0 (0)

*AIDS indicates acquired immunodeficiency syndrome; and ARC, AIDS-related complex.
†P < .006 (Fisher's exact test).

Drug use patterns are shown in table 7-2. All groups were similar in drug use patterns. Heroin and cocaine, either alone or in combination, were universally used by patients and "healthy" controls. Most patients and controls were daily users of IV drugs, had used drugs for more than 5 years, and were actively using drugs at the time of the study. There were no differences in the use of IV drugs between homosexual and heterosexual drug abusers. Moderate to heavy use of alcohol and marijuana was common in all groups, but the use of inhaled nitrites was infrequent. Only six

Table 7-3

Needle Sharing Among Intravenous (IV) Drug Abusers

	No. (%)				
	AIDS* Patients (n = 16)	ARC* Patients (n = 24)	Total Patients (n = 40)	AIDS/ARC Homosexual Men (n = 7)	"Healthy" IV Drug Abuser Controls (n = 14)
Share needles	14/16 (88)	21/24 (88)	35/40 (88)	7/7 (100)	14/14 (100)
Share needles with homosexual men	9/14 (64)	11/21 (52)	20/35 (57)	5/7 (71)	4/13 (31)†
Attend "shooting galleries"	12/14 (86)	16/21 (76)	28/35 (74)	6/7 (86)	10/14 (71)

* AIDS indicates acquired immunodeficiency syndrome; and ARC, AIDS-related complex.
† Information not available in one control.

(15%) of 40 AIDS and ARC patients and three (21%) of 14 healthy controls had used nitrites. However, there were significant differences in the use of these agents related to sexual orientation. Only 2 (6%) of 33 heterosexual IV drug abusers with AIDS or ARC used nitrites, whereas 4 (57%) of 7 homosexual IV drug abusers with AIDS or ARC used nitrites ($P < 0.006$). A similar difference was found between homosexual and heterosexual IV drug abuser controls. There were no other significant differences between heterosexual and homosexual men with respect to drug use.

Needle-sharing experience is recorded in table 7-3. The sharing of needles among IV drug abusers was extremely common in all groups, and included all homosexual male patients and 7 of 8 female patients. Needle-sharing with men thought to be homosexuals was commonly reported. Although this was reported more frequently among AIDS patients (9/16, 64%) than "healthy" controls (4/13, 31%), this difference was not statistically significant ($p = 0.12$). Attendance at "shooting galleries," where anonymous, multiple-partner needle-sharing took place, was frequent in all groups.

"Shooting galleries" were described as transient or semipermanent sites, such as apartments, storefronts, basements, or burned-out buildings. They were usually managed by a proprietor who both sold drugs and rented needles, syringes, and other drug apparatus. After drugs were administered, the rented needle and syringe were returned to the proprietor. The same needle and syringe were then sequentially rented to other IV drug abusers.

Comments

Although AIDS was initially thought to be confined to homosexual men, IV drug abuse was soon recognized to be a risk factor for AIDS acquisition. We noted the appearance of AIDS among IV drug abusers at the same time the syndrome was first noted in homosexual men (Small, Klein, and Friedland 1983). Intravenous drug abusers now constitute the second largest AIDS risk group. Of the 3,000 patients with AIDS reported through December 1983, 510 (17%) were recorded by the Centers for Disease Control as IV drug abusers (Centers for Disease Control 1983). Therefore, approximately 25% of the total AIDS population use IV drugs. In our patient population, 76% of AIDS or ARC patients are IV drug abusers. The presence of AIDS in female sexual partners of IV drug-abusing men with AIDS (Harris, Small, and Klein 1983) and in children whose parents are IV drug abusers (Moll, Emeson, and Small 1983) has focused attention on IV drug abusers as an important population in whom questions of AIDS risk and transmission require further investigation.

IV abuse of opiates in the United States became common in the 1920s (O'Donnel and Jones 1968). There was a marked increase in the use of IV opiates in the northeastern cities in the 1960s and early 1970s and again in the late 1970s to the present (Des Jarlais and Uppal 1980). It is estimated that there are approximately 200,000 IV drug abusers in New York City and 750,000 nationally (Des Jarlais 1983). Despite the size of this population and the well-recognized medical complications of IV drug abuse (Louria, Hensle, and Rose 1967), there has been little written about the details of drug administration and the demographic characteristics of drug abusers. This information is central to our understanding of the appearance and transmission of AIDS in this population.

In this preliminary study of IV drug abusers in the Bronx, interesting and important information about the population at risk and drug use practices emerged. Contrary to commonly held belief, we found that our patients generally admitted to IV drug abuse and discussed their use of IV drugs openly. This is reflected in the high proportion of positive responses about drug use in our total AIDS population. This risk factor could be identified in 41 of 42 heterosexual men and in 10 of 16 women with AIDS or ARC.

This study has shown that IV drug abusers in the Bronx with and without AIDS are a homogeneous population of young, poor men and women who are members of minority groups, have a remarkably similar pattern of drug use, and who are restricted geographically. These demographic characteristics support those reported among IV drug abusers with AIDS by Guinan, Thomas and Pinsky (1984). Our IV drug abuser patients remain in the Bronx and rarely travel out of New York City. This fact explains the relative infrequency of AIDS among IV drug abusers living outside of the New York metropolitan area. Although drugs travel widely throughout the country, drug users do not. In this lack of mobility, IV drug users differ from homosexual men with AIDS, who tend to be white, middle class (Jaffe, Bregman, and Selik 1983a; Jaffe, Choi, and Thomas, 1983b; Guinan, Thomas and Pinsky 1984), and may travel between areas in which AIDS is now heavily concentrated. Indeed, case-finding studies have directly associated homosexual men with AIDS in different cities with each other (Auerbach, Darrow, and Jaffe 1984).

There appeared to be a uniform pattern of drug use among IV drug abusers in this study. Heroin and/or cocaine use was universal in our sample. Most IV drug abusers with or without AIDS used heroin and/or cocaine daily and had used these drugs for over 5 years. Although alcohol and marijuana use were frequent, nitrite use was uncommon. The use of inhaled nitrites was initially highly correlated with AIDS in homosexual men and thought to be of etiologic significance (Marmor, Friedman-Kien, and Laubenstein 1982). More recent studies have confirmed the frequent use of nitrites in homosexual men but suggest that nitrite use is a marker for promiscuity rather than of etiologic significance (Jaffe, Bregman, and Selik 1983a; Jaffe, Choi, and Thomas 1983b; Marmor, Friedman-Kien, and Zolla-Pazner 1984). In the present study, nitrite use was significantly less common among heterosexual IV drug abusers with AIDS or ARC then among homosexual IV drug abusers. Nitrites could not be of etiologic significance in the development of AIDS if only 6% of the IV drug abusers with AIDS or ARC use them. The presence of AIDS in diverse and seemingly unrelated populations has been among the strongest arguments favoring a transmissible biologic agent as the cause of AIDS. This epidemiologic observation is now supported by evidence etiologically associating a newly described human retrovirus with AIDS (Barre-Sinoussi, Chermann, and Rey 1983; Gallo, Salahuddin, and Popovic 1984). The existence of large homosexual and IV drug abuser populations with AIDS in New York City, as well as the appearance of the syndrome in both populations at the same time, suggest that these two largest groups with AIDS are epidemiologically connected. It is noteworthy that 14% of patients nationally with AIDS and 17% of our patients with AIDS or ARC were both IV drug abusers and homosexual men. Individuals belonging to both major risk groups are the likely connection between the two groups.

What feature(s) of drug use might result in the spread of AIDS among IV drug abusers and between heterosexual and homosexual populations? Inoculation of blood via the sharing of contaminated needles appears to be the most likely. We found a remarkably high frequency of needle-sharing among IV drug abusers. The high prevalence of hepatitis B markers as well as outbreaks of malaria in IV drug-abusing populations have been assumed to be the result of the communal use of unsterile needles (Louria, Hensle, and Rose 1967). However, the striking ubiquity of needle-sharing among present-day IV drug users has not been previously recorded (Des Jarlais, Jainchill, and Friedman 1986; Lewis and Galea 1986). In this study, all categories of patients and controls routinely shared needles with others during drug administration. Importantly, needle-sharing often took place in "shooting galleries." It is noteworthy that the number of "shooting galleries" has apparently markedly increased during the past decade in New York City, and it is now estimated that there are close to 1,000 "shooting galleries" in the New York metropolitan area (Des Jarlais, 1984, unpublished data). In "shooting galleries," needles and syringes were sequentially and anonymously shared by multiple IV drug abusers. This process provides a logical explanation for the presence of a blood-borne infectious disease among IV drug abusers and for the remarkably high rate of antibody (58% to 87%) to human immunodeficiency virus, the presumed AIDS etiologic agent, among New York City drug abusers (Centers for Disease Control 1984). Needle-sharing is also the likely epidemiologic connection between the homosexual and heterosexual AIDS populations, since homosexual IV drug abusers admit to using "shooting galleries" and sharing needles at the same high rate of heterosexual IV drug abusers. In this connection, it is of interest that, in our study population, over half of the heterosexual IV drug abusers with AIDS or ARC were aware of sharing needles with men they thought to be homosexuals.

It remains unclear why some IV drug abusers get AIDS and others do not, since the majority appear to have been exposed to the putative etiologic agent. In this preliminary study, we did not identify risk factors among drug users related to demographic characteristics or drug use practices. This may be a function of the small "healthy" IV drug abuser control group and/or insufficient detail in our drug abuse histories. Quantification of needle-sharing episodes and partners, "shooting gallery" use, and more detailed exploration of specific drug use practices might uncover differences between those IV drug abusers who develop AIDS and those who do not. More likely, differences in individual host susceptibility may well be of greatest significance. For example, IV drug use itself results in immunologic abnormalities in some drug abusers (Brown, Stimmel, and Jaub 1974; McDonough, Madden, and Falek 1980). Case-control studies employing larger numbers of subjects as well as prospective longitudinal studies of IV drug abusers will be necessary to define risk factors and to more fully understand transmission in this second largest AIDS at-risk population.

References

Auerbach, D. M., W. Darrow, and H. Jaffe. 1984. Cluster of cases of the acquired immunodeficiency syndrome. *Am. J. Med.* 76:487-91.

Barre-Sinoussi, F., J. Chermann, and F. Rey. 1983. Isolation of T-lymphotropic retrovirus from a patient at risk for acquired immunodeficiency syndrome (AIDS). *Science* 220:868-71.

Brown, S. M., B. Stimmel, and R. Jaub. 1974. Immunologic dysfunction in heroin addicts. *Arch. Intern. Med.* 134:1001-6.

Centers for Disease Control. 1982. Update on acquired immune deficiency syndrome (AIDS) among patients with hemophilia A. *M.M.W.R.* 1982; 31:644-52.

———. 1983. Update: acquired immunodeficiency syndrome (AIDS). *M.M.W.R.* 1983; 32-688-90.

———. 1984. Antibodies to a retrovirus etiologically associated with acquired immunodeficiency syndrome (AIDS) in populations with increased incidences of the syndrome. *M.M.W.R.* 1984; 33:377-79.

Curran, J., D. Lawrence, and H. Jaffe. 1983. Acquired immunodeficiency syndrome (AIDS) associated with transfusions. *N. Engl. J. Med.* 310:69-75.

Des Jarlais, D. 1983. *Heroin influx update.* New York: New York State Division of Substance Abuse Services, Bureau of Research.

Des Jarlais, D., and G. Uppal. 1980. Heroin activity in New York City, 1970-1978. *Am. J. Drug Alcohol Abuse* 7:335-46.

Des Jarlais, D. C., N. Jainchill, and S. Friedman. 1986. AIDS among IV drug users: epidemiology, natural history and therapeutic community experiences. *Proceedings of the 9th World Conference of Therapeutic Communities*, 69-73. San Francisco, California.

Gallo, R. C., S. Salahuddin, and M. Popovic. 1984. Frequent detection and isolation of cytopathic retroviruses (HTLV-III) from patients with AIDS and at risk for AIDS. *Science* 224:500-3.

Guinan, M., P. Thomas, and P. Pinsky. 1984. Heterosexual and homosexual patients with the acquired immunodeficiency syndrome. *Ann. Intern. Med.* 100:213-18.

Harris, C., C. Small, and R. Klein. 1983. Immunodeficiency in female sexual partners of men with acquired immunodeficiency syndrome. *N. Engl. J. Med.* 308:1181-84.

Jaffe, H. W., J. Bregman, and R. Selik. 1983a. AIDS in the United States: the first 1,000 cases. *J. Infect. Dis.* 148:339-45.

Jaffe, H. W., K. Choi, and P. Thomas. 1983b. National case-control study of Kaposi's sarcoma and *Pneumocystis carinii* pneumonia in homosexual men. I. Epidemiologic results. *Ann. Intern. Med.* 99:145-51.

Lewis, B. F., and R. Galea. 1986. A survey of the perceptions of drug abusers concerning the acquired immunodeficiency syndrome (AIDS). *Health Matrix* 4: 14-17.

Louria, D., T. Hensle, and J. Rose. 1967. The major medical complications of heroin addiction. *Ann. Intern. Med.* 67:1-22.

Marmor, M., A. Friedman-Kien, and L. Laubenstein. 1982. Risk factors for Kaposi's sarcoma in homosexual men. *Lancet* 1:183-87.

Marmor, M., A. Friedman-Kien, and S. Zolla-Pazner. 1984. Kaposi's sarcoma in homosexual men. *Ann. Intern. Med.* 100:809-15.

McDonough, R. J., J. Madden, and A. Falek. 1980. Aberration of T and null lymphocyte frequencies in the peripheral blood of human opiate addicts: in vivo evidence for opiate receptor sites on T lymphocytes. *J. Immunol.* 125:2539-43.

Moll, B., E. Emeson, and C. Small. 1983. Inverted ratio of inducer to suppressor T-lymphocyte subsets in drug abusers with opportunistic infections. *Clin. Immunol. Immunopathol.* 24:417-23.

O'Donnel, J. A., and J. Jones. 1968. Diffusion on the intravenous technique among narcotic addicts in the United States. *J. Health Soc. Behav.* 9:120-89.

Rubinstein, A., M. Siclick, and A. Gupta. 1983. Acquired immunodeficiency with reversed T4-T8 ratios in infants born to promiscuous and drug addicted mothers. *J.A.M.A.* 289:2350-56.

Sherlock, S. 1981. *Diseases of the liver and biliary system.* Oxford, England: Blackwell Scientific Publications.

Small, C. B., R. Klein, and G. Friedland. 1983. Community-acquired opportunistic infections and defective cellular immunity in heterosexual drug abusers and homosexual men. *Am. J. Med.* 74:433-41.

8
Human Immunodeficiency Virus Infection in Hetero- sexual Intravenous Drug Users in San Francisco

Richard E. Chaisson, MD; Andrew R. Moss, PhD; Robin Onishi, MD; Dennis Osmond, MA; and James R. Carlson, PhD.

Introduction

The acquired immunodeficiency syndrome (AIDS) has occurred in specific high-risk groups in the United States consistently since 1981. Homosexual or bisexual men and intravenous (IV) drug users constituted 72% and 17%, respectively, of all AIDS cases reported to the Centers for Disease Control through 13 January 1986 (Centers for Disease Control 1986) and represent the largest populations of infected individuals, including an 8% overlap of cases involving both homosexuality and drug abuse. A human retrovirus, human T-lymphotrophic virus type III/lymphadenopathy-associated virus or ARV (now referred to as human immunodeficiency virus [HIV]), has been established as the causative agent of AIDS and related conditions (Barre-Sinoussi, Chermann, and Rey 1983; Gallo, Salahuddin, and Popovic 1984; Levy, Hoffman, and Kramer 1984).

Reprinted from "Human Immunodeficiency Virus in Heterosexual Intravenous Drug Users in San Francisco," by Richard E. Chaisson, Andrew R. Moss, Robin Onishi, Dennis Osmond, and James R. Carlson, *American Journal of Public Health* 77:169-72, 1987, by permission of the publisher.

Serologic surveys of asymptomatic members of risk groups have revealed a high prevalence of infection with HIV, ranging from 40% to 70% of homosexual men in San Francisco and 50% to 60% of IV drug users in New York and northern New Jersey (Anderson and Levy 1985; Jaffe, Darrow, and Echenberg 1985; Novick, in press; Osmond et al. 1985; Weiss, Ginzburg, and Goedert 1985). In the metropolitan New York area, the prevalence of HIV infection is extremely high in both IV drug users and homosexual men, and an overlap in exposure to the virus in these two groups has been reported (Friedland, Harris, and Butkus-Small 1985).

San Francisco has a high incidence of AIDS but, unlike eastern cities, the AIDS epidemic in San Francisco has been confined almost exclusively to homosexual men. As of 31 January 1987, there had been 2,853 cases of AIDS in San Francisco, of which 97% were homosexual or bisexual males and 1% was heterosexual IV drug users (San Francisco Department of Public Health 1986). San Francisco also has a large population of IV drug users (10-12,000: 1.5% of the population), the majority of whom are heterosexual opiate users (Newmeyer 1985). To investigate the prevalence of HIV infection in this population, we conducted a seroepidemiologic survey of heterosexual IV drug users in San Francisco. To avoid selection bias that may have overestimated the prevalence of infection, we recruited nonhospitalized IV drug users in community-based settings.

Methods

We studied heterosexual IV drug users enrolled in five major opiate addiction treatment programs, representing the majority of treatment facilities in San Francisco, and a sample of addicts who were not undergoing treatment, from December 1984 to October 1985. Subjects in treatment were receiving either acute heroin detoxification or chronic methadone maintenance. All subjects had reliable histories of opiate addiction. Eligibility for detoxification programs included a documented history of needle use and a positive urine opiate test. To enroll in methadone maintenance, a two-year history of opiate addiction must be documented. Potential subjects were approached in the clinic and informed of the purpose of the study and asked to participate. Recruitment rates ranged from 54% to 79% of clients approached, and varied from clinic to clinic.

Refusing clients most often cited lack of time as the reason for not participating. Out-of-treatment subjects were recruited from community settings in high drug use areas of San Francisco using a chain-referral technique. All gave histories of chronic IV drug use and had stigmata of needle use. Informed consent was obtained from all subjects agreeing to be studied, and an anonymous identification code was generated for each subject. The study was approved by the Human Subjects Committee of the University of California, San Francisco.

Each subject was interviewed with a standard questionnaire to obtain demographic, sexual, drug use, and behavioral information. The number of persons with whom needles were usually shared during drug injection was obtained for the last 209 subjects. Following interview, serum was collected from each subject and stored at -70°C prior to testing for HIV antibodies. Testing for antibody to HIV was performed in duplicate by enzyme-linked immunosorbent assay (ELISA), as previously described (Carlson, Bryant, and Hinrich 1984). Sera positive by ELISA (subject/control optical density ratio $\geq$ 2) were confirmed by Western blot. Sera with bands at the p24 and/or gp41 region were considered positive; only sera positives by both ELISA and Western blot were analyzed as positives.

Data analysis was performed using the chi-square or Fisher's exact test for univariate measures; the Mantel-Haenszel adjustment was used to assess independence of risk factors found significant by univariate analysis. A logistic regression analysis of weighted needle-sharing data was used to analyze risk associated with this practice.

Results

During the 10-month course of this study, 291 IV drug users were enrolled in the study and underwent interview and antibody testing. Ten men who gave a history of homosexual behavior were excluded from analysis; one of these men was seropositive. The subjects had a median age of 34 years, and 54% were male. Fifty-one percent were white, 21% were black, and 28% were of other racial-ethnic origin, primarily Latino. The median duration of IV drug use was 13 years.

Of the 281 heterosexual IV drug users studied, 28 or 10% (95% confidence interval: 6.8% to 14.2%) were positive by ELISA and

Western blot for antibodies to HIV (table 8-1). The distribution of seropositives did not significantly differ by sex, age, or duration of drug use. There was no difference in prevalence of antibody among subjects in treatment by type of treatment program (detoxification vs. methadone maintenance); however, the small sample of subjects (N = 47) recruited from out-of-treatment programs included only one seropositive (2%), thus differing from the in-treatment group. Other factors for which no significant differences could be detected include history of prostitution (4/40 subjects reporting a recent history of prostitution were seropositive), number of sexual partners, and travel to metropolitan New York in the previous 5 years. Two subjects reported having had sex with AIDS cases; one of these was seropositive. Small numbers of subjects reported regularly cleaning needles with alcohol or by boiling; no significant differences in seroprevalence were detected between those who did and did not clean needles regularly.

A clear difference in seroprevalence was detected by history of regularly sharing needles when injecting drugs (table 8-2). Of a subset of 209 subjects for whom needle-sharing data were available, seroprevalence was 3% (2/65) for those who did not regularly share needles vs. 15% (10/68) for those who regularly shared with two or more persons. The odds ratio for seropositivity was 5.43 (95% confidence interval: 1.1% to 52.5%) for subjects sharing with two or more persons.

Of 143 whites studied, 8 (6%) were seropositive compared to 20 of 138 (14%) blacks, Latinos, and others (odds ratio = 2.9; 95% confidence interval: 1.15% to 7.77%). Analysis of seroprevalence by race controlling for needle-sharing showed persistence of the racial difference (adjusted odds ratio = 2.8; 95% confidence interval: 0.84% to 8.59%) with the difference most pronounced in blacks and Latinos who regularly shared needles with two or more persons. Moreover, whites had a higher mean number of persons with whom needles were regularly shared.

Discussion

We found a 10% prevalence of antibody to the HIV among 281 heterosexual IV drug users in San Francisco during late 1984 and 1985. Because our sample was taken at random, subjects may not be representative of the entire IV drug-using population in San Fran-

Table 8-1

Prevalence of HIV Antibodies in 281 Heterosexual IV Drug
Users in San Francisco, 1984 - 85

Characteristics	Number Tested	Number Positive	% Positive
All subjects	281	28	10
Sex*			
Male	152	17	11
Female	128	11	9
Race			
White	143	8	6
Black	60	9	15
Latino/Other	78	11	14
Program Type			
Detoxification	115	12	10
Methadone Maintenance	119	15	13
Out-of-treatment	47	1	2
Age† (years)			
≤ 25	30	2	7
26 - 35	130	12	9
36 - 45	76	13	17
≥ 46	27	1	4
Duration of Heroin Use** (years)			
≥ 5	38	3	8
6 - 10	57	7	12
11 - 15	68	8	12
16 - 20	48	2	4
> 20	48	8	17
History of Prostitution (Females)			
Yes	40	4	10
No	88	7	8

* Sex missing for 1 subject
† Age missing for 18 subjects
** Unable to determine for 22 subjects

Table 8-2

Seropositivity for Antibodies to HIV by Number of Persons
with Whom Needles Are Usually Shared for 209 IV Drug Users

No. Persons Needles Shared with	Number Tested	Number Positive (%)	Odds Ratio (95% C1)
0	65	2 (3)	1
1	76	7 (9)	3.2 (.58-32.4)
≥ 2	68	10 (15)	5.4 (1.08-52.5)

cisco. However, there is no indication that individuals at increased risk of HIV infection either preferentially volunteered for or avoided this study. These data, while in distinct contrast to the prevalence of infection among homosexuals in San Francisco (Anderson and Levy 1985; Jaffe, Darrow, and Echenberg 1985; Osmond et al. 1985), suggest an emerging epidemic of AIDS among drug users in San Francisco. AIDS cases in IV drug users in San Francisco are now being reported at the rate of several per month (San Francisco Department of Public Health 1987). This is closely comparable to the situation in homosexual men in 1982. It is likely that growth of the epidemic in IV drug users in San Francisco will parallel the epidemic in homosexual men, as has occurred nationally (Goedert 1985).

Retrospective studies of sera from other populations of IV drug users suggest that once HIV is introduced into a community, it spreads rapidly to infect the majority of drug addicts. In New York City, the prevalence of HIV antibody in a sample of IV drug users increased from 11% in 1977 to 27% in 1979 to 58% in 1984 (Novick, Kreek and Des Jarlais in press). In Edinburgh, similar changes have been documented among drug users, with seroprevalence rising to more than 50% in a 2-year period (Robertson, Bucknall, and Welsby 1986). In Italy and Spain, rapid increase in the proportion of seropositives from nil to one-half to three-fourths of all addicts tested have been documented in the space of several years (Angarano et al. 1985; Rodrigo et al. 1985). The striking increases in seroprevalence seen in these subpopulations appear to reflect the introduction and rapid spread of HIV in at-risk populations as a whole.

Previous studies in IV drug users have demonstrated an increased risk of seropositivity in addicts who report regularly sharing needles (Cohen, Marmor, and Des Jarlais 1985; Robertson, Bucknall, and Welsby 1986). Our data expand these findings by demonstrating increased risk of seropositivity with increasing number of persons with whom needles are regularly shared. We were unable to document a protective effect of needle-cleaning prior to injection. However, although almost all subjects who shared needles reported rinsing with water, only 16% and 19% of subjects, respectively, usually or always boiled or rinsed needles in alcohol.

HIV infection in San Francisco's IV drug users is significantly more prevalent in blacks and Latinos than in whites (table 8-3). This

Table 8-3

Prevalence of HIV Antibodies by Race in 281 IV Drug Users

Race	Number Tested	Number Positive (%)	Odds Ratio (95% C1)
White	143	8 (6)	1
Black, Latino, Others	138	20 (14)	2.9 (1.5-7.77)

Adjusted Odds Ratio = 2.8 (95% confidence interval 0.84-8.59) controlled for needle sharing using Mantel-Haenszel adjustment for 209 subjects for whom data were available

racial difference has also been reported in New York and New Jersey (Weiss, Ginzburg, and Goedert 1985), although not in European surveys. There are no evident behavioral or demographic characteristics that readily explain the alarming prevalence of infection in this population. While needle-sharing is no more prevalent among blacks and Latinos than among whites, the risk of infection is clearly greater for individuals who share needles with minority group members due to the higher prevalence of infection in this group.

Several factors may explain why HIV infection in San Francisco drug users lags behind homosexual men by 4 years. First, there appears to be little overlap between the homosexual and heterosexual drug-using populations in San Francisco. In one cohort of homosexual men at risk for AIDS, 26% had a history of IV drug use but only 2% had ever used heroin. Hence, heterosexual heroin users have little opportunity to share needles with homosexual men who may be seropositive. The majority of heterosexual IV drug users with AIDS or AIDS-related complex in one New York study, on the other hand, had shared needles with homosexual men (Friedland, Harris, and Butkus-Small 1985). Nationally, 8% of AIDS cases are traced to both sexually active homosexual/bisexual men and IV drug categories. In addition, the use of "shooting galleries," areas where addicts gather to purchase and inject drugs with used and shared needles and other paraphernalia, is common in New York City but less so in San Francisco. The social isolation of addicts and lack of "shooting galleries" in San Francisco may have provided a protective barrier to early introduction of HIV to drug users here. Now that the virus is established among IV drug users, the rate of increase in prevalence may parallel changes seen in other populations of addicts in the eastern United States and Europe.

These data have several important implications. The potential of an epidemic of AIDS in IV drug users in San Francisco will necessitate changes in the city's medical care system for AIDS and in AIDS prevention programs, both of which are oriented to a predominantly white, middle-income homosexual population. The most effective strategy to prevent HIV infection in IV drug users is to eliminate IV drug injection altogether. For individuals who continue to inject drugs, a cessation of needle-sharing and the use of sterile needles and syringes are essential. Overcoming a number of educational, legal, and financial barriers to the use of sterile needles by addicts unable to stop injecting may be the most effective means of halting the spread of the AIDS epidemic in IV drug users.

The situation of IV drug users in San Francisco presents a unique challenge to public health officials, substance abuse professionals, and health care providers. With a small minority of IV drug users infected currently, aggressive intervention efforts can be instituted to prevent further transmission of the virus to uninfected individuals. With knowledge of the cause of AIDS and of the mechanisms of transmission of the HIV at hand, it is imperative that immediate action be taken. While it is not clear which strategies will be most effective, it is certain that failure to act will result in large-scale infection of at-risk individuals and a new wave of deaths from a now preventable epidemic.

References

Anderson, R. E., and J. Levy. 1985. Prevalence of antibodies to AIDS-associated retrovirus in single men in San Francisco. *Lancet* 1:217.

Angarano, G., G. Pastore, L. Monno, T. Santanio, N. Luchena, and O. Schiraldi. 1985. Rapid spread of HTLV-III infection among drug addicts in Italy. *Lancet* 2:1302.

Barre-Sinoussi, F., J. Chermann, and F. Rey. 1983. Isolation of a T-lymphotropic retrovirus from a patient at risk for acquired immunodeficiency syndrome. *Science* 220:868-71.

Carlson, J. R., M. Bryant, and S. Hinrich. 1984. AIDS serology in low- and high-risk groups. *J.A.M.A.* 253:3405-8.

Centers for Disease Control. 1986. Update: acquired immunodeficiency syndrome

—United States. *M.M.W.R.* 35:17-21.

Cohen, H., M. Marmor, and D. Des Jarlais. 1985. Behavioral risk factors for HTLV-III/LAV seropositivity among intravenous drug abusers. In *The International Conference on Acquired Immunodeficiency Syndrome: Abstracts.* American College of Physicians, Philadelphia, Pennsylvania.

Friedland, G. H., C. Harris, and C. Butkus-Small. 1985. Intravenous drug abusers and the acquired immunodeficiency syndrome: demographic, drug use, and needle-sharing patterns. *Arch. Intern. Med.* 145:1413-17.

Gallo, R. C., S. Salahuddin, and M. Popovic. 1984. Frequent detection and isolation of cytopathic retroviruses (HTLV-III)

from patients with AIDS and at risk for AIDS. *Science* 224:500-3.

Goedert, J. J., and W. Blattner. 1985. The epidemiology of AIDS and related conditions. In *AIDS Etiology, diagnosis, treatment and prevention*, eds. V. T. DeVita, S. Hellman, and S. A. Rosenberg, 1-30. Philadelphia, Pennsylvania: J. B. Lippincott.

Jaffe, H. W., W. Darrow, and D. Echenberg. 1985. The acquired immunodeficiency syndrome in a cohort of homosexual men: a 6-year followup study. *Ann. Intern. Med.* 103:210-14.

Levy, J. A., A. Hoffman, and S. Kramer. 1984. Isolation of lymphocytopathic retrovirus from San Francisco patients with AIDS. *Science* 225:840-42.

Newmeyer, J. 1985. Drug abuse in the San Francisco Bay area: June 1985. In *Patterns and Trends in Drug Abuse, a National and International Perspective*. Bethesda, Maryland: National Institute on Drug Abuse.

Novick, D., M. Kreek, and D. Des Jarlais. Antibodies to LAV in New York City, historical and ethical considerations. In *Proceedings of the 46th Annual Scientific Meeting, Committee on Problems of Drug Dependence*, ed. L. Harris. Bethesda, Maryland: National Institute on Drug Abuse. In press.

Osmond, D., A. Moss, P. Bachetti, P. Volberding, F. Barre-Sinoussi, and J. Chermann. 1985. A case-control study of risk factors of AIDS in San Francisco. In *The International Conference on the Acquired Immunodeficiency Syndrome: Abstracts*. American College of Physicians, Philadelphia, Pennsylvania.

Robertson, J. R., A. Bucknall, and P. Welsby. 1986. Epidemic of AIDS related virus (HTLV-III/LAV) infection among intravenous drug abusers. *Br. Med. J.* 292:527-29.

Rodrigo, J. M., M. Serra, E. Aguilar, D. Del Olmo, V. Gimeno, and L. Aparisi. 1985. HTLV-III antibodies in drug addicts in Spain. *Lancet* 2:156-57.

San Francisco Department of Public Health. May 1986. San Francisco AIDS cases by age group, race/ethnicity and patient group through 4/30/86. San Francisco, California.

San Francisco Department of Public Health. 1978. AIDS in IV drug users, San Francisco, 1979-1986. *San Francisco Epidemiol. Bull.* 2:1-2.

Weiss, S. H., H. Ginzburg, and J. Goedert. 1985. Risk of HTLV-III exposure and AIDS among parenteral drug abusers in New Jersey. In The International Conference on the Acquired Immunodeficiency Syndrome: Abstracts. American College of Physicians, Philadelphia, Pennsylvania.

9

Risk Reduction for the Acquired Immunodeficiency Syndrome among Intravenous Drug Abusers

Don C. Des Jarlais, PhD; Samuel R. Friedman, PhD; and William Hopkins, MA.

Intravenous drug users are the second largest risk group for the acquired immunodeficiency syndrome (AIDS) and a bridge to two other groups: children and heterosexual partners. In the absence of effective treatment or vaccines, control of the epidemic among drug users will rely on efforts to reduce needle-sharing. However, the traditional image of intravenous drug users leads one to expect little or no risk reduction. In this article, we review characteristics of AIDS as a disease that impedes efforts at risk reduction among drug users and report on current risk reduction among intravenous drug users in New York City. There has been a sustained increase in the demand for new, unused needles, as shown in the emergence of "resealed" needles and in interviews with persons selling needles in illicit drug-purchasing areas.

The second largest group of persons at risk for AIDS is intravenous drug users. Of the 33,482 cases of AIDS reported to the Centers for Disease Control (CDC) through 30 March 1987, 5,540 (17%) have had intravenous drug use as their primary risk factor.

Reprinted with permission from "Risk Reduction for the Acquired Immunodeficiency Syndrome among Intravenous Drug Users," by Don C. Des Jarlais, Samuel R. Friedman, and William Hopkins, *Annals of Internal Medicine* 103:755-59, 1985.

Another 2,535 cases (8%) have had both intravenous drug use and male homosexual activity as risk factors (CDC). These percentages have been relatively stable throughout the epidemic (Selik, Haverkos, and Curran 1984).

The cases of AIDS in intravenous drug users have been concentrated in the New York City metropolitan area. Of the current cases in which drug use is the primary risk factor, a high percentage are in the northeast and in other AIDS "hot spots," such as Florida and California. However, evidence shows a slow spread to other cities with large numbers of intravenous drug users; both San Francisco and Chicago show approximately 10% seroprevalence for antibody to the human immunodeficiency virus (HIV) among such persons (Spira, Des Jarlais, and Bokos 1985).

Transmission of AIDS within this group is believed to occur through the transfer of small amounts of blood during the sharing of needles. Data from studies directly examining relationships between antibody prevalence, drug injecting, and needle-sharing are now becoming available (Cohen, Marmor, and Des Jarlais 1985; Weiss, Ginzburg, and Goedert 1985).

Intravenous drug users appear to be a bridge to two other groups at increased risk for developing AIDS. Of the 108 cases of AIDS in children reported to the CDC through 5 April 1985, 55 (51%) have occurred in children for whom at least one parent was an intravenous drug user (A. Hardy, CDC, personal communication). For these children, the transmission of human T-lymphotrophic virus type III/lymphadenopathy-associated virus is likely to occur in utero (Thomas, Jaffe, and Spira 1985). The second risk group, "heterosexual partners," is composed of persons whose only known risk factor for AIDS is heterosexual activity with members of a previously identified risk group. In 53 of 73 (73%) cases currently reported to the CDC, the heterosexual contact was with an intravenous drug user (K. Castro, CDC, personal communication).

Public health control of the AIDS epidemic must include control within the intravenous drug use group, because of both the large numbers of intravenous drug users at risk and the possibility of outward spread to nondrug users. In the absence of effective treatment or vaccines, control of the epidemic must be attempted through reducing transmission-related behavior.

Because of the long-term intractability of much drug-taking behavior at the individual level (Simpson, Savage, and Sells 1978) and traditional descriptions of drug addiction as psychopathologic (Kuehnle and Spitzer 1981), there are doubts as to whether risk reduction behavior will occur in this risk group. These doubts are based on the traditional image of the heroin addict's behavior as completely dominated by the desire for the drug (Califano 1982).

This article first examines selected aspects of AIDS among intravenous drug users that affect perception of risk and thus motivation for changes in behavior. (In examining possible risk perception, we are implicitly following cognitive models of health-related behavior [Rosenstock 1966].) We then report on the current risk reduction efforts occurring among intravenous drug users in New York City.

Epidemiologic Impediments to Perceptions of Risk

The newness and the high fatality rate of AIDS contribute to its psychological saliency among all risk groups and increase the likelihood that it will be perceived as a major threat to health. Several aspects of the disease, however, have served to limit perceptions of risk by intravenous drug users. The first is the relatively long "latency" period between exposure to HIV and the development of diagnosable AIDS (Curran, Lawrence, and Jaffe 1984). Antibody studies of sera collected in drug treatment centers in Manhattan before the AIDS epidemic show that the initial spread of HIV occurred before 1979. Approximately one-third of the samples collected in that year contained antibody to the virus (M. J. Kreek et al., unpublished data). This spread of the virus preceded all known cases of AIDS among intravenous drug users. From retrospective diagnoses, the first cases of AIDS in intravenous drug users in New York City appeared in 1980 in 9 intravenous drug users, 4 of whom were homosexual men. The incidence in drug users then increased rapidly, with 29 new cases in 1981, 148 in 1982, and 324 in 1983 (Thomas, personal communication).

Because the historically collected sera were not from random samples of intravenous drug users in New York City, and because an unknown number of early cases may have been missed in the retrospective surveillance efforts, care must be taken in interpreting these trends. It does seem safe to conclude, however, that the average latency period between viral exposure and development of diagnosable AIDS for drug users is probably three or more years.

This long latency undoubtedly delayed any risk reduction efforts among this group in New York. It also suggests that risk reduction in other cities may have to begin before even moderate numbers of cases appear.

Another impediment to the perception of AIDS as a health risk by intravenous drug users is the difficulty in distinguishing AIDS as a singularly important cause of death compared with the many other causes of death in the group. Coincident with the spread of HIV among drug users in New York, there has been a great increase in "narcotic-related" deaths, including large increases in pneumonias other than *Pneumocystis carinii* pneumonia (Stoneburner, Breuer, and Friedman 1984). Exhibit 9-1 shows the number of narcotic-related deaths and the number of cases of AIDS among intravenous drug users in New York City (all sexual preferences included) from 1978 to 1983. Allowing for a minimum average survival of 1 year between diagnosis and death from AIDS, AIDS had not become a dominant cause of death in intravenous drug users through 1983.

The increase in these other narcotic-related deaths raises questions about possible causal relationships between HIV exposure and susceptibility to "nonopportunistic" infections in drug users. Antibody to HIV in drug users without AIDS is associated with lowered serum B-cell counts, increased serum immunoglobulin levels, and abnormal T-cell counts (Des Jarlais, Friedman, and Spira 1985) (table 9-1). Altered humoral immune functioning, in conjunc-

Exhibit 9-1

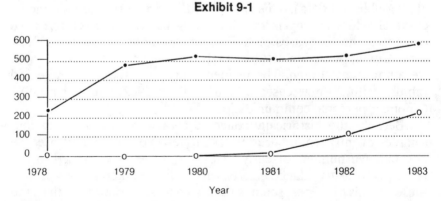

Narcotic-related deaths *(solid circles)* and deaths from the acquired immunodeficiency syndrome *(open circles)* among intravenous drug users in New York City.

tion with frequent nonsterile drug injections, might increase susceptibility to various infections. Preliminary analysis of our data from New York City indicate significantly raised risk for endocarditis among intravenous drug users with exposure to HIV. Other researchers have also found possible links between HIV and susceptibility to nonopportunistic infections (Duncanson, Hewlett, and Maayan 1985; Stoneburner and Kristal 1985; Shine, Moll, and Emeson 1985).

If the information that HIV increases susceptibility to various severe nonopportunistic infections was communicated to intravenous drug users, it could dramatically alter the risk they associate with an "AIDS virus." Linkage of an AIDS virus to these other common ways of dying could lead them to see the virus as a predominant cause of death, rather than merely as one cause among

Table 9-1

Serum Lymphocyte and Immunoglobulin Levels Among
Intravenous Drug Users in New York City

	Persons Seropositive for Antibody HTLV-III/LAV*		*p* Value†
	Negative (*n* = 110)	Positive (*n* = 160)	
Total lymphocytes, /*mL*	2910 ± 855	2617 ± 1203	0.02
B cells, /*mL*	314 ± 197	225 ± 187	0.01
T3 (total T cells), /*mL*	2199 ± 671	2079 ± 980	NS
T4 (helper cells), /*mL*	1099 ± 406	790 ± 455	0.001
T8 (suppressor cells), /*mL*	890 ± 390	1084 ± 627	0.001
T4/T8 ratio	1.39 ± 0.69	0.87 ± 0.62	0.01
IgG, *mg/dL*	1636 ± 548	2175 ± 1015	0.001
IgA, *mg/dL*	247 ± 115	269 ± 130	NS
IgM, *mg/dL*	327 ± 179	369 ± 206	NS

* Subjects were recruited from drug detoxification and methadone maintenance centers. Data are mean ± SD. Antibody status was determined with an enzyme-linked immunosorbent assay done at the Centers for Disease Control; lymphocyte subsets were determined with a Coulter EPICS C flow cytometer (Coulter Electronics, Inc., Hialeah, Florida) and Ortho OKT3, OKT4, and OKT8 (Ortho Diagnostics, Inc., Raritan, New Jersey) and Coulter B1 monoclonal antibodies (Coulter Electronics) at the New York City Department of Health; immunoglobulins were measured with a Beckman rate nephelometer and anti-IgG, anti-IgA, and anti-IgM (Beckman Instruments, Inc., Fullerton, California) at Beth Israel Medical Center. HTLV-III/LAV = human T-lymphotropic virus type III/lymphadenopathy-associated virus.

† Analysis of variance was used to determine statistical significance. NS - not significant.

many. Such a change in perception could greatly increase the probability of sustained risk reduction behavior.

A perception of HIV exposure and AIDS as health risks for intravenous drug users need not be based on deaths. It might also be based on observation of symptoms of the AIDS-related complex. The symptoms can be seen both as indications of AIDS and as health risks in their own right. Preliminary analysis of data from a survey we conducted of 59 intravenous drug users in treatment programs in New York City during the summer of 1984 showed that 36 (61%) of them could properly identify one of more AIDS-related symptoms.

We examined the self-reported prevalence of AIDS-related symptoms for the previous 5 years in 82 HIV/antibody-negative and 136 antibody-positive intravenous drug users. The symptoms included lymphadenopathy, weight loss, unexplained fever, night sweats, diarrhea, and mouth infections. Table 9-2 shows the prevalence of one or more AIDS-related symptoms among antibody-negative drug users and among antibody-positive drug users grouped by their number of HIV-related immunologic abnormalities. Symptoms are common even among drug users who have not been exposed to HIV, and they rise to significantly higher levels only in one-third of the antibody-positive drug users who have several immunological abnormalities.

Weight loss (of 4.5 kg or more) accounted for approximately 90% of the AIDS-related symptoms in all groups listed in Table 9-1. In the antibody-negative group and in the antibody-positive persons with less than two immunological abnormalities, the weight loss is presumably a result of intensive cocaine use or poor nutrition. Thus, whereas intravenous drug users appear to be reasonably well informed about AIDS-related symptoms, the symptoms do not provide a clear basis for their linking exposure to an AIDS virus and increased health risks.

The epidemic history and selected disease characteristics of AIDS in intravenous drug users present special problems for motivating risk reduction behavior. The long latency period, the background of other causes of death, and the ambiguity of AIDS-related symptoms all impede the perception of a high personal risk from AIDS. Despite these problems, we are finding almost universal awareness of AIDS among intravenous drug users in New York and a sustained reduction in needle-sharing.

Table 9-2

Percentage of Intravenous Drug Users with at Least One
Symptom of the Acquired-Immunodeficiency-Syndrome-Related
Complex

Immunologic Status	Persons with at Least One Symptom
	n/n(%)
HTLV-III/LAV antibody negative	49/82 (60)
HTLV-III/LAV antibody positive*	89/136 (65)
No immunologic abnormality	26/41 (63)
One immunologic abnormality	24/47 (51)
Two immunologic abnormalities	16/22 (73)
Three immunologic abnormalities	14/16 (88)
Four immunologic abnormalities	9/10 (90)

*The immunologic abnormalities (T4/T8 ratio < 1.0, T4-cell count ≤ 491/mL, total lymphocyte count ≤ 1745/mL, B-cell count ≤ 73/mL) form a cumulative order within the antibody-positive group. A subject who has a specific abnormality will also typically have all preceding abnormalities. Thus, a subject with a low total lymphocyte count will also have a low T4-cell count and a low T4/T8 ratio (11). HTLV-III/LAV = human T-lymphotropic virus type III/lymphadenopathy-associated virus.

Awareness and Risk Reduction

The data presented up to this point primarily have been from studies of persons in treatment for substance abuse, AIDS, or other drug-related health problems. The data presented in the rest of this article are primarily behavioral data about intravenous drug users who were not in any form of drug-abuse or health-care treatment at the time of data collection. Data on the behavior of drug users out of treatment are probably more relevant to public health control of the AIDS epidemic but clearly require different methods for collection. A brief description of how we collected these data will be useful.

The Bureau of Research of the New York State Division of Substance Abuse Services operates a "Street Research Unit" to monitor drug activity in New York City. The unit is composed of persons very knowledgeable about drug activity on the street; most are former intravenous drug abusers. They can blend inconspicuously with the quasi-public street drug activities found in the city without actually purchasing or using drugs. They are able to learn the "news" within the street drug subculture and conduct informal interviews with the many drug users and dealers who hang out in the major "copping" (drug sale) areas.

Narcotic and Drug Research, Inc., is a not-for-profit corporation affiliated with the Division of Substance Abuse Services. It maintains an ethnographic research storefront in a New York City neighborhood with a high level of intravenous drug abuse. Drug users are recruited for various research projects at the storefront. It provides a setting for conducting extensive interviews that could not be conducted in public places. Subjects are usually paid small fees, about $15 per hour, for their time. The operation of the ethnographic storefront has been described previously (Johnson, Goldstein, and Preble 1985). Both the Street Research Unit and the storefront are examples of the "street ethnography" tradition in drug abuse research (Weppner 1977). As such, they often provide data from the perspective of the current drug user, which may be quite different from that of drug users in treatment.

The Street Research Unit first heard concern about AIDS in the late spring of 1983, at the time of the widespread media attention to AIDS. Since then, there has been continuing concern about AIDS in the streets, with observations of increased sales of "new" needles (not previously used for injecting illicit drugs). Over this time, the unit has also heard increased concerns about other health problems on the streets, notably an illness called "walking pneumonia."

In the fall of 1983, we used the storefront to conduct extensive interviews with 18 intravenous drug users who were not in treatment at the time. They had all heard of AIDS and believed that it was spread through the sharing of needles used for drug injection. They also reported an increased demand for "new" needles among intravenous drug users as a result of AIDS.

In response to questions, the respondents were not certain whether the increased use of new needles would be sustained or whether the situation would revert to the previous level. They stated that the critical factors in sustaining increased use of new needles were not only the intentions of the drug users but also the ready availability of new needles. In their opinion, intravenous drug users typically obtain needles at the same time or after obtaining drugs. The period after drugs have been obtained is characterized by an intense desire to use the drugs. If new needles are readily available during this period, they will be used; if not, whatever needles are handy are likely to be used. Thus, the extent of increased use of new needles would depend not only on the person's general intentions to avoid sharing needles, but also on market supply mechanisms for providing new needles at the appropriate times.

The intensity of the desire to inject once drugs have been obtained should not be thought of as simple impatience; evidence shows that the situation of having drugs to inject can provoke or intensify physical withdrawal symptoms (Wikler 1980). Although withdrawal is rarely life-threatening, it can be quite uncomfortable and serves a strong motivation for short-term behavior.

One indication that the demand for new needles had been sustained came in the summer and fall of 1984, when we heard reports of the selling of "resealed" needles. Needle sellers were placing used needles back in the original packaging, resealing the packaging, and then selling the needles as new. The resealing is done with heatsealing machines that can be purchased in local hardware stores. This phenomenon had not been reported before the emergence of AIDS. (The resealing is often not perfect, and careful examination of the package by the buyer may lead to discovery.)

Since the fall of 1984, the reports of resealed needles have been confirmed by various sources: patients in drug treatment programs, intravenous drug users interviewed for other purposes at our research storefront, and even intravenous drug users in private psychotherapy (M. Chernoff, personal communication). The demand for new needles has reached a point where it can now support a supply of counterfeit new needles.

To study the demand for new needles in greater depth, our Street Research Unit conducted interviews with persons "hawking" needles on the street during the spring of 1985. A major advantage in studying changes in needle use by interviewing the sellers is that their answers should be relatively free of the social desirability effects that might influence responses to questions about a user's own risk reduction behavior. Brief in-the-street interviews were held with needle sellers in major "copping" areas in the city.

Eighteen of 22 (82%) needle sellers reported that new needle sales had increased over the last year. They reported an average profit of $2 on each new needle sold, based on an average cost to them of $1 per new needle and an average selling price of $3. When asked the reasons for the increased business in new needles, 6 of the

18 reported increased demand in general terms, 5 reported it was now easier to obtain new needles, and 4 specifically mentioned AIDS as the reason for the increased sales. When asked if they had ever sold used needles as new, 10 of 21 reported that they had. Seven of these 10 stated that they had resealed used needles and sold them as new.

The Street Research Unit also observed the use of AIDS in "advertising" for new needles. One seller was chanting "Get the good needles, don't get the bad AIDS" as a sales pitch for his wares.

The data from our street observations and interviews with the needle sellers are consistent with the reports obtained from our storefront and from persons in drug treatment programs. The demand for new needles has increased, and the increase is linked to concerns about AIDS. One final aspect of the increase in use of new needles is worth noting. This increase has been sustained without any positive feedback that using new needles does any good. The same characteristics of AIDS that hinder perception of risk also hinder any perception of the effectiveness of risk reduction.

Conclusions

AIDS poses a major threat to the health of intravenous drug users, their sexual partners, and their potential children. Because we currently have neither effective treatment nor vaccines, control of the disease must be through changes in transmission-related behavior. Several characteristics of the disease hinder perception of risk and thus limit motivation for behavior change.

Despite these problems, we have observed a sustained increase in the use of new needles among drug users in New York City. The data clearly contradict the stereotype of intravenous drug users as incapable of modifying their behavior and as unconcerned with their health.

We must also distinguish conceptually between the individual level of analysis and the group level. The behavior of an individual drug user, particularly in the time between drug purchase and injection, may be hard to modify by changes in health beliefs. Interactions between individual beliefs and group processes, such as supply and demand, may lead to a greater behavioral change.

We cannot yet tell either the percentage reduction in needle-sharing or its distribution in the population of drug users. Further research is needed on the specific sources of information used by drug users in their perception of risk for AIDS, the market mechanisms for supplying new needles, and methods to facilitate risk reduction efforts in other cities. Resolution of whether HIV exposure increases susceptibility to the various serious infections common among intravenous drug users (and communication of the results to the group) could also dramatically change perceptions of AIDS-related risks. Finally, research is needed to estimate the effectiveness of the observed risk reduction in altering the spread of the disease among drug users, their sexual partners, and their children.

Despite the many unknowns regarding risk reduction among intravenous drug users, the present evidence clearly indicates that risk reduction has occurred in response to the AIDS epidemic. Increased public health efforts at facilitating risk reduction among drug users should be undertaken, particularly in areas where the epidemic is still in an early stage.

References

Califano, J. A. 1982. *Report on drug abuse and alcoholism.* New York: Warner Press.

Cohen, H., M. Marmor, and D. Des Jarlais. 1985. Behavioral risk factors for HTLV-III/LAV seropositivity among intravenous drug abusers. In *The International Conference on the Acquired Immunodeficiency Syndrome: Abstracts.* Philadelphia, Pennsylvania: American College of Physicians.

Curran, J. W., D. Lawrence, and H. Jaffe. 1984. Acquired immunodeficiency syndrome (AIDS) associated with transfusions. *N. Engl. J. Med.* 310:69-75.

Des Jarlais, D. C., S. Friedman, and T. Spira. 1985. A stage model of HTLV-III/LAV in intravenous drug users. In *Problems of drug dependence,* ed. L. Harris. Rockville, Maryland: National Institute on Drug Abuse.

Duncanson, F. P., D. Hewlett, and S. Maayan. 1985. Tuberculosis and the acquired immunodeficiency syndrome in non-Haitian intravenous drug abusers. In *The International Conference on the Acquired Immunodeficiency Syndrome: Abstracts.* Philadelphia, Pennsylvania: American College of Physicians.

Johnson, B. D., P. Goldstein, and E. Preble. 1985. *Taking care of business: the economics of crime by heroin abusers.* Lexington, Massachusetts: Lexington Books.

Kuehnle, J., and R. Spitzer. 1981. DSM-III classification of substance use disorders. In *Substance abuse: clinical problems and perspectives,* ed. J. Lowinson and R. Ruiz. Baltimore, Maryland: Williams and Wilkins.

Rosenstock, I. M. 1966. Why people use health services. *Milbank Mem. Fund Q.* 44(suppl):94-124.

Selik, R. M., H. Haverkos, and J. Curran. 1984. Acquired immune deficiency syndrome (AIDS) trends in the United States, 1978-1982. *Am. J. Med.* 76:493-500.

Shine, D., B. Moll, and E. Emeson. 1985. Serologic, immunologic, and clinical features of I.V. drug abusers without AIDS. In *The International Conference* on the *Acquired Immunodeficiency Syndrome: Abstracts.* Philadelphia, Pennsylvania: American College of Physicians.

Simpson, D. D., L. Savage, and S. Sells. 1978. *Data book on drug treatment outcomes.* Fort Worth, Texas: Institute of Behavioral Research.

Spira, T. J., D. Des Jarlais, and D. Bokos. 1985. HTLV-III/LAV antibodies in intravenous (IV) drug abusers—Comparison of high and low risk areas for AIDS. In *The International Conference on the Acquired Immunodeficiency Syndrome: Abstracts.* Philadelphia, Pennsylvania: American College of Physicians.

Stoneburner, R., B. Breuer, and S. Friedman. 1984. Trends in pneumonia mortality and their possible relationship to acquired immunodeficiency syndrome in New York City. Paper presented at the Thirty-Third Annual Epidemic Intelligence Service Conference, April, Atlanta, Georgia.

Stoneburner, R. J., and A. Kristal. 1985. Increasing tuberculosis incidence and its relationship to acquired immunodeficiency syndrome in New York City. In *The International Conference on the Acquired Immunodeficiency Syndrome: Abstracts.* Philadelphia, Pennsylvania: American College of Physicians.

Thomas, P. A., H. Jaffe, T. Spira, R. Reiss, I. Guerrero, and D. Auerbach. 1985. Unexplained immunodeficiency in children: a surveillance report. *J.A.M.A.* 252:639-44.

Weiss, S. H., H. Ginzburg, and J. Goedert. 1985. Risk for HTLV-III exposure and AIDS among parenteral drug abusers in New Jersey. In *The International Conference on the Acquired Immunodeficiency Syndrome: Abstracts.* Philadelphia, Pennsylvania: American College of Physicians.

Weppner, R. S., ed. 1977. *Street ethnography.* Beverly Hills, California: Sage.

Wikler, A. 1980. A theory of opioid dependence. In *Theories on drug abuse*, eds. D. J. Lettieri, M. Sayers, and H. W. Pearson. Rockville, Maryland: National Institute on Drug Abuse.

PART III

Psychiatric and Psychosocial Aspects of AIDS

AIDS is a disease whose treatment involves mental health issues, not only because of the neurological complications of the virus and opportunistic infections, but also because of the stress placed on AIDS patients by their families, friends, and society. These patients, and especially intravenous drug users with AIDS, are often cut off from the networks of support that help other terminally ill patients.

"Psychosocial Issues in AIDS" by Grace Christ, Lori Wiener, and Rosemary T. Moynihan addresses the effect of this debilitating and fatal illness on people in their 20s and 30s, and the stresses that face AIDS patients at the time of diagnosis, with the onset of symptoms, during the course of treatment, and when treatment is terminated. Patients with AIDS, the authors note, must not only deal with the "asynchrony" of terminal illness at what is normally the most active stage of life, but they also face discrimination in unemployment and insurance, lack the support of families, and may be unable to obtain care and help because they live alone.

Dilley et al. look at the denial, fear, and mourning of the dying patient as concomitants of the physical symptoms of AIDS. They also discuss the depression, anxiety, mood swings, and agitation of the AIDS patients, which may be symptoms of neurological dysfunction caused either by the human immunodeficiency virus infection of the central nervous system or by other opportunistic infections associated with AIDS.

Nichols' article, "Psychosocial Reactions of Persons with Acquired Immunodeficiency Syndrome" details the author's clinical work with AIDS patients needing psychiatric help. He finds that the response of these patients is one of "situational distress" and is precipitated by a number of crises throughout the course of the illness: fear of death, vulnerability to infection and disfiguration, and loss of independence are a few of these factors. Patients with AIDS must confront such issues again and again, which, the author says, creates the "emotional roller coaster" of AIDS.

10
Psychosocial Issues in AIDS

Grace H. Christ, MSW; Lori S. Wiener, MSW; and
Rosemary T. Moynihan, MSW.

The complexity of problems confronting people with acquired
immunodeficiency syndrome (AIDS) and the terror it engenders
sets this disease apart from virtually every other contemporary
public health problem. Its onset affects every aspect of a patient's
life: it may cause serious problems for those with whom the patient
has personal, intimate, familial, or occupational ties; it produces difficult patient-management issues for health care institutions and
community agencies; and it raises basic ethical issues for the health
care community as long as the contagion potential of the disease
remains uncertain.

Although treatments are currently available for specific opportunistic infections, Kaposi's sarcoma, and other diseases associated
with AIDS, the patient is confronted with the fact that there are no
treatments for the underlying immunodeficiency. The disease and
its sequelae are overwhelmingly physically debilitating. For a young,
vigorous person, becoming a debilitated, symptom-racked, possibly
dying person often within a few weeks or months requires a massive
adjustment.

Reprinted from "Psychosocial Issues in AIDS," by Grace H. Christ, Lori S. Wiener, and
Rosemary T. Moynihan, *Psychiatric Annals* 16(3):173-79, 1986, by permission of Slack, Inc.

The purpose of this article is to increase understanding and facilitation of this adjustment. The clinical characteristics of the disease, its mortality rates, and distribution have been covered in detail elsewhere (Krown 1984; DeVita, Hellman, and Rosenberg 1985), and the anxiety that the disease has engendered in the general public as well as in high-risk groups is common knowledge. The four groups at highest risk of contracting AIDS continue to be homosexual and bisexual men, intravenous drug users and their children, and hemophiliacs.

Stress and Its Treatment

This section addresses the psychosocial impacts of the stresses associated with: (1) diagnosis of AIDS, (2) its specific clinical syndromes, (3) treatment, and (4) termination of treatment. The overwhelming nature of emotions caused by these stresses often interferes with compliance with treatment, impedes social functioning, and thus obstructs the provision of patient care.

Diagnosis

Diagnosis is an especially stressful event for AIDS patients and has been identified as a critical, but often neglected, time for psychosocial intervention (Malyon and Pinka 1983; Nichols 1983; Grossman 1984). Because of the high mortality rate associated with the disease, patients are confronted not only with the threat to their long-term survival, but also with the need to make immediate changes in their lifestyle.

Denial can be a useful and necessary defense for patients with a potentially fatal illness because it gives them some control over when and how they will confront their own mortality. For AIDS patients, however, denial is less likely to be effective because of all the publicity the disease has received. In addition, patients are often demoralized by the deaths of other AIDS patients that they have known.

The age at which AIDS strikes is another traumatic factor. Most AIDS patients are between 25 and 49 years old—an age group that does not expect to develop a potentially fatal illness. As Rossi (1980) pointed out, stress is often "a manifestation of asynchrony in the timing of life events. It is the unanticipated event, not the anticipated, which is likely to represent the traumatic event."

Patients are also confronted with the issue of their being contagious. For example, they must worry about transmitting the disease to others, protecting themselves from opportunistic infections, and dealing with the fears of lovers, friends, family, and the public about AIDS. Because the public is ambivalent, at best, about the disease and its victims, some of the psychological benefits of the sick role that other seriously ill patients receive tend to be withheld from AIDS patients. Instead, these patients are socially rejected and are often denied benefits, employment, and care.

Finally, at diagnosis, many patients are confronted with the prospect of having to reveal their homosexuality to family, friends, and colleagues. (Four of five urban gay men interviewed for a 1982 market survey had not told their families about their homosexuality [Coppola and Zabarsky 1983].)

Malyon and Pinka noted that, at diagnosis, many health care providers fail to recognize the AIDS patient's immediate and long-term need for psychological support (Nichols 1983). And "if these (needs) are identified, a referral is usually made to yet another individual or agency. At this point, the coordination of services starts to become unmanageable." Therefore, although referrals to community support services may be appropriate over the course of the illness, psychosocial intervention by mental health professionals working closely with the patient's physician should begin immediately. Early intervention is also important to resolve practical problems such as how the patient will support himself if he cannot work, how his medical treatment will be paid for, and how he will communicate about the disease with his family and friends.

Clinical Syndromes

The debilitating and, at times, disfiguring effects of AIDS also cause stress. Many patients have central nervous disease, which is often characterized by a slowly progressive dementia that can become severely incapacitating (Snider, Simpson, and Nielson 1983; Fauci, Macher, and Longo 1984; Lowenstein and Sharpstein 1984). Some become confused and disoriented and have short-term memory deficits; some experience severe weight loss, weakness of the legs, and blurred vision or blindness, while others may also demonstrate psychiatric symptomatology. These patients often need extensive help with the basic activities of daily living and help in traveling to and from the hospital because they become confused about directions. These cognitive changes also have a tremendous impact on patients' relationships with people close to them. When one patient accused his friends of stealing from him, they became reluctant to enter his apartment to provide the care he so desperately needed. Taking care of patients who have these behavior problems is especially difficult when the caretakers are unaware of the organic cause or are confused and frightened by the effects of the illness. As the signs and symptoms of the illness progress, the patient often requires an amount of home care that is difficult to provide by friends, family, and health care workers.

Unlike cancer patients, AIDS patients with opportunistic infections have no structured treatment regimen to follow that will help them cope with the fear of the progressive effects of their disease. Infections must be treated as they occur, and cure does not represent a remission of the underlying disease. Multiple reinfections become increasingly relentless, and the patient is chronically tired and uncomfortable and rarely experiences the signs of improvement of the plateaus experienced by the cancer patient.

Patients with Kaposi's sarcoma live with a constant visual reminder of the disease. Although the treatment regimen for this manifestation of AIDS is intense and has many side effects, the regular involvement of the hospital staff that it requires provides patients with emotional support, encourages the hope of remission, and provides patients with opportunities to ventilate their fears, obtain information, and learn new ways of coping with the disease.

Patients who have chronic lymphadenopathy syndrome of AIDS-related complex, a possible prodrome of AIDS, are stressed by the lack of clarity about the relationship between the condition and AIDS. Because the ambiguities of this condition create tremendous anxiety, support groups are conducted separately from those for patients with a diagnosis of AIDS. This seems to help lymphadenopathy patients better cope with fears of developing AIDS.

Treatment

Some treatments have side effects such as weakness and depression, which only add to the AIDS patient's dysphoric state. Furthermore, treatments often require multiple clinic visits, painful tests and procedures, and prolonged hospitalizations with isolation precautions. Isolation is particularly stressful because the patient is confronted with sensory deprivation at a time when closeness to others is especially comforting. Finally, the complex nature of treatment for AIDS means that a broad range of consultants is involved. Thus, the patient risks losing the emotional security of having one central physician to rely on.

Termination of treatment is another particularly stressful time for the AIDS patient. Stopping an activity that apparently controls the disease and no longer being under intense medical surveillance greatly increases fears of renewed progression of the disease.

Special Problems of Patients and Families

Special problems of AIDS patients have been identified from clinical experience and from a pilot study involving psychosocial assessments of 42 of the first 58 patients treated at Memorial Sloan-Kettering Cancer Center between April 1981 and December 1982. The study highlighted certain characteristics of AIDS patients that make them more vulnerable than other patients to social and psychological dysfunctions.

Employment and Insurance

The patients in the pilot study represented a broad range of occupations and professions, such as architecture, education, finance, health care, interior design, and skilled labor. Many were self-employed and thus had less financial and job security than those who worked for an organization. However, early in the epidemic, many patients were fired from long-standing, secure jobs in organizations because of pervasive social fear of contracting AIDS. Now, legal organizations challenge many of these situations in court.

The lack or limited amount of insurance is also a major problem for AIDS patients. Over one-third of the patients in the pilot study either had no insurance, or their insurance had been terminated when they were fired from their jobs after diagnosis or when they were no longer able to afford private coverage. Applying for Medicaid and Social Security disability are new processes for many patients, and the requirement that they divest themselves of most resources to be eligible for some of these benefits often means leaving familiar surroundings and drastically changing their lifestyle.

Support Network Limitations

Young adult patients with life-threatening illnesses, such as leukemia, generally become intensely reinvolved with their families of origin and rely on the family as well as spouses and friends for financial and emotional support. For AIDS patients, the family is less available; thus, they are more dependent on lovers and/or the wider network of friends. In the initial pilot study, over 62% of the AIDS patients had minimal or no contact with their families.

We have found that some AIDS patients live in what can be called a "family reconstitution" with close friends. However, about one-third of the patients in the pilot study lived alone and lacked a support network they could count on for help. For such patients, drug rehabilitation or gay organizations and hospital staff support structures often become vital to the patient's ability to cope with the stresses of AIDS.

Among patients who keep in contact with their families, communication is typically most open with siblings and least open with the father. This pattern of communication often causes confusion, ambivalence, and further isolation at a time of great emotional need. Family secrets concerning who knows and who does not know about the patient's lifestyle often limit the family's ability to respond and provide the needed support.

Living Alone

Almost three-fourths of the patients in the pilot study said that they lived alone. About half of these said that neighbors and acquaintances could help them with daily chores if necessary; the other half said they had no one to help them.

Agencies such as visiting nurse services serve AIDS patients, but are limited in what they can provide, e.g., they usually cannot always give 24-hour nursing care or provide free care. Although the "buddy system" developed by the New York City gay community and gay service agencies in other cities offer shopping, housekeeping, and other practical and supportive services to patients at home, the patient who lives alone is less certain of immediate care and help when he needs it.

Families

In many cases, the families of AIDS patients also are in great need of supportive care. They, too, face the threat of social rejection in a frightened society. In addition, many must confront the crisis of learning of a child's, sibling's, or spouse's drug use or homosexuality at the same time they must cope with the possibility of his death. Furthermore, the family may get into conflict with the patient's reconstituted family because they are perceived as having more control in vital treatment decisions. Finally, the family must cope with the patient's death and the many unresolved emotional and social issues.

A Psychosocial Intervention Model

The Social Work Department at Memorial Sloan-Kettering Cancer Center developed a psychosocial intervention program for patients, their friends and relatives, and the center's staff in 1982. In addition to the patient-related problems described earlier, this study revealed a major lack of home and supportive care resources as well as a lack of coordination between acute care facilities and community groups. Furthermore, it was clear that activities designed to reduce emotional, social, and physical stress among AIDS patients and their caregivers and to foster public attitudes that facilitated patient management would result in more effective delivery of treatment and strengthen preventive efforts. The following is a model program to provide comprehensive services to AIDS patients within an acute care center.

Orientation to the Center

A social worker meets each patient on his first visit to the hospital, preferably before a physician sees him—a sequence that has proved to be the most effective way of dealing with the patient's initial panic and mistrust of the institution. The purpose of this initial meeting is to engage the patient with the hospital in a way that meets his needs for information and personal acceptance and meets the staff's need for information. The social worker prepares the patient for what will happen that day, gives him a booklet that answers many of his questions, and describes the services and resources available to his/her friends and family. These services include financial resources, community support services, and counseling. At this time, the patient also is introduced to the clinic nurse who facilitates the management of his treatment and systems negotiations.

The worker also briefly assesses the patient's need for psychosocial intervention in the future. This assessment includes: information about the demographics; the nature and stability of the patient's living and occupational arrangements; the quality of his relationships with family, partners, and significant others; the amount of emotional support these individuals can provide; the patient's behavior patterns; his knowledge of and reactions to the disease; beliefs, attitudes, and expectations about treatment and outcome; and preliminary information about the patient's ability to cope. This information is shared with the treating physician.

Depending on information obtained before or during the medical examination, the social worker may begin individual counseling immediately to resolve urgent problems. If a patient seems to have severe psychopathology, is potentially suicidal, or asks to see a chaplain because of urgent religious conflicts, the worker makes the appropriate referrals. The worker also makes referrals to appropriate community resources such as support organizations, Social Security, public assistance, Medicaid, and legal services, and invites the patient to join a weekly support group conducted at the center.

Ongoing Interventions and Support

The same social worker provides the patient with practical and counseling services throughout his treatment. Knowing that someone will direct his questions and concerns to the appropriate staff and help the patient obtain financial and other concrete services greatly reduces the patient's anxiety, conserves the physician's time, and results in more continuous care.

In addition to immediate crisis intervention and individual counseling, the program provides the following ongoing psychosocial support activities: (1) support groups for patients, lovers, and families; (2) patient education; (3) instruction in relaxation and other behavioral techniques; and (4) liaison with community resources such as drug treatment programs, gay service agencies, cancer counseling agencies, and the Social Security Administration.

Support Groups

After the AIDS patient's basic needs have been met and his individual problems have been addressed, support groups are highly effective. The center currently conducts three psychoeducationally-oriented support groups for AIDS patients: one for lymphadenopathy patients, one for AIDS patients and their partners, and one for patients with Kaposi's sarcoma. Conducting a separate support group for lymphadenopathy patients seems to help them cope better with fears of contracting AIDS. This group has been expanded to include human immunodeficiency virus seropositive "worried-well."

New patients have an immense need for reassurance and for a chance to observe and speak with other patients who are experiencing the same illness. A support group reduces the patient's feelings of isolation and loneliness, enables the sharing of experiences, and offers wide range of people with whom he can interact and solve problems. A professional skilled in group dynamics serves as facilitator. The self-help approach is an acknowledgment that experiential knowledge is different from professional knowledge and offers a unique contribution. Individual group members not only serve as models for others, but also reinforce their own self-perceptions as people capable of controlling their own lives and situations.

Although all groups have a flexible membership and attendance, patients are encouraged to attend regularly. A support group is vitally important, cost-effective intervention, but it should not be viewed as the only ongoing intervention (Weinberg and Williams 1984). Some patients are reluctant to participate in groups or do so only when they are not acutely upset; others use the group continuously for encouragement and support. Individual crises and a vast range of practical problems usually cannot be handled adequately in a group.

The death of a group member is a special problem in groups of potentially terminally ill patients. The group facilitator informs the members of the patient's death during the subsequent group meeting rather than allowing them to hear about it informally, tells them about the care the patient received, who was with the patient when he died, and other pertinent information. The group facilitator encourages the group to discuss their reactions and to ask questions; then the group refocuses on the present and how members can cope with the disease.

Patient Education

Education is an integral part of the group treatment program. At times, group facilitators adopt an active educative technique or use outside speakers to present information on topics such as medical and psychiatric AIDS research studies, legal issues, relaxation techniques, infectious diseases, etc. The group process gives members an opportunity to ask questions in an informal and supportive atmosphere, have contact with physicians, and gain information that can be relayed to their friends and family. The emphasis on education gives them a greater sense of control through improved access to information.

Individual Instruction

Individual instruction and printed materials have proved to be of vital importance in helping patients cope. The printed materials cover information about: the disease, its symptoms, and its treatment; self-care and ways of preventing the spread of the disease; and methods of obtaining appropriate medical and nonmedical services.

Methods of cognitive control over anxiety, such as relaxation techniques, help patients cope with extreme anxiety related to medical procedures, pain, and chronic stress of the illness. These methods can be taught individually or in groups and are especially helpful to patients who previously relied on drugs or compulsive sexual behavior to reduce tension.

Staff

Physicians, nurses, and others involved in patient care are prone to occupational stress, fear and anxiety, prejudices, and guilt feelings as a result of working with AIDS patients. Thus, education, multidisciplinary patient care rounds, crisis intervention, and ongoing stress reduction groups have proved to be effective with the center's staff.

Educational materials and programs for physicians and other professionals present detailed information about the disease. For example, information that will help sensitize staff to the drug-using or gay lifestyle is presented, and complementary measures to improve communication between staff and patients are taken. Poor communication contributes to staff discomfort with AIDS patients—a problem related, in part, to the extreme anxiety exhibited by many patients and their tremendous need for contact, encouragement, and reassurance. These factors, together with the different lifestyles of the two groups, often lead to mutual suspicion and uneasiness.

Crisis intervention for staff members is also available. Staff crises are usually precipitated by a sudden resurgence of acute fear about contracting AIDS, by pressure from a spouse about contagion, by pregnancy, by pressure from social contacts, or by a confrontation with a patient's lifestyle, deteriorating condition, or death. Either time-limited or ongoing staff support groups that focus on emotional reaction, problem solving, and development of mutually supportive relationships have been used to reduce stress and increase productivity.

Future Directions

The AIDS crisis has had several positive consequences. One important one is that traditional and nontraditional service agencies, government groups, and organizations for gay and drug-addicted nongay people have been collaborating on an ongoing basis. One hopes that this new collaboration will continue and that these groups can be mobilized to address creatively not only future crises, but also currently unresolved service delivery problems. If this can be done, the result should be optimism and increased collaboration.

References

Coppola, V., and M. Zabarsky. 1983. Coming out of the closet. *Newsweek*, 8 August.

DeVita, V. T., S. Hellman, and S. Rosenberg, eds. 1985. *AIDS: etiology, diagnosis, treatment and prevention.* Philadelphia, Pennsylvania: J. B. Lippincott.

Fauci, A. S., M. Macher, and D. Longo. 1984. Acquired immunodeficiency syndrome: epidemiologic, clinical, immunologic and therapeutic considerations. *Ann. Intern. Med.* 100:92-106.

Grossman, R. J. 1984. Psychosocial support in AIDS: a practitioner's view. In *AIDS*, eds. A. Friedman-Kien and L. J. Lauberstein. New York: Masson, Inc.

Krown, S. E. 1984. Kaposi's sarcoma and AIDS: clinical manifestations and treatment. *J. Psychosocial Oncol.* 2:1-17.

Lowenstein, R. J., and S. Sharpstein. 1984. Neuropsychiatric aspects of acquired immune deficiency syndrome. *Int. J. Psychiat. Med.* 13:255-60.

Malyon, A. K., and A. Pinka. 1983. Acquired immune deficiency syndrome: a challenge to psychology. *Profess. Psychol.* 7:1-10.

Nichols, S. E., Jr. 1983. Psychiatric aspects of AIDS. *Psychosomatics* 24:1083-89.

Rossi, A. S. 1980. The middle years of parenting. In *Life-span development and behavior*, vol. 3, eds. P. Baltes and O. Brim Jr. New York: Academic Press.

Snider, W. D., D. Simpson, and S. Nielson. 1983. Neurological complication of acquired immune deficiency syndrome: analysis of 50 patients. *Ann. Neurol.* 14:403-18.

Weinberg, S., and C. Williams. 1984. *Male homosexuals: their problems and adaptations.* New York: Oxford University Press.

11
Psychiatric and Ethical Issues in the Care of Patients with AIDS

James W. Dilley, MD; Earl E. Shelp, PhD; and
Steven L. Batki, MD.

Our purpose is to highlight the clinical management and ethical issues confronting the consultation-liaison psychiatrist asked to see a patient with acquired immunodeficiency syndrome (AIDS). We will approach these issues in the following manner. First, we comment on the general psychological and social milieu surrounding a patient diagnosed with AIDS. Second, we describe common medical complications of the disease as they pertain to psychiatric assessment. Third, we draw on the implications of the previous material to identify special ethical considerations in the care of patients with this disease.

The psychological and social climate surrounding an individual diagnosed with AIDS can be summarized as follows:

1. Because AIDS is a relatively new and complex disease, well-intentioned but inadequately informed persons may be confused about the risk of infection and thus overreact to someone with AIDS.

Reprinted, with changes, from "Psychiatric and Ethical Issues in the Care of Patients with AIDS," by James W. Dilley, Earl E. Shelp, and Steven L. Batki, *Psychosomatics* 27:562-66, 1986, by permission of the Academy of Psychosomatic Medicine.

2. Since AIDS is acquired primarily through sexual contact or through intravenous drug use, and because both of these activities may incur moral judgments, some persons may "blame the victim" for the illness.

3. Historically, intravenous drug users and homosexual men have been stigmatized on the basis of social prejudices concerning homosexuality, and drug abuse (Larsen, Reed, and Hoffman 1980).

4. AIDS is seen as a terminal disease.

These factors must be viewed in relation to the likely or common course of illness experienced by an individual with AIDS. To do so, the consultant needs to be aware of the different prognostic implications of the various presentations of AIDS. For example, individuals first diagnosed with Kaposi's sarcoma may be essentially healthy from a subjective point of view and may remain so for several years. On the other hand, the patient whose AIDS diagnosis is first brought about by the appearance of *Cryptococcal meningitis* has a life expectancy of less than six months (Rivin, Monroe, and Hubschuman 1984).

While 86% of the first 1,065 AIDS patients cared for in New York City between 1981 and 1984 survived their initial hospitalization, their quality of life was severely compromised. Forty-six percent of those survivors spent at least 30% of their remaining weeks or months in a hospital, and 32% of them required hospitalization for at least half of their remaining lifetime (Rivin, Monroe, and Hubschuman 1984). The most common course of the disease, then, is the intermittent development of illnesses not usually seen in the general, immunocompetent public. Sometimes, these illnesses can be treated, while leaving the patient with the underlying disorder largely unable to return to his/her usual level of activities. Most often, this intermittent development of illnesses is additive and progressive, leading to both physical and emotional exhaustion.

Additionally, each of the factors outlined previously is significant because of the attitudes of nonpatients as well as the patient's own attitudes toward these issues. Thus, persons with AIDS may blame themselves for their illness, at times perceiving the disease as retribution for such behaviors as drug abuse or homosexuality.

Neuropsychiatric Complications

It is important for the consultant to be aware of the high incidence of neurologic complications in this group of patients. Studies (Snider, Simpson, and Nielson 1983; Britton and Miller 1984; Levy, Bredesen, and Rosenblum 1985) have found that 30% to 40% of all AIDS patients will develop some neurologic dysfunction. Also, in a controlled study in New York of neuropsychological functioning in 80 patients with AIDS, 50% of them evidenced some cognitive impairment on formal testing. Deficits were noted in the speed of processing new information, memory, and ability to complete several step tasks (Tross, Price, and Sidtis 1985).

The nonspecific nature of psychiatric presentations in persons with AIDS can also be problematic. A review of published case studies of neuropsychiatric presentations in these patients reveals no pathognomonic signs or symptoms that are of particular value in assessment. Patients most often present with depressive or anxious syndromes marked by motor retardation or agitation, sadness, mood swings, or generalized apathy. Alternatively, psychiatric sequelae of organic brain syndromes, e.g., deficits in verbal and visual memory, disorientation, decreased attention or concentration, apathy, or thought disorders, grandiose delusions, and bizarre behavior, have been reported. Although laboratory and physical findings are usually nonspecific, they can provide important corroborative information. Common laboratory findings include mild to moderately dilated ventricles and/or cerebral atrophy on CT scans, and generalized slowing or normal results on the EEG. Protein may be elevated in the cerebrospinal fluid or lumbar puncture (Lowenstein and Sharfstein 1983-84; Kemani, Drob, and Alpert 1984; Ochitill, Perl, and Dilley 1984-85; Hoffman 1984).

The absence of clear findings in the laboratory work-up, potential central nervous system involvement by AIDS-associated virus (Shaw, Harper, and Hahn 1985), and the significant psychosocial stressors previously mentioned combine to complicate psychiatric evaluation in this group.

What then are likely intrapersonal reactions to this disease? It is important to note that following the initial psychological reactions to the diagnosis of a life-threatening illness, which usually involve existential searching (Weisman and Worden 1976-77), the immediate needs of the patient are educational and supportive. At later stages, often after the second or third episode of illness, the consultant can expect a greater emphasis on the patient's need to grieve, as the adaptive denial probably seen in the earlier stage begins to crumble under the weight of physical deterioration. Difficult diagnostic questions again arise for the consultant: when does normal grieving become psychopathology, and what role do organic factors play in a particular patient's presentation?

Ethical Considerations

The interplay of the medical, psychological, and social factors outlined generates important ethical issues that should not be overlooked by the consultant striving to provide quality care for patients with this disease. For ease of discussion, important issues are presented in a sequence based on the course of the illness (exhibit 11-1). Many of these issues are equally applicable to members of both groups at highest risk for AIDS (intravenous drug users and homosexual and bisexual men).

New Diagnosis

Because of the social implications of an AIDS diagnosis, the issue of confidentiality is paramount. Caregivers and their patients need to agree clearly about what information is to be disclosed and who is to receive it. A clear understanding of these matters can help to protect a physician from inadvertently disclosing information that could result, for example, in the needless loss of employment, insurance benefits, or emotional support. Furthermore, truthful com-

Exhibit 11-1

Selected Ethical Issues In the Care of AIDS Patients

New diagnosis	Mid-stage	Terminal care
Confidentiality	Power of attorney	Patient's choices
Truthfulness	for health care	regarding treatment
Informed consent	Suicidal ideation	Scope of care
		and loyalty
		Life supports

munication between patient and physician is critically important. Honest and complete disclosures by patients can contribute to proper diagnosis and appropriate therapy. Similarly, disclosure by the physician will enhance constructive and responsible decision-making on the part of the patient. Accurate medical information on current studies, treatment options, and prognosis will enable a patient to make informed judgments about conventional or experimental treatments for the multiple complications associated with AIDS. Medical personnel are, of course, ethically bound to abide by the decisions of competent patients regarding their medical care.

Discussion with patients about life supports should occur early in the illness so that the possible sudden development of cognitive impairment owing to central nervous system pathology does not deprive the patient of the ability to participate in treatment decisions. In this regard, it is especially important to inform the patient about use of a power of attorney to delegate health care decisions to a person of his choice, should the time come when the patient is no longer able to make such decisions.

At Midstage

The assessment of suicidal ideation can also be problematic in this group of patients. Few physicians would deny a legal or ethical duty to intervene with the physically healthy patient who expresses suicidal intent. Generally accepted as a cry for help, suicidal ideation in this group motivates physicians to take an active, even aggressive stance: patients are hospitalized against their will and at times even are physically restrained to prevent them from harming themselves. The rationale for these measures to a large extent derives from belief in the patient's chances for improvement: the depression or despair will lift and the person will return to a productive life. In the case of AIDS or other terminal diseases, however, medical and legal scholars continue to debate whether suicide is a moral wrong and/or whether intervention by physicians or the police is warranted (Perlin 1975; Schneidman 1981; Wallace and Eser 1981; Battin 1982). No clear medical, moral, or legal consensus exists that suicide is always wrong in this group. Consequently, AIDS patients who express suicidal intent can pose particularly dif-

ficult professional and personal problems for the psychiatric consultant asked to intervene.

Terminal Care

When a patient enters the terminal phase of the illness, it is important to recall the principle of respecting his/her right to participate in treatment decisions. Although a medical, legal, and ethical consensus has been reached (President's Commission For the
Study of Ethical Problems in Medicine and Biomedical Problems in
Medicine and Biomedical and Behavioral Research 1983; Lo and
Steinbrook 1983; Jonsen, Siegler, and Winslade 1982) that life-sustaining treatment may be limited when further therapy is medically
futile, the patient's participation in treatment decisions should be
solicited. We believe, additionally, that the scope of the physician's
responsibility also includes a duty to provide care to significant
others identified by the patient. Furthermore, physicians have an
ethical duty not to abandon patients or their families during the
course of dying. Finally, it may be possible to moderate contentious
issues regarding the withholding or withdrawing of life supports if
the patient or legal surrogate is well-informed and encouraged to
participate in treatment decisions.

Intravenous Drug Users with AIDS

The dual diagnosis of intravenous drug use and AIDS compounds treatment problems. Treatment of drug use in these patients
is fraught with difficult choices for the clinician. It is generally
agreed that continued intravenous drug use by AIDS patients not
only endangers the patient's health by offering new avenues for opportunistic infection, but also may endanger other such drug users
and eventually the community-at-large through needle-sharing and
sexual contact. Concerns about public health, therefore, inevitably
intrude into the treatment of the individual drug user and can raise
unique ethical issues for the consultant.

For example, how strenuously does the clinician address the
treatment of drug use in the patient? One view is that the treatment
of drug use is integral to the rest of AIDS treatment. This view holds
that treatment, such as methadone maintenance for opiate users,
must be provided as a matter of course for the AIDS patient in

order to reduce the likelihood of continued drug use. An extreme form of this view takes the position that methadone treatment should be mandatory for opiate users with AIDS. A differing viewpoint places individual patient rights above public health concerns. The patient is encouraged to seek treatment for drug use but the consultant does not require it.

Even after an AIDS patient has entered treatment for drug use, ethical problems may persist. Drug programs generally use techniques such as close monitoring, firm limit-setting, confrontation, and the use of sanctions to help patients refrain from illicit drug use. In addition, these programs are generally designed for patients who are able to generate some degree of motivated effort to remain drug-free. However, motivation may be difficult to develop among drug users with AIDS who may lack the orientation to future possibilities that is important for recovery in chemical dependence. Intravenous drug users with AIDS are also likely to have other emotional and physical discomfort that may contribute to continued illicit drug use even if they are receiving methadone through a treatment program. An additional stressor is potential ostracism of such a patient by other patients and perhaps staff members at the treatment center because of the AIDS diagnosis. This may prove to be a further impediment to the patient's assimilation into the therapeutic environment.

The ethical problems confronting the psychiatric consultant involved in substance abuse treatment may include the question of how firm to be in setting behavioral limits for the AIDS patient. Does the patient receive more lenient treatment than other patients? Are usually firm drug treatment principles compromised? Are treatment program rules suspended? What are the possible deleterious effects on the treatment program if "special" rules apply to certain patients? Ordinarily, drug users who continue illicit use while in treatment are not allowed to continue in programs such as methadone maintenance. However, the enforcement of typical drug treatment rules may become very difficult for the clinician concerned about the consequences of ending treatment and sending the drug-using AIDS patient "back on the street."

Conclusions

We have identified psychiatric and ethical issues in the care of patients with AIDS. Many of the issues raised here are also potentially present in the care of other chronically or terminally ill patients. However, because of the unique psychosocial ramifications of AIDS, these issues take on particular urgency.

A comprehensive analysis of the psychiatric and ethical issues involved in the care of AIDS patients is beyond the scope of this brief report. However, by highlighting some of these special issues, we hope that a more detailed discussion will ensue. The psychiatric consultant can provide a service to both patients and staff by prompting discussions of these issues before they actually present a clinical crisis.

References

Battin, P. 1982. *Ethical issues in suicide.* Englewood Cliffs, New Jersey: Prentice-Hall.

Britton, C. B., and J. Miller. 1984. Neurological complications in acquired immune deficiency syndrome (AIDS). *Neurol. Clin.* 2:315.

Hoffman, R. S. 1984. Neuropsychiatric complications of AIDS. *Psychosomatics* 25:393-400.

Jonsen, A. R., M. Siegler, and W. Winslade. 1982. *Clinical ethics.* New York, Macmillan.

Kemani, E., S. Drob, and M. Alpert. 1984. Organic brain syndromes in three cases of AIDS. *Comp. Psychiat.* 25:292-97.

Larsen, K. S., M. Reed, and S. Hoffman. 1980. Attitudes of heterosexuals toward homosexuality. *J. Sex Res.* 16:245-49.

Levy, R. M., D. Bredesen, and M. Rosenblum. 1985. Neurological manifestations of the acquired immune deficiency syndrome (AIDS): experience at UCSF and review of the literature. *J. Neurosurg.* 62:475-95.

Lo, B., and R. Steinbrook. 1983. Deciding whether to resuscitate. *Arch. Intern. Med.* 143:1561-63.

Lowenstein, R. J., and S. Sharfstein. 1983-84. Neuro-psychiatric aspects of AIDS. *Int. J. Psychiat. Med.* 13:255-61.

Ochitill, H., M. Perl, and J. Dilley. 1984-85. Case reports of psychological disturbances in patients with AIDS. *Int J. Psychiat. Med.* 14:259-63.

Perlin, S., ed. 1975. *A handbook for the study of suicide.* New York: Oxford University Press.

President's Commission for the Study of Ethical Problems in Medicine and Biomedical Problems in Medicine and Biomedical and Behavioral Research. 1983. *Deciding to forego life-sustaining treatment.* A Report on the Ethical, Medical and Legal Issues in Treatment Decisions. Washington, D.C.: Government Printing Office.

Rivin, B. E., J. Monroe, and B. Hubschuman. 1984. AIDS outcome: a first follow-up (letter). *N. Engl. J. Med.* 311:857.

Schneidman, E. S. 1981. *Suicide thoughts and reflections, 1960-1980.* New York: Human Sciences Press.

Shaw, G., M. Harper, and B. Hahn. 1985. HTLV-III infection in brains of children and adults with encephalopathy. *Science* 227:177-81.

Snider, W. D., D. Simpson, and S. Nielson. 1983. Neurological complications of acquired immune deficiency syndrome: analysis of 50 patients. *Ann. Neurol.* 14:403-18.

Tross, S., R. Price, and J. Sidtis. 1985. Psychological and neuropsychological function in AIDS spectrum disorder patients. Paper presented at the International Conference on the Acquired Immune Deficiency Syndrome (AIDS), 14-17 April, Atlanta, Georgia.

Wallace, S. E., and A. Eser, eds. 1981. *Suicide and euthanasia: the rights of personhood.* Knoxville, Tennessee: University of Tennessee Press.

Weisman, A. D., and J. Worden. 1976-77. The existential plight in cancer: significance of the first 100 days. *Int. J. Psychiat. Med.* 7:1015.

12
Psychosocial Reactions of Persons with the Acquired Immunodeficiency Syndrome

Stuart E. Nichols, MD.

Since late 1981, I have evaluated clinically the psychosocial problems of several hundred patients with the acquired immunodeficiency syndrome (AIDS). Distinguishing between the two primary problems, one a result of the disease itself, the other societally induced, is important in understanding and perhaps dismantling some of the damaging psychosocial aspects of AIDS.

The psychological effect on patients has been described as an adjustment reaction in which the stress is severe enough to be considered catastrophic (Haussman 1983; Morin 1984). Catastrophes often produce situational distress that elicits similar emotional responses in almost everyone subjected to the stress (Tyhurst 1951; Parkes 1971; Weiss 1976). Situational distress occurs in three phases: crisis, transitional state, and deficiency state. Reactions to AIDS follow this pattern with the frequent addition of a fourth stage, the preparation for death (Nichols, in press).

Reprinted, with changes, from "Psychosocial Reactions of Persons with the Acquired Immunodeficiency Syndrome," by Stuart E. Nichols, *Annals of Internal Medicine* 103:765-67, 1985, by permission of the publisher.

Initial Crisis

Studies of the effects of life-threatening illnesses on patients (Hackett and Cassem 1970; Horowitz 1974) and others have shown an acute response of denial alternating with periods of intense anxiety. The denial may be so complete that the patient will adopt an attitude of indifference, possibly leading to a dangerous disregard of medical advice. If medical advice is followed, however, the denial should be considered an equilibrium-preserving response to the crisis, and no attempts should be made to dislodge it. Patients may be overwhelmed by emotion or increase their denial, and perhaps engage in life-threatening behavior if the denial becomes more prominent. Outlining at this stage the usual emotional reactions to AIDS, which include shock, denial, guilt, fear, anger, sadness, bargaining, and acceptance (Nichols 1984), can help patients to feel that their own reactions to AIDS are understandable and normal.

One of the most disruptive complications of AIDS is its impact on supportive relationships. The physician should ascertain whether the family knows about the patient's drug addiction or accepts his homosexuality. The onset of AIDS also may force disclosure of previously disguised drug use in drug-addicted patients, which may weaken familial support. The stigma attached to AIDS affects all patients, including children, women, and military service personnel.

Patients in the crisis stage typically have difficulty retaining information and may distort what they are told regarding their illness. Contact with support services such as crisis counseling, legal and financial assistance, and therapy – usually available through drug treatment programs or the gay community for the homosexual/bisexual addicts who comprise 8% of the cases – should begin as early as possible. Because of their emotional numbness, some patients in severe shock may appear unperturbed by experiences such as discriminatory or unprofessional treatment that otherwise would greatly trouble them.

Transitional State

The transitional state begins when alternating waves of anger, guilt, self-pity, and anxiety supersede denial. Patients may obsessively review their past in an attempt to understand what they may have done to "deserve" AIDS.

The transitional period is a time of distress, confusion, and disruptiveness. Social rejections are deeply felt, aggravating the situation. Changes in self-esteem, identity, and values, estrangement from families and community, the occurrence of more drug use, and considerations of suicide may occur. However, despite the dangers present, or because of them, patients are especially accessible to psychosocial intervention at this time.

Severe withdrawal, a dangerous reaction in which patients refuse to deal with the disease and avoid friends, family, and physicians, may also occur. Some patients may displace their anger in continued drug using or sexual behavior, endangering others as well as themselves.

Due to frequently impaired comprehension, another person should accompany a patient on medical visits to ensure adherence to instructions. Patients may magnify differences in medical opinion. Slightly different advice about "clean needles" or "safe sex" practices, for example, may cause them to panic or conclude that the medical profession is incompetent.

Additional stress in the transitional stage may include discharge from a drug treatment program, infecting a sexual partner, the loss of job, income, and even one's home. The bargaining reactions, in which patients may believe they will be cured by promising to "be good," may prevent the expression of the tremendous anger they feel. Consequently, they are likely to exhibit fear and depression, rather than anger.

Persons in the transitional state must form new values, a new sense of self, and a new community; often they must restructure altered relationships with loved ones and families. Participation in a social group, a support group, a drug treatment program, or individual counseling, may help new patients to become comfortable talking about AIDS and to accept their own reactions to the disease. However, counselors should be aware that seeing persons at advanced stages of the illness can often be overwhelming to patients who are just beginning to adjust to AIDS.

The Deficiency State: Acceptance

Formation of a new, stable identify occurs upon reaching the stage of acceptance. Others have labeled this state supportive denial (Dilley 1984), but acceptance better describes the attendant adjustment and the extent of identity shifting that occurs. Patients in this stage learn to accept the limitations imposed on them by AIDS, but also realize that they can still manage their lives by reacting to the disease with more reason than emotion. In making a conscious effort to live each day fully, these patients: examine sources of pain and pleasure; reassess the value of courage, commitment, affection, and concern for others; and learn to appreciate quality rather than quantity in living. Some patients also may embrace spiritual concepts for hope and relief.

Patients begin to feel less victimized by life, become less egocentric, and find satisfaction in altruistic and community activities – often involving themselves with issues and pursuits previously ignored. They take more responsibility for their own health, sometimes experimenting with holistic medical practices such as positive imaging, macrobiotic diets, and meditation. A fighting spirit develops toward their illness and their physicians.

Reaching the state of acceptance is facilitated by contact with other patients who serve as role models. That acceptance is a deficiency state, however, as is evidenced by losses of health, energy, income, and independence. Under these circumstances, the human spirit's ability to marshal such inner resources is remarkable.

Special Features of Situational Distress

Application of the situational distress model must allow for the different, sometimes simultaneous, crises patients are likely to experience – acceptance is not a permanent state. New crises may force renegotiation of transitional states to reach acceptance again. This feature has been tagged by patients as the roller coaster of AIDS.

Patients may benefit from medication for insomnia, anxiety, depression, hypomania, or preexisting conditions exacerbated by their diagnosis, e.g., methadone maintenance for drug abusers. Because of the rapid shifts in emotional states, antianxiety agents are often chosen first for depressive symptoms of short duration, but antidepressant drugs may be needed if there is no improvement. Antipsychotic medication may help patients whose illness is complicated by organic psychotic reactions.

Patients face additional adjustments which may trigger a situational distress reaction such as the fear of death and dying, the sense of vulnerability to opportunistic infections, the threat of disfiguration, the continued loss of independent function, prejudice of others, the loss of friends who die of AIDS, and, finally, the need to prepare for one's own death.

Preparation for Death

The fear of becoming totally dependent on others usually supersedes the fear of death. Many patients feel that overdosing or suicide would be preferable to such dependency, yet they continue to fight for life despite increasing disability. The final stage of adjustment, however, is spent primarily in preparing for death.

In the early stages of the disease, patients may benefit from completing unfinished business, such as asking for or granting forgiveness, seeing or speaking to certain persons once again, or finishing a drug treatment program or creative project. When patients are comfortable talking about death, they should be encouraged to share their feelings about how and where they would prefer to die, as well as how they would prefer arrangements handled after their death. Patients' desires may be difficult to honor, however: hospitals may require more medical intervention than patients wish, and hospices may refuse them admittance. Drug addicts and homosexual patients may find problems between friends and family exacerbated as death approaches, due to friends being addicts.

Problems Resulting From Societal Reactions

It is frequently discovered that family dynamics contribute to the psychological symptoms experienced by AIDS patients; indeed, the maintenance of family equilibrium often necessitates their presence. Therefore, resistance to change among nonpatient family members may be the most difficult problem of therapy; the family often refuses to accept its role in the production and maintenance of the symptoms.

Social prejudice may play an analogous role in the development of psychological symptoms in the AIDS patient. Prejudice distorts judgment with negativism and insensitivity; victims of discrimination are seen as fundamentally different from other persons, less deserving of basic human rights, and deserving of the treatment they receive.

Although casual contact has not been shown to transmit AIDS, many health care professionals also continue to display prejudice against AIDS patients. They may protect themselves from patients in inappropriate ways, such excessive masking and gowning, handling patients' documents with tweezers, and calling for quarantines. Prejudice in health care may interfere with confidentiality and consideration of the patients' emotional well being (Haussman 1983; Morin 1984). The public does not believe the data on transmission and continues to act and react with fear, anger, and an absence of reason (Haussman, 1983).

During the outbreak of the disease, the medical community was preoccupied with trying to determine its prevalence, cause, and possible treatment. The emotional impact of AIDS on patients and the discrimination to which they were subjected was barely noticed. Popular reports, however, headlined society's panic and actions taken against persons it considered dangerous or repugnant (Morin 1984).

A contributing factor in this absence of justice is the lack of natural advocates for AIDS risk groups (Parkes 1971). Although some hospitals have established programs for staff education, they frequently emphasize contagion control rather than social prejudice. In addition, these programs also often lack the support of strong administrative policy that disciplines personnel who engage in unprofessional behavior. Patient complaints of inappropriate conduct are usually referred to patient liaison or social work staffs; physicians rarely handle these problems (Parkes 1971).

Health care professionals often rationalize that such problems are beyond the scope of medicine. However, when prejudice results in patient harm, as in the case of AIDS, it must be addressed by the medical profession. Fearing discrimination, patients with AIDS may be reluctant to seek help for their illness or to receive AIDS education to help them lessen their high-risk behaviors.

Psychosocial reactions to AIDS have made it clear that taboo remains a powerful societal force. Taboos, primitive social devices designed to discourage behavior deemed harmful, should have no validity in modern times.

Even in modern times, however, the investigation of drug addicts and sexuality has met with strong resistance. Freud was ejected from his medical society because of his studies on infantile sexuality. Kinsey's work on male sexuality was once compared by the president of Princeton University of "toilet wall inscriptions," and it provoked a professor at Columbia University to call for "a law against doing research exclusively with sexuality" (Tripp 1975). Once again, because of the outbreak of AIDS, society is examining the behavioral and sexual practices of certain groups, an undertaking that is altering previous concepts and causing a backlash. However, when the new information uncovered by AIDS is integrated into our general store of knowledge, increased understanding of drug addicts and human sexuality will result.

The study of the effect of taboo on society is made possible by the AIDS epidemic; as in family therapy, only after exposure of the dynamics of a problem can healing and the discovery of solutions begin. When a taboo is broken, society goes through a transition, searching for new concepts and behavioral standards appropriate to new knowledge. All members of society, including those in healing professions, should participate in this search.

Summary

AIDS causes two types of psychosocial crises: one among patients, the other in the general population—both yield opportunities and pitfalls. Medicine and allied professions can help marshal intelligent responses to regressive societal forces unleashed by the AIDS dilemma, as well as help patients stave off their sense of impending doom and hopelessness, and accept the losses imposed on them by the disease. Persons with AIDS can serve as models of adjustment to a progressive and devastating illness.

References

Dilley, J.W. 1984. Treatment interventions and approaches to care of patients with acquired immune deficiency syndrome. In *Psychiatric implications of acquired immune deficiency syndrome*, eds. S.E. Nichols and D.G. Ostrow. Washington, D.C.: American Psychiatric Press, 62-80.

Hackett, T.P., and N. Cassem. 1970. Psychological reactions to a life-threatening illness. In *Psychological aspects of stress*, ed. H. Abram. Springfield, Illinois: Charles C. Thomas, 29-43.

Haussman, K. 1983. Treatment victims of AIDS poses challenge to psychiatrists. *Psychiatric News*, 5 August.

Horowitz, M.T. 1973. *Stress response syndromes*. New York: Jason Aranson.

Morin, S.F. and W. Batchelor. 1984. Responding to the psychological crisis of AIDS. *Public Health Report* 99:4-9.

Nichols, S.E. 1983. Psychiatric aspects of AIDS. *Psychosomatics* 24:1083-9.

———. 1984. The social climate when the acquired immune deficiency syndrome developed. In *Psychiatric implications of the acquired immune deficiency syndrome*, eds. S.E. Nichols and D.G. Ostrow. Washington, D.C.: American Psychiatric Press, 85-92.

———. Psychotherapy and AIDS. In *Avenues to understanding psychotherapy in gay men and lesbians*, eds. T.S. Stein and C.J. Cohen. New York: Plenum Press. In press.

Parkes, C.M. 1971. Psychosocial transitions; a field for study. *Soc. Sci. Med.* 5:101-15.

Tripp, C.A. 1975. *The homosexual matrix.* New York: McGraw-Hill.

Tyhurst, J.S. 1951. Reactions to community disaster: the natural history of psychiatric phenomena. *Am. J. Psychiat.* 107:765-69.

Weis, R.S. 1976. Transition states and other stressful situations: their nature and programs for their management. In: *Support systems and mutual help*, eds. G. Caplan and M. Killilea. New York: Grune & Stratton, 213-32.

13
Findings in Psychiatric Consultations with Patients with Acquired Immune Deficiency Syndrome

James W. Dilley, MD; Herbert N. Ochitill, MD;
Mark Perl, MBBS; and Paul Volberding, MD.

Since it was first described in 1979, acquired immune deficiency syndrome (AIDS) has become a health problem of epidemic proportions (Durack 1981; Macek 1982; Desforges 1983). Although primarily occurring within discrete at-risk subgroups (sexually active gay men, Haitians, intravenous drug users, and hemophiliacs), the disease does appear in other groups (Joncas, Delage, and Chad 1983; Oleske, Minnefor, and Cooper 1983). The clinical characteristics are by now well known: the disease is probably mediated by an as yet unidentified agent that is transmitted by sexual contact and blood-borne contamination. The agent brings about a reduction in cellular immunity, leaving the individual susceptible to overwhelming opportunistic infections and Kaposi's sarcoma. There is no treatment for this underlying immune deficiency, and the mortality rate of all diagnosed patients at any given time is 41% (Offenstadt, Pinta, and Hericord 1983).

Reprinted, with changes, from "Findings in Psychiatric Consultations with Patients with Acquired Immune Deficiency Syndrome," by James W. Dilley, Herbert N. Ochitill, Mark Perk, and Paul A. Volberding, *American Journal of Psychiatry* 142:82-86, 1985, by permission of the American Psychiatric Association. Copyright 1985.

San Francisco is one of the centers in the United States with a high prevalence of AIDS (Centers for Disease Control 1982). It is culturally, racially, and ethnically diverse and has a large population of mobile gay men. In the inner city there are substantial numbers of poor and homeless persons; substance abuse is prevalent. San Francisco General Hospital is a 400-bed hospital serving much of the city and county of San Francisco. The hospital is a clinical campus of the University of California, San Francisco, School of Medicine. Seventy-five AIDS patients have been treated at this hospital, of whom 40 were inpatients at some point in their illness.

In this report we detail the psychiatric profiles of those hospitalized AIDS patients who were referred for psychiatric consultation. We discovered recurrent psychological issues specific to the AIDS patient as well as other issues held in common with other severely ill patients.

Method

Patients were seen by the psychiatric consultation-liaison service following referral from the general medical wards of the hospital. Consultations were prompted by the patient's request, by the primary physician's perception that the patient's emotional or behavioral state was unusual, or by the patient's presenting a management problem on the ward. Patients' medical and psychosocial histories were reviewed, and semistructured interviews and mental status examinations were performed. When appropriate, recommendations were made for further physical and psychological work-up, medications, or other therapy. Diagnoses were made according to DSM-III.

Results

Thirteen of the 40 inpatients were seen over a 9-month period. Eleven were gay and two were bisexual men; their average age was 33.8 years (range: 24 to 42 years). One patient was black and one was Hispanic; the remainder were white. As a group, the patients were well educated—six held college degrees. Eleven of the 13 were unemployed at the time of consultation; seven were receiving some form of public assistance or long-term disability payments because of this illness. Seven were living alone.

The medical status of the patients is summarized in exhibit 13-1. The most common presenting symptoms were fever, cough, and weight loss. All patients required one or more major diagnostic procedures: lumbar puncture, bronchoscopy, and lung biopsy were the most frequent. Patients with respiratory complications were administered oxygen and other appropriate supportive measures. Those with *Pneumocystis carinii* pneumonia received intravenous trimethoprim-sulfisoxazole, pentamidine, or both. Six patients had previously been hospitalized at least once with an AIDS-related complication. The mean length of stay in the hospital at the time of consultation was 29.6 days (range 3 to 64 days). Five patients died in the hospital; the others were discharged home.

Psychiatric consultations were requested an average of 6.8 days into the hospitalization (range: 1 to 11 days). Nine requests were for evaluation of "depression" or "anxiety and depression." Other reasons for consultation were to distinguish a functional illness from dementia, to evaluate acute delirium, to assess acute anxiety attacks, and to intervene with an angry patient demanding to leave the hospital against medical advice. Three consultations were requested by the patients themselves.

Twelve of the 13 received psychiatric diagnoses. The most common psychiatric diagnosis (N-7) was adjustment disorder with depressed mood, thought to be a reaction to the patients' present illness. Only two patients fulfilled DSM-III criteria for a diagnosis of major depressive disorder. Both of these patients had histories of depression that were responsive to antidepressant medications. Other diagnoses were dementia (N-1), delirium (N-1), and panic disorder (N-1). None of the patients had had previous psychiatric hospitalizations, and none was judged to be at risk for suicide. Three patients were intravenous drug users, and two others had used hallucinogens and cocaine in the past. One patient was a controlled alcoholic.

Case Report

Mr. A, a 42-year-old white man who had been employed as a health care professional for many years, presented with fever and shortness of breath. Diagnoses of *Pneumocystis carinii* pneumonia

Exhibit 13-1 Medical Profiles of 13 Patients With Acquired Immune Deficiency Syndrome Referred for Psychiatric Consultation

Patient	Presenting Complaint	Medical Complications	Treatment and Procedures
1	Diarrhea, weakness	Gastrointestinal-tract herpes, *P. carinii* pneumonia	Antibiotics
2	Fever, chills, weight loss	Herpes, cytomegalovirus pneumonia	Respiratory support
3	Decreased visual acuity, dental abscess	Cytomegalovirus retinitis, cytomegalovirus pneumonia	None
4	Fever, cough, weight loss, diarrhea	Candidiasis, cryptococcal pneumonia	Antifungals
5	Fever, chills	*P. carinii* pneumonia, candidiasis	Respiratory support, antibiotics
6	Dyspnea, cough, fever, night sweats	*P. carinii* pneumonia	Respiratory support, antibiotics
7	Bruising	Idiopathic thrombocytopenic purpura	Steroids
8	Fever, cough, wasting, vomiting	Kaposi's sarcoma, cytomegalovirus pneumonia, histoplasmosis	Antifungals, respiratory support
9	Cough, fatigue, weight loss, painful rash	Erythema multiforme, thrush	Steroids, respiratory support, antibiotics, antifungals
10	Dyspnea, cough	*P. carinii* pneumonia	Respiratory support, antibiotics
11	Confusion, memory loss, ataxia, incontinence	Decubiti, history of *P. carinii* pneumonia	Wound care, antibiotics
12	Skin lesion, cough, fever, malaise	Tuberculosis, Kaposi's sarcoma	Antibiotics
13	Shortness of breath, cough, fever	*P. carinii* pneumonia, idiopathic thrombocytopenic purpura	Steroids, antibiotics

and idiopathic thrombocytopenic purpura were made on hospital day 4. He was started on intravenous trimethoprim-sulfisoxazole and corticosteroids. After the development of a rash due to the intravenous antibiotic, the patient was switched to pentamidine, an experimental drug that he said he "hated. The Federal Drug Administration hasn't even approved it."

Psychiatric consultation was requested on the 16th hospital day. Mr. A was hostile and angry and was demanding to leave against medical advice. He had multiple complaints about his physicians and his treatment. He felt the doctors "knew next to nothing" about his disease and that they "didn't really care anyway." He admitted to crying spells and terminal insomnia; he felt abandoned by his friends, and he worried about his family's reaction to his disease. He admitted to withdrawing from others and to feeling that his illness represented punishment for being a "bad person." He also reported a past hospitalization for a major depression that had been relieved by antidepressant medication.

The patient lived alone and reported that he had always been emotionally distant from others. He had had a series of brief and unsatisfying sexual encounters. He said that all his life he had "been there for others, but no one has been there for me." He worried about his two dogs, who had given him "more love than any human being ever had," and he wanted to take care of them at home. He thought his friends were afraid of "catching something" so they stayed away from him and even stopped telephoning. He disliked being in isolation and having to wear a mask when leaving his room. He dreaded telling his family of his illness because "they've never accepted my lifestyle, and this will only convince them they were right." He also felt the need to confide in them, as he "didn't want to die alone."

A diagnosis of major depression was made. A liaison meeting with the house staff was productive, as they were able to hear Mr. A's concerns in the light of his depression and no longer felt personally affronted by his anger. He was started on trazodone, 50 mg at night, which was gradually increased to 250 mg at night. He was seen in brief, daily follow-up interviews. He was encouraged to ventilate his feelings of frustration, and a positive therapeutic alliance was rapidly achieved. As the intensity of his feelings diminished, he was able to view his situation more rationally. He was able to accept that his physicians labored under many of the same frustrations as he did. He benefited from the interpretation that some of his anger stemmed from his feelings about his friends' lack of support. He decided to stay in the hospital for the remainder of his treatment. He was discharged home a week later and was followed as an outpatient by the consultant.

Psychological Themes

During the course of the diagnostic and follow-up interviews, the patients elaborated on several recurring themes. We will delineate those reactions which seemed to arise specifically from the diagnosis of AIDS and those which seemed representative of a more general response to life-threatening illness.

Uncertainty

Perhaps the most pervasive feelings voiced by our patients were anxiety and anger over the uncertainty surrounding their illness and treatment. Their questions about etiology, course, treatment, and lifestyle modifications following acute illness were generally met with incomplete and unsatisfactory answers. Such answers were largely reflective of the current lack of information about AIDS, although at times the patients reported that their physicians failed to attend to their questions. Patients reported disappointment, fear, and in some cases, anger at this lack of information. Not infrequently, their anger was directed at their caregivers. This was especially true in patients hospitalized for long periods and in those unresponsive to treatment, e.g., those undergoing a trial of pentamidine after a poor response to the trimethoprim-sulfisoxazole. Many patients also experienced anger and fear over "being experimented upon," feeling that they were being used as "medical guinea pigs." Not infrequently, this anger was aimed at their caregivers and was expressed in both direct and indirect ways. Some staff reported being the objects of verbal outbursts; more commonly, issues were dealt with in passive-aggressive ways, e.g., by struggling over medications, refusing to comply with treatment, and repeatedly calling nurses to perform small tasks that the patient himself was capable of performing.

Isolation

Although fears of social abandonment are common in those facing a life-threatening illness, our patients were immediately confronted with this reality. By the time of admission, many patients had not worked for several months, had diminished their sexual contacts, and had become socially withdrawn. They were given a diagnosis wryly described by one as "not very socially acceptable" and placed in isolation rooms. Isolation precautions magnified their sense that others would not be available for them. Many spoke of feeling "unclean" as they watched their caretakers enter their rooms masked, gowned, and gloved. Furthermore, several patients saw their worst fears mirrored in the exaggerated behavior of some of the staff: doctors standing at arm's length when talking to them and nurses shying away from anything but brief physical contact. Some patients even became aware of staff members who at times refused to come into their rooms at all.

Additionally, several patients saw their friends fail to support or visit them during their hospitalization. Patients were often convinced that their friends feared they might "catch something." Sometimes, too, there had been longstanding problems with others' acceptance of their patients' sexual orientation. Many patients were already geographically isolated from their families, in part because of conflicts over these same issues. Some now failed to notify family or friends of their illness, fearing a rekindling of old conflicts: it would mean disclosing their sexual orientation and dealing with the anticipated negative reaction.

Illness as Retribution

Patients' fears were compounded by the thought of the illness being sexually transmitted. Several patients who had had multiple sexual partners expressed considerable guilt over their behavior, blaming themselves for the development of the illness. They overgeneralized their feelings, expressing guilt about homosexuality in any form. They found in their sexual orientation an easy answer to the question "Why me?" In effect, this group experienced their illness as punishment. Such patients experienced the greatest discomfort, requiring more support and psychotherapeutic intervention than did the others; guilt and depression were common.

General Responses to Life-Threatening Illness

The reactions of our patients were in many ways typical of others with severe illnesses, for example, cancer (Derogatis, Morros, and Fetting 1983) or burn patients (Moos 1977). In more recently diagnosed patients, feelings of numbness and anger and a sense of betrayal were typical. There was also a tendency to search relentlessly for an explanation. Patients struggled with fears related to their illness—fears of disability, loss of body control, pain, and death. Sadness and depression were common: patients faced multiple losses of health, employability, income, and, at times, relationships. They mourned their loss of physical stamina and tried to maintain an attitude of optimism in the face of grim prognosis. There was a sense of "unfinished business" in contemplating interpersonal and family problems; time to ameliorate problems was running out. Many conducted a "life review," taking stock of past achievements, failures, and relationships and reevaluating them in the light of a disabling illness associated with a shortened life span.

Conclusions

We have presented the psychiatric profiles of 13 AIDS inpatients referred for psychiatric consultation. A majority of the patients lived alone, a demographic factor that may reduce the ability to withstand the stress of illness (Cobb 1976). The most common reason for referral was a request from the primary care provider to evaluate the patient's mood and coping abilities. Assessment of a mood disorder is a frequent reason for obtaining mental health consultation (Shortell and Daniels 1974; Karasu 1978). The more frequent psychiatric diagnosis was adjustment disorder with depressed mood; only two of our patients were found to have a major mood disturbance. This is similar to the findings of one study of cancer patients (Derogatis, Morros, and Fetting 1983). Although psychiatric help was requested in all phases of the illness, newly diagnosed patients were often seen within a few days, suggesting that learning the diagnosis is itself particularly stressful. Our findings, as well as those of others (Plumb and Holland 1977; Goldberg 1981), suggest that those patients who have had previous depressive episodes may be at risk for experiencing a recurrence when faced with severe illness.

Our patients faced complex issues related to their illness. We have separated those common to persons coping with a severe life-threatening illness from issues that seem specific to AIDS. To summarize the most prominent:

1. There was marked uncertainty surrounding the etiology, course, and treatment of this disease, leading many patients to feel anger and resentment toward their caregivers.

2. There was social isolation, both within the hospital, and in the patients' social networks. Because of the uncertain transmissibility and high mortality rate of the disorder, patients were often aware that friends, lovers, or family were failing to visit or to sustain contact, and that at times even health care professionals were withdrawing from them.

3. For some patients, a diagnosis of AIDS stimulated conflicts over their sexual orientation. They experienced the illness as "a just punishment" for their homosexuality. These patients struggled with guilt about their lifestyle and blamed themselves for their illness. At a time when they most needed a stable sense of self-worth, they were assailed by self-hatred. Sometimes these feelings were mirrored in the reactions of others who also had conflicts about the patient's lifestyles. When guilt and self-blame were present, more time was needed to explore and question these beliefs. A cognitive approach proved useful, in which staff discussed the difference between causation and association and pointed out the occurrence of the disease in other groups.

Our findings suggest a number of recommendations for the primary care staff and psychiatric consultant.

1. Health care providers should review their attitudes and feelings in several areas; specifically, they must confront damaging stereotypes of homosexual or drug-abusing patients and their own personal apprehensions about the illness, including their own potential susceptibility to it. Failure to address these issues can magnify the patient's anxiety and the physician's withdrawal from the patient.

2. Care providers need to openly recognize the frustrations associated with treatment of the disorder. A provider's sense of helplessness in the face of a lethal disorder can be the most disturbing element of care.

3. The psychiatrist needs to review personal doubts or anxieties about working closely with patients having a transmissible, life-threatening condition, although no cases of patient-to-staff transmission have been documented.

4. The psychiatrist should be clear about the nature of his or her involvement with the patient, given the all-too-frequent social isolation experienced by the AIDS patient. The consultant must be clear about the potential for extended work with the patient. Ideally, he or she should be willing to follow the patient on an outpatient basis. At times the situation is further complicated when the staff has withdrawn from the patient and the consultant is implicitly promoted as the primary care provider.

5. The psychiatrist should be particularly thorough and adept in the assessment of mood and cognitive disturbances. The consultant must have a special appreciation for the factors contributing to organic mental disorder and its manifestations.

6. The small group of patients with more severe disturbance, and perhaps histories of mood disorder, requires direct ongoing intervention by the consultant.

7. Lay volunteers can be very helpful. The psychiatrist and medical staff can assist them in clarifying their appropriate role in working with AIDS patients. In some treatment settings, the psychiatrist determines what their involvement should be, relating it to the magnitude of the volunteer pool and the consultant's assessment of the patient. Sometimes the psychiatrist assumes important supervisory and didactic functions with the volunteer group.

8. There is, of course, no room in the care of the AIDS patient for moral posturing. The patient should be offered information about contributing factors and the disease's transmissibility in a secure, nonjudgmental fashion.

References

Centers for Disease Control. 1982. Update on acquired immune deficiency syndrome (AIDS)—United States. M.M. W.R. 31:507-14.

Cogg, S. 1976. Social support as a moderator of life stress. *Psychosom. Med.* 28:300-14.

Derogatis, L.R., G. Morros, and J. Fetting, 1983. The prevalence of psychiatric disorders among cancer patients. *J.A.M.A.* 249:751-57.

Desforges, J.F. 1983. AIDS and preventive treatment in hemophilia. *N. Engl. J. Med.* 308:94-95.

Durack, D.T. 1981. Opportunistic infections and Kaposi's sarcoma in homosexual men. *N. Engl. J. Med.* 305:1465-67.

Goldberg, R.J. 1981. Management of depression in the patient with advanced cancer. *J.A.M.A.* 246:373-76.

Joncas, J.H., G. Delage, and Z. Chad. 1983. Acquired (or congenital) immuno-deficiency syndrome in infants born of Haitian mothers (letter). *N. Engl. J. Med.* 308:842.

Karasu, T.B. 1978. Utilization of a psychiatric consultation service. *Psychosomatics* 19:467-73.

Macek, C. 1982. Acquired immunodeficiency syndrome cause(s) still elusive. *J.A.M.A.* 248:1423-31.

Moos, R., ed. 1977. *Coping with physical illness.* New York: Plenum.

Offenstadt, G., P. Pinta, and P. Hericord. 1983. Multiple opportunistic infection due to AIDS in a previously healthy black woman from Zaire (letter). *N. Engl. J. Med.* 308:775.

Oleske, J., A Minnefor, and R. Cooper. 1983. Immune deficiency syndrome in children. *J.A.M.A.* 249:2345-49.

Plumb, M.M., and J. Holland. 1977. Comparative studies of psychological function in patients with advanced cancer. *Psychosom. Med.* 39:264-75.

Shortell, S.M., and R. Daniels. 1974. Referral relationships between internists and psychiatrists in fee-for-service practice. *Med. Care* 12:229-40.

PART IV

AIDS—The Therapeutic Community and Health Education

At this time, education remains the most promising means of preventing the transmission of the human immunodeficiency virus. In the case of the intravenous drug user, the development of educational modules is particularly critical since, unlike sexually active homosexual and bisexual men, the drug user "on the streets" lacks a community network to spread prevention information. As the authors contributing to Part IV note, behavior change can be difficult for intravenous drug users, because of their addiction and because of the ritualistic nature of certain behaviors, such as sharing needles.

Here, the authors look at AIDS education in treatment settings and in the community. Chapter 14, "A Biopsychosocial Approach to AIDS," discusses the treatment of intravenous drug users with AIDS in the general hospital, considering the behavior problems drug users present for medical staff unaccustomed to working with them. In chapters 15 and 16, the treatment setting considered is the drug-free, residential therapeutic community. Robak looks at actual cases of AIDS-related complex in clients and the development of therapeutic groups to help them deal constructively with the medical and psychological uncertainties of their diagnosis. Lewis and Galea report on the perceptions of intravenous drug users—what they know about AIDS symptoms, the cause of the disease, and their own ability to stop behaviors that put them at risk.

In chapters 17 to 19, the contributing authors consider drug users who are "on the streets." Their findings are surprising in the light of commonly held beliefs about intravenous drug users, e.g., the authors find evidence of both knowledge about AIDS and attempts at behavior change to lessen transmission among drug users in New York City and San Francisco.

153

14
A Biopsychosocial Approach to AIDS

Mary Ann Cohen, MD; and
Henry W. Weisman, MD.

The Multidisciplinary AIDS Program (MAP), a comprehensive team approach, has been developed at Metropolitan Hospital Center, a 600-bed municipal hospital. The goal has been to improve the care of persons with AIDS by means of a biopsychosocial approach (Engel 1977; Kimball 1981; Engel 1982) to the multiple aspects of AIDS—an approach that views these individuals as deserving coordinated care and dignified treatment. Additional goals of the program have been to diminish the patient's sense of alienation and expendability, improve communication, and further staff education.

Alienation and Expendability

The MAP has involved approximately 300 persons with AIDS and AIDS-related complex (ARC). Of these, 70% were intravenous drug abusers, 22% were gay or bisexual men, and the remaining 8%, both men and women, had contracted ARC/AIDS from other sour-

Reprinted, with changes, from "A Biopsychosocial Approach to AIDS," by Mary Ann Cohen and Henry W. Weisman, *Psychosomatics* 27:245-49, 1986, by permission of the Academy of Psychosomatic Medicine.

ces. Subjects were followed for an average of ten months, and/or the duration of the illness, whenever possible. A consistent theme of alienation and expendability was evident (Sabbath 1969). Based on their lifestyles, many persons with AIDS have been given overt and covert messages by employers, families, and communities that they are unwanted. Many had isolated themselves and felt unloved, unwanted, and expendable even before developing AIDS. Some were subjected to discrimination because they were members of risk groups initially associated with AIDS.

Intravenous drug abusers with ARC/AIDS may be premorbidly depressed and self-destructive individuals who have effectively severed the bonds that linked them with their families and communities. Based on their antisocial behavior, they may have incurred the anger of loved ones and been ostracized because of crimes associated with buying or selling drugs. Gay or bisexual men with ARC/AIDS may have had recent losses of lovers and others so that they also may feel isolated, alienated, or rejected. Paradoxically, persons with AIDS may have maintained contact with friends and families without informing their families about their AIDS diagnosis. A mother may learn on the same day that her son is gay and has AIDS. One mother reacted to this with hostility and openly maintained a prayer vigil outside the intensive care unit, praying that her son would die because of the shame he had caused her.

The sense of expendability experienced by the cohort studied suggested that the dynamic could be reflected verbally or nonverbally by rejection of friends and loss of employment. Some patients have no place to go, having previously lost their homes and lived at shelters for the homeless. Once they are found to have AIDS, they are no longer eligible for the shelters. Other facilities, such as nursing homes, chronic care hospitals, and homes for the terminally ill, do not accept persons with AIDS. The attitudes of families, funeral directors, prison guards, and employers are compounded by fears and anxieties about the possibility of contagion. These attitudes are also reflected in hospital staff members. As a result, persons with ARC/AIDS have problems obtaining health care, finding a place to live while they can still care for themselves, and finding a chronic care facility or ultimately a place to die.

Repercussions of the Illness

The experience of the MAP has been that patients upon learning of the diagnosis of AIDS experienced severe anxiety, fear of the multiple illnesses, and fear of death (Nichols 1983). We learned that persons with AIDS may not seek medical care until the associated illnesses have progressed overwhelmingly. This may be a result of denial, lack of access to medical care for those who are homeless and without resources or insurance, and/or because decreased cognitive functioning can make the individual less aware of and concerned about symptoms. The diminished cognitive capacities have been associated with focal brain lesions (Snider, Simpson, and Neilson 1983) (toxoplasmosis, cytomegalovirus, and microabscesses) and generalized encephalopathy. Unexplained dementia has now been attributed to the presence of human immunodeficiency virus infection in the brains of persons with AIDS (Shaw, Harper, and Hahn 1985).

Psychological Reactions

A natural concomitant of the consistent themes of alienation and expendability is the thought of suicide, often compounded by severe illness, terminality, lack of impulse control, lack of adequate support systems, depression, organicity, and frequent lengthy hospitalization. One individual expressed the idea that he would electrocute himself in the bathtub upon discharge if he survived his first episode of *Pneumocystis carinii* pneumonia, and other persons have contemplated poisoning themselves, overdosing, continued drug-taking behavior, jumping from windows, or wrist-slashing at various points in their course of treatment. As the illnesses progress, hospital stays lengthen and profound dependency, withdrawal, and regression may ensue, further alienating and disturbing staff and other patients (Holtz, Dobro, and Palinkas 1983).

Psychiatric diagnoses include delirium, dementia, organic delusional syndrome, organic affective syndrome, bereavement, major depression, antisocial personality disorder, and borderline personality disorder, in addition to the various medical diagnoses and social problems possible. Many persons with AIDS manifest organic mental syndrome whether or not evidence for brain lesions or encephalopathy can be established (Shaw, Harper, and Hahn 1985).

Exhibit 14-1

Biopsychosocial Aspects of Diagnosis of AIDS

"Bio"	"Psycho"	"Social"
Pneumocystis carinii pneumonia	Organic metal syndrome	Recent separation
Toxoplasmosis	Delirium	Recent losses
Cryptococcal meningitis	Major depression	Lack of social
Cryptococcal pneumonia	Bereavement	support network
Disseminated herpes zoster	Substance abuse disorder	Lack of family
Esophageal candidiasis	Dysthymic disorder	network
Disseminated candidiasis	Borderline personality disorder	Homelessness
Kaposi's sarcoma	Antisocial personality disorder	Unemployment
Mycobacterium avium	Organic affective syndrome	Financial problems
intracellulare	Organic delusional syndrome	Illegal alien status
End-stage renal disease		Distance from home
CNS lymphoma		and family
Cytomegalovirus retinitis		Language barrier

As individuals lose both strength and cognitive functioning, cortical inhibitions may be released, leading to outbursts of violence or severe regression. One severely ill and emaciated young man repeatedly assaulted staff members, including nurses, physicians, and dietary workers. Another made repeated attempts to hug and kiss staff members, touching and clinging in desperation.

In addition, we found that individuals are disturbed by the contagious nature of the illness. They may see themselves as contaminated. They need support, psychological care, individual and family therapy, and at times psychotropic medications.

Staff Reactions

Apart from the frustrations inherent in treating patients who almost certainly will die, AIDS takes a psychological toll on the hospital staff. Intravenous drug abuse, homosexuality, and sexual promiscuity run counter to many staff members' belief systems. Intravenous drug abusers may be the most disliked patients in the general hospital. They are seen as manipulative, demanding, and ungrateful. In the case of both intravenous drug abusers and gay men, many staff members believe that "these people brought this illness on themselves."

The fear of developing AIDS themselves is also quite prevalent among staff members, reflected in reluctance to touch a patient or enter his room, in increased absenteeism, and in requests for transfers. Some house officers are very uneasy about needle sticks with contaminated blood, and may consider it a matter of time until one of them develops AIDS.

Patient account representatives have refused to interview people with AIDS and obtained union backing for their position. Staff attitudes reflected not only anxiety about AIDS, but also discrimination against intravenous drug abusers, and homophobia, and discrimination against gay men (Deuchar 1984). Interestingly, this homophobia is also reflected in the attitudes of many intravenous drug abusers. It was based on the above dynamics that MAP was undertaken.

Multidisciplinary AIDS Program

The sense of alienation and expendability felt by persons with AIDS can be overwhelming. The MAP addressed these feelings through increasing the staff's understanding of AIDS patients and decreasing fragmentation of care (Cohen and Merlino 1983; Landesman, Ginzburg, and Weiss 1985). As a complicated syndrome with multiple treatments, AIDS requires involvement of many services with multiple admissions over time. In view of the characteristics of the illnesses and the needs of the hospital, the director of consultation-liaison psychiatry, in conjunction with the director of infectious disease and a social work supervisor, and in cooperation with the chief of medicine and the hospital's executive director, undertook organization of a program to provide a comprehensive approach to AIDS. The organization chart (exhibit 14-2) show the multiple services involved.

The goals and objectives of the program were as follows.

Goals: To improve care of the person with AIDS by means of a biopsychosocial approach that maintains a view of each individual as deserving coordinated care and treatment with dignity, and to improve communication and diminish alienation and a sense of expendability.

Enabling objectives: (1) identification of volunteers from all areas of the hospital; (2) formation of a multidisciplinary team; (3) development of a comprehensive program for clinical care of patient-staff education, faculty development, liaison with outside

Exhibit 14-2

Components of the Multidisciplinary AIDS Program.

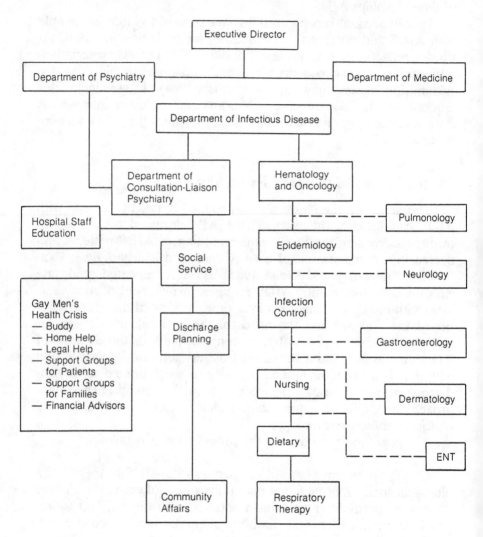

agencies, and research; and (4) development of methods to provide comprehensive care, with regular rounds for persons with AIDS, special AIDS rounds on a weekly basis for meeting with all staff members involved, and identification of psychological and social problems frequently encountered in those with AIDS.

Terminal objectives: (1) heightened awareness of psychological problems encountered in persons with AIDS and ARC and in their families; (2) greater understanding by staff members of psychological reactions to individuals with AIDS; (3) improvement in physician-patient communication; (4) opening avenues of communication among health professionals dealing with AIDS; (5) a humane approach to those with AIDS by both professional and nonprofessional hospital staff members; and (6) identification and treatment of psychological problems through individual, couples, family, group, and psychopharmacologic therapy.

Team Organization and Functioning

The MAP was comprised of two liaison psychiatrists, two liaison psychiatry fellows, two epidemiologists, two directors of infectious disease, an infectious disease specialist, a head nurse, a dietary director, a respiratory therapist, a discharge planner, a social work supervisor, two social workers, and a hematologist-oncologist.

The team began meeting in 1983 for 1 1/2 hours each week to share and review new information about AIDS and to discuss patients. During the meeting, each patient was presented briefly and discussed among team members who participated in care of the patient.

The following case is an example of how the MAP impacted on treatment. A husband, who was known to be an intravenous drug abuser with AIDS, had not told his wife of his diagnosis because he was afraid of losing her. His wife, the mother of a 9-year-old from a prior marriage, had systemic lupus erythematosus and was then 5 months pregnant. By accident, while visiting the hospital with her husband she saw his diagnosis on a desk. She was frightened as to the implications of the diagnosis for herself, her son, and her unborn child. Her husband panicked and denied knowing that he had AIDS, although he had known of the diagnosis for one year. He began to increase drug abuse in a futile effort to escape from the inevitability of his wife's learning the truth.

The team acted to moderate the crisis. The patient's therapist and a social worker supervisor arranged for an emergency meeting with the couple, the director of infectious disease, the obstetrician and pediatrician involved, and with liaison psychiatrists. As a result, the couple's fears were allayed. They became more open with each other and functioned better through the pregnancy, birth of the child, and death of the husband.

The MAP provides a nucleus of permanent staff members who meet weekly and know each other well. It has fostered communication between disciplines and enables them to interact efficiently. The program is visible throughout the hospital, and house officers, attending physicians, and nurses frequently utilize bedside consultations or refer patients to it. The fact that MAP consists of permanent staff members with whom the patient can relate and who are familiar with the problems offsets, at least partially, the alienation experienced when house officers rotate to other services, or when the patient is transferred to another unit, such as intensive care.

A major aspect of MAP is staff education, by means of seminars, conferences, and workshops on AIDS. Finally, MAP serves as a link between the hospital and outside agencies also assisting persons with AIDS. Appropriate referrals have enabled individuals with AIDS to return home to be reunited with their families while still receiving continued and appropriate medical attention.

The program has emphasized the concept of determining the patient's understanding of the illness so as to facilitate communication at the appropriate level of understanding and to better obtain compliance. House officers have called on MAP members for help in telling a patient about the diagnosis of AIDS. A few house officers have asked liaison psychiatrists or other MAP members to so inform the patient. The liaison psychiatrist goes over the approach with each house officer, explaining and enabling the physician to discuss feelings. House officers are advised to rehearse their opening questions and statements, to sit down with the patient, and to provide realistic encouragement and the reassurance that care in the form of a program specifically organized for the purpose will continue to available.

The MAP thus provides a support network to patients and staff, and also serves as a model for improving patient care, for improving communication among patients and health professionals, and for providing educational programs for staff members.

References

Cohen, M.A., and J.P. Merlino. 1983. The suicidal patient on the surgical ward: a multidisciplinary case conference. *Gen. Hosp. Psychiat.* 5:65-71.

Deuchar, N. 1984. AIDS in New York City with particular reference to psychosocial aspects. *Br. J. Psychiat.* 145:612-19.

Engel, G.L. 1977. The need for a new medical model: a challenge for biomedicine. *Science* 196:129-36.

———. 1982. The biopsychosocial model and medical education: who are to be the teachers? *N. Engl. J. Med.* 306:802-5.

Holtz, M., J. Dobro, and R. Palinkas. 1983. Psychological impact of AIDS. *J.A.M.A.* 250:167.

Kimball, C.P. 1981. *The biopsychosocial approach to the patient.* Baltimore, Maryland: Williams & Wilkins.

Landesman, S.H., H. Ginzburg, and S. Weiss. 1985. The AIDS epidemic. *N. Engl. J. Med.* 312:521-25.

Nichols, S.E. 1983. Psychiatric aspects of AIDS. *Psychosomatics* 24:1083-89.

Sabbath, J. 1969. The suicidal adolescent: the expendable child. *J. Am. Acad. Child Psychiat.* 8:272-89.

Shaw, G.M., M. Harper, and B. Hahn. 1985. HTLV-III infection in brains of children and adults with AIDS encephalopathy. *Science* 277:177-82.

Snider, W.D., D. Simpson, and S. Neilson. 1983. Neurological complications of AIDS: an analysis of 50 patients. *Ann. Neurol.* 14:403-8.

15

The Development of Support Groups for ARC-Diagnosed Clients at Daytop Village

Ross Robak, PhD, and Joseph E. Caffrey, CSW.

Daytop Village, a long-term residential therapeutic community, initiated the development of a support group for recovering addicts suffering from AIDS-related complex (ARC). Therapists leading the group utilized a conceptual model developed by Elisabeth Kubler-Ross in her book *On Death and Dying*, since anecdotal evidence indicated that this model had been found particularly appropriate in work with AIDS patients by New York Gay Men's Health Crisis.

According to Kubler-Ross, an individual cannot be at peace with his or her own death as long as any "unfinished business" remains. It is most important, in the achievement of the acceptance of death, that the sense of denial be overcome. For those individuals who continue to deny the reality of their impending death, "the more difficult it will be for them to reach this final stage of acceptance with peace and dignity" (Kubler-Ross 1962). For the individual diagnosed with ARC, overcoming denial and achieving a sense of completion can be particularly difficult because of the ambiguity of the diagnosis itself—the ARC patient is not dying, yet just the same

Reprinted, with changes, from a presentation on "The Development of Support Groups for ARC-Diagnosed Clients at Daytop Village," by Ross Robak and Joseph E. Caffrey, by permission of the authors. Presented at the Annual Conference of the World Federation of Therapeutic Communities, Eskilstuna, Sweden.

must face the fear and anxiety associated with the possible development of full-blown AIDS. Estimates on the number of ARC patients who will eventually develop AIDS vary between 6% and 20% (National Academy of Sciences 1986). In addition, the health problems often associated with ARC, such as lymphadenopathy, fevers, and extreme fatigue, can prove both painful and debilitating.

At the time the ARC support group was initiated, public anxiety about the AIDS "epidemic," enhanced by coverage given the disease in the media, was quite high. This mood was exacerbated within many therapeutic communities by the growing realization that intravenous drug users belong to one of two groups at greatest risk for AIDS. The risk of contracting AIDS through the use of contaminated needles, or "works," may have existed as far back as the 1970s (Friedman, Des Jarlais, and Sotheran 1986; Moore 1986). Since research has found rates of seropositivity among intravenous drug users of up to 60% in New York City (Des Jarlais, Jainchill, and Friedman 1986), and of 50% in metropolitan New Jersey (Weiss et al. 1985), with lower rates of 2% in southern New Jersey, it is possible that a significant number of therapeutic community residents from the New York/New Jersey area may have been exposed to the virus. Staff concern about the development of ARC/AIDS cases within the program, and their own fears and anxieties regarding the disease, leads to a program of staff training and the eventual development of therapeutic groups for program clients.

Goals of the group included emotional support for clients diagnosed with ARC, and the development of an educational forum that could bring people together to share medical and health-related information. It was hoped that the group would serve to lessen feelings of isolation and powerlessness among the ARC-diagnosed clients, as well as to allow them to express their frustrations, anxiety, and anger in a supportive and understanding setting.

The Kubler-Ross Model: Its Applicability and Limitations

The conceptual model developed by Kubler-Ross outlines a series of emotional stages through which the dying person passes, ending with the eventual acceptance of his/her impending death. These stages are: denial, isolation and withdrawal, anger, depression, and, finally, acceptance (Kubler-Ross 1962). The use of the Kubler-Ross model poses some problems in work with ARC patients; given the relative "newness" of the disease, the lack of medical knowledge about its eventual clinical course, and the uncertainty over how many ARC patients will actually develop AIDS, these ambiguities necessitated some alteration of the model. The nature of this ambiguity was described by one group member who said, "I am not denying, but I don't know what to accept."

Although the Kubler-Ross stages appeared to occur in close sequence when a client first learned of his/her diagnosis, acceptance was only tenuously achieved. A remission of physical symptoms in clients often prompted a return to the initial stage of denial and a subsequent "recycling" through stages.

Early in the group process, it was found that concentration on the stage of "acceptance" produced a sense of powerlessness and fear of an unknown future. Quite often, this sense of not being in control led to anxiety in the group members and, if unresolved, to depression. However, successful mastery of this anxiety resulted in "activation," a return of the sense of internal control. Observation of this process in members of the ARC support group resulted in a revision of the Kubler-Ross model to the following:

$$\text{Denial} \rightarrow \text{Isolation} \rightarrow \text{Anger} \rightarrow \text{Anxiety} \rightarrow \genfrac{}{}{0pt}{}{\text{Activation}}{\text{Depression}}$$

The group's emphasis on activation/control resulted in an acceptance of the ambiguity of the ARC diagnosis. The resulting therapeutic effect was reflected in a change from isolation and withdrawal to a greater involvement in the community.

This process was particularly helpful based on the limited ability of the newly recovered addicts to identify their feelings and mobilize their anger to produce change. This mode of adaption, historically marked by denial, made it necessary to help each individual attain acceptance of this life crisis.

Existential Issues

Confrontation with the diagnosis of ARC was, for group members, an urgent experience outside the realm of usual conscious experience. It was no longer possible for them to ignore their mortality or to live, as Heidegger (1962) put it, in a state of "forgetfulness of being." Concentration on issues such as living a full life, coming to terms with loved ones, and intimacy helped to lessen their preoccupation with physical symptoms (a reactive stance) and left the group open to consider issues that were more under their control.

Discussions occurred around reasons each member gave for living and what each one wanted to do with the rest of his/her life. These discussions helped group members frame their lives in a positive way. For example, one client was able to distinguish between "sad" periods, when he moved toward isolation, and those times when he was happy, performing music and enjoying the company of his friends.

The issue of self-esteem seems central in working with ARC patients. A member who was self-affacing and closely identified with a former lifestyle saw herself as unattractive and unwanted because of her age, telling the rest of the group that she could no longer even be a good prostitute. Shortly afterward, her health began to deteriorate rapidly; she died after her first episode of *Pneumocystis carinii* pneumonia.

This episode emphasized the importance of the will to live and feel good about oneself in the face of the ARC diagnosis; it also raised the possibility that the group member's death involved issues of self-worth.

The group's experience also underscored the question as to whether intravenous drug users who contract AIDS may succumb more quickly to the progression of the AIDS virus than members of other identified high risk groups. Intuitively, the author feels that this may be so, and that it should, perhaps, become a hypothesis for future research.

The Humanistic Perspective

In the therapeutic community, the enhancement of self-esteem is a major goal, and it is achieved, in large measure, by community recognition for positive attainments in the course of treatment. The extent to which ARC-diagnosed residents become identified with this process is crucial to their building of self-esteem and, therefore, to their will to live. Members of the group may doubt their own ability to complete their treatment program. A major effort of the group was to overcome their doubts about completing anything. The implementation of more staff training helped to minimize the clients' sense of being different and isolated from the rest of the community, and allowed them to benefit from the public approval and esteem that are hallmarks of a residential drug treatment program.

The major initial dynamic of each member entering the group had been the conflict between feeling isolated, and yet at the same time, wishing to withdraw even further. In some cases, group members' support of each other was the only opportunity for unconditional positive regard and acceptance. Therefore, the group became a curative experience with group acceptance fostering continued self-disclosure and ultimately, self-acceptance.

Another issue for group members was their need for physical contact and sexual relationships. One member described, vividly, his need for physical affection and sexual fulfillment. He had ruled out any possibility of these needs being met; in fact, he had resigned himself to a life of celibacy and isolation.

When the group began to explore and validate his needs, he was finally able to conceive of himself having an intimate relationship. He wondered if he could find a woman with a similar medical condition, and finally even considered the possibility of "safe sex" in a relationship once he had taken the risk of becoming involved with another person.

According to Rogers (1974), an individual's potential for self-understanding can emerge if given the right psychological climate. The climate described by Rogers includes unconditional positive regard and acceptance by therapists and other group members. This humanistic orientation was maintained by the therapists throughout the group process.

One member who attained such self-understanding was Michael, a young man with a great capacity for denial. During his slow course of gaining trust in the group, he revealed that he had been abused as a child. Further examination of his admission showed that he had been sodomized by an older adolescent in a city park. He had hidden the experience from everyone; in fact, he had never spoken of it until the evening of this group session, 20 years later.

Michael's admission gave the group a powerful metaphor for the way he handled his diagnosis of ARC. He recognized the similarity of his reactions to both crises, and that his denial of ARC was developmentally identical to the denial of the earlier abuse. To

Michael's surprise, he was not rejected by the group as a consequence of his admission; rather, the group's increased acceptance helped him to accept both himself and his symptoms.

The group's facilitation of gains in self-understanding complements the approach of most therapeutic communities. The isolation and withdrawal that result from a resident's ARC diagnosis can "short circuit" the therapeutic process within the program: instead of participating actively in the therapeutic community, group members tended to focus on the negative aspects of their lives, refusing to accept their own positive attributes. This lack of acceptance, projected on the psychological environment, can limit the effectiveness of treatment. The focus on each group member's self-acceptance complements the larger environment and helps to make treatment more effective.

Case Study

Bob C. is a 33-year-old, divorced man in Daytop treatment for 1 year. Within his family of origin, he seemed overly close to his mother, and distant from his father, a New York City policeman.

Bob was one of the original group members and for the first several months he presented as withdrawn and unable to share with the rest of the group. He had to be pulled into the group repeatedly by the therapists and often verbalized the idea that he had to "do it alone."

Before entering the group, Bob had been consistently mildly depressed. When he was told that his cluster of symptoms represented ARC, he became even more depressed and morbid in demeanor.

For the first few weeks in the group, his ability to relate to other group members was vague and ineffectual. He spoke in a self-centered way of fulfilling his lifelong dream, while he still could: going to Ireland and visiting his family there. He telephoned his mother and ex-wife, trying to enlist their nurturance. His efforts to make contact with his wife were marked by scapegoating of her and acting out of anger when she did not respond. Generally, his efforts seemed haphazard and without direction.

Bob showed a marked lack of self-esteem and self-direction. While this may not have been an issue for him prior to entering treatment, or even during the early phases of his treatment, the added stress of his ARC diagnosis precipitated an identity crisis. He could no longer identify himself in terms of his mother or his wife, and because of the nature of his medical condition, he felt truly alone. Other group members would not allow him to avoid facing his loneliness and his need to learn to perceive himself without relying on past defense mechanisms, in particular the projection of blame onto his wife and mother.

In the earliest phases of the group, involving the examination of medical information about ARC, Bob was able to continue his old pattern of projections. However, as the group became less informational and more dynamic, the members' scrutiny helped lead to Bob's attempts at self-definition. He began to stop focusing on his past relationship with his wife and focused more on his experience of the here and now—and of the future. The group helped him to identify feelings about the way he viewed himself and how he was viewed by others. In time, Bob was forced to express his anger and anxiety directly within the group. When he reverted to self-pity, group members often told him "we hear you getting ready to die but not getting ready to live."

While Bob was struggling with these issues, another group member died. Her death profoundly changed the experience of the entire group, especially Bob's. He had strongly identified with her and had, in some ways, used her as a vehicle for expressing his own anger. He often said he did not like the way she was treated because of her illness and came to her defense in spite of his difficulty in expressing his anger on his own behalf.

The group member's death brought an immediacy to the group. The philosophical possibilities that had been discussed abstractly had turned, instead, to an emotional confrontation with mortality.

Before she died, Bob visited her on a hospital isolation unit, an event that left him shaken. Afterwards, when he reported his visit to the group, he seemed to have ended his intellectualization, his last line of defense was gone. When she died minutes before a scheduled group session, leaving the group members vulnerable and in touch with their immediate feelings, the opportunity for a powerful catharsis was provided. The stage was set for the group members to support each other in the most profound sense.

Bob went to the viewing of his fellow group member at the funeral home with a great deal of trepidation, although he said he felt it was something he had to do in order to confront his own mortality. Afterward, he said he felt the experience lifted "a great burden" from him. He told the group that he was unable to see himself in the casket; he was afraid of death. Group discussion of this admission helped Bob see that, although he was afraid of dying, he could still determine his own future. He could maintain control of his life for as long as he lived.

Summary

Initially, Daytop's ARC group was supportively oriented, but the focus of group discussions quickly became existential in nature. The Kubler-Ross model was seen as applicable, although use of the model with this group required some modification. Its application was found to facilitate initial acceptance of the clients' ARC diagnosis.

The focus on existential issues of death and the meaning of individual life afforded the group members a sense of integrity and control, and seemed to prevent regression to the stage of denial. In particular, the degree of self-worth the ARC patients felt and the resulting will to live were seen as crucial factors in surviving this condition, and perhaps as factors that differentiate the intravenous drug-using population from the gay community.

Another important focus of therapy with ARC clients was the power of the group in helping the individual attain both self-disclosure and self-acceptance. Given their low self-esteem and their conflicting urges to withdraw from the community and attain more acceptance, this was particularly difficult for these clients.

Indications for further research may lie in the differential use of the Kubler-Ross model for ex-intravenous drug users and other groups at high risk for AIDS.

References

Des Jarlais, D., N. Jainchill, and S. Friedman. 1986. AIDS among IV drug users: epidemiology, natural history and therapeutic community experiences. *Bridging Services* 69-72.

Freidman, S., D. Des Jarlais, and J. Sotheran. 1986. AIDS health education for intravenous drug users. *Health Education Quarterly* 13:383-93.

Heidegger, M. 1962. *Being and time.* Translated by J. Macquarrie and E. Robinson. New York: Harper and Row.

Kubler-Ross, E. 1962. *On death and dying.* New York: MacMillan Publishing Co.

Moore, J. 1986. HTLV-III seropositivity in 1971-1972 parenteral drug users: a case of false positives or evidence of viral exposure. *N. Eng. J. Med.* 314:1387-88.

National Academy of Sciences. 1986. *Mobilizing against AIDS*. Cambridge, Massachusetts: Harvard University Press.

Rogers, C.R. 1974. In retrospect: 46 years. *Am. Psychol.* 29:115-23.

Weiss, S.H., H. Ginzburg and J. Goedert. 1985. Risk for HTLV-III exposure and AIDS among parenteral drug abusers in New Jersey. Paper presented at the International Conference on Acquired Immunodeficiency Syndrome (AIDS), 14-17 April, Atlanta, Georgia.

16

A Survey of the Perceptions of Drug Abusers Concerning the Acquired Immunodeficiency Syndrome (AIDS)

Benjamin F. Lewis, EdD; and
Robert P. Galea, PhD.

Intravenous (IV) users of illicit drugs and members of their social networks are the second largest and most rapidly growing group of persons "at risk" for the acquired immunodeficiency syndrome (AIDS). When IV drug use is isolated in the nonhierarchical presentation of AIDS data by the Centers for Disease Control, IV drug abusers represent more than 25% of all reported AIDS cases (Ginzburg, 1984b). In addition, because of (1) transmission of the virus from infected mothers to infants, (2) the compounding of IV drug abuse by bisexual activity, and (3) the limited but growing threat, that transmission from females to males may occur through prostitution, the IV drug-abusing community may be a critical bridge for transmission of the epidemic from male and female drug abusers to the general population of nondrug abusers (Marmor 1984).

Treatment programs for IV and other drug users face a number of issues in regard to the threat of AIDS. These include medical, clinical, legal, and ethical questions. By the same token, these programs are in a unique position to develop and test out detection,

Reprinted, with changes, from "A Survey of the Perceptions of Drug Abusers Concerning the acquired Immunodeficiency Syndrome," by Benjamin F. Lewis and Robert P. Galea, *Health Matrix* 4(2):14-17, 1986, by permission of the authors.

counseling, education, and preventive prototypes, given the nature and needs of this population and the likelihood that a large percentage of those prematurely discharged from treatment programs will most likely use IV drugs in the future.

Questions about the degree of aggressiveness with which screening, counseling, and education should be carried out are currently being debated by government agencies, public health departments, and residential and outpatient drug programs.

A review of the literature regarding AIDS reflects a phenomenal increase in knowledge from 1981-87, covering the seroprevalence and socioepidemiological patterns of the disease. In addition, however, as early identified cases have taken their clinical course and mortality rates have been calculated (over 50%), the popular press and media have spread epidemic fears, considerable misinformation, melodrama, and outrage. Often a punitive response has been communicated to both the general as well as the IV drug-abusing population.

In order for the drug treatment community's response to be appropriate and effective, as much information from as many sources as possible, including the perspectives of IV drug users themselves, as well as service providers, must be developed.

Spectrum House, Inc., a comprehensive drug treatment program located in Westboro and Worcester, Massachusetts, conducted a survey in January 1986 of clients in its drug-free residential program to get a better idea of the knowledge, beliefs, and attitudes of IV drug users regarding AIDS and to solicit from this "at-risk" population their ideas and suggestions for intervening in and limiting the spread of this disease among both the IV drug-using network and the general population.

This was felt to be important in order to develop appropriate staff training and develop, disseminate, and target information and education interventions to this "at-risk" population and their network of needle-sharers, sexual partners, family, and friends.

The population surveyed was 49 adult clients in a drug-free residential treatment program (therapeutic community) who have been in treatment from one week to one year. The general demographics of those surveyed, including medical, socioeconomic, psychological, legal, and drug use profiles, are similar to clients entering the program's Detoxification Center, reflecting that the responses are reasonably typical of the IV drug-using population "on the street." Forty percent of those surveyed were female.

Clients were informed of the voluntary and anonymous nature of this survey, and they were asked to respond candidly to questions having to do with their knowledge about AIDS, the extent of their contact with individuals suspected of having the disease, and what they thought could be done to prevent the spread of the disease. The respondents were also asked for any additional thoughts, feelings, or ideas about AIDS.

Previous studies of drug abusers regarding their concerns about AIDS have looked at factors in risk reduction behavior (Des Jarlais, Friedman, and Hopkins 1985) and level of knowledge and concern about AIDS (Ginzburg, 1984a). Both studies suggest that knowledge about AIDS has some influence on the behavior of IV drug abusers and that future research is needed regarding methods for risk reduction and the type of information useful for substantial change in the behavior of IV drug abusers.

The results of this study (1) support and refine some of the previous findings regarding high degrees of knowledge about AIDS, (2) reflect considerably higher degrees of felt concern and anxiety regarding the respondents' risk of contracting AIDS, and (3) provide a look at IV drug users' perceptions of the devastating effects of AIDS in the IV drug user's social network. In addition, the population surveyed stressed the importance of information and education regarding AIDS for the IV drug community in order to prevent the spread of the disease.

Specifically, a number of questions asked respondents to indicate their knowledge about ways AIDS can be contracted by the general public and specifically by drug addicts. Virtually 100% indicated that the use of dirty needles was the most likely manner for AIDS to be transmitted.

Heterosexual contact was seen to be the second most common manner of transmission in both groups, with transmission by homosexual activity mentioned for the general population often but practically not at all for the drug-addicted population. However, promiscuous heterosexual contact was mentioned third most frequently as a vehicle for transmission of the virus in the drug-addicted subgroup. There was nobody who could not list at least two medically acknowledged manners of transmission.

A wide range of other responses mirroring accurate information as well as misinformation portrayed in the media and "on the street" were provided.

Of interest is that of the women surveyed (20% or 41%) felt that drug-abusing women might contract AIDS from prostitution and/or promiscuous sex, a perception which is not borne out in Centers for Disease Control statistics.

While 40% of the population believed that AIDS was treatable and 20% "didn't know" if it was, 85% did not believe that AIDS was curable. Fifteen percent thought that AIDS "might be" curable. It is unclear as to whether these responses are typical in the general population or whether an element of denial and/or hope is reflected in their perspective on treatability and recovery.

A number of questions were aimed at identifying the extent to which respondents felt they might have had exposure to actual AIDS victims or perceived AIDS carriers. In response to the question, "Do you know anyone who you believe has been exposed to AIDS," almost 1 of 3 respondents believed they personally knew individuals who have been exposed to AIDS.

In regard to the extended network of associations of IV drug users, slightly over 50% of the respondents believed that their extended social network (friends of friends) involved contact with individuals who they believed had been exposed to AIDS. While 70% said they would continue to associate with a person they suspected was exposed to AIDS, 100% indicated that they would not engage in sexual relations with someone they suspected of being exposed to AIDS, and 96% said they would not "shoot dope" with a person they suspected of being exposed to AIDS.

It is of significance and concern that (1) 45% felt that the odds were "pretty good" that they as IV drug users might get AIDS, (2) an additional 40% felt that the odds were in the range of between 1 in 10 and 5 in 10 that they might contract AIDS, and (3) that in response to the question, "Do you believe that you could contract AIDS based on your past activity?", 80% felt that they might have been exposed to and be vulnerable to human immunodeficiency virus (HIV) infection.

These findings are particularly alarming in that the respondents generally felt that, if they were "shooting drugs," they would "hardly ever" be able to exercise enough self-control not to "shoot" with a dirty needle (85%). For the remaining 15%, self-control was also "somewhat" problematic.

When those surveyed were asked how they felt about the public concern regarding AIDS, no one felt that there was overconcern and 63% felt that "too little" concern was being evidenced. Eighty-five percent felt that the government had a responsibility to do something to help prevent AIDS.

When asked about the type of activities that should be undertaken to help prevent the spread of AIDS: (1) the most frequently given response (56%) involved the need for information and education to heighten awareness of AIDS both for drug abusers themselves and also for the general public. (2) The second most frequently given response was some variation of the need to "keep works clean" (35%). Based, however, on misconceptions regarding techniques for "sterilizing works," combined with the stated inability to forestall "shooting up" even knowing that their "works" may be contaminated, it does not seem that this response would actually be carried out by most IV drug addicts. Related to this the responses involving using a clean needle or not sharing a needle appeared with slightly less frequency (31%). (3) The third most popular response (31%) involved the development of some type of screening or testing program. One of the threads woven through many of the responses given in the survey appears to be a belief that screening and testing will aid in identification of individuals who have been exposed to HIV, thus reducing personal anxiety and permitting better targeting of resources.

In response to the question, "Would you be interested in being tested at no cost to see if you have been exposed to HIV?", 90% of the respondents indicated that they would like to be tested. This finding is interesting in relation to the large percentage who identified screening and testing as important prevention activities.

The following responses were also given: (4) check before heterosexual sex—15%, (5) stop using drugs—14%, (6) legalize needles—12%, (7) spend more money on research—12%, and (8) some variation on the theme of eliminating homosexual encounters and/or isolating and ostracizing homosexuals. Most of the responses, but particularly this last response, often reflecting a blaming attitude, were magnified when those surveyed were asked to hypothetically put themselves in the position of a Commissioner of Public Health and indicate what they might do in that role to help prevent the spread of HIV among drug abusers. The frequency of responses clustered around certain categories as follows: (1) more programs of public awareness and information (38%); (2) more clinics/sites for testing and screening (38%); (3) making syringes legally available (31%); (4) controlling AIDS victims through – (a) registration (8%), (b) isolation (10%), or (c) incarceration (15%); (5) more money for research (8%); (6) more drug treatment facilities (5%); and (7) more drug maintenance programs (4%).

At the end of the questionnaire, those surveyed were given the opportunity to add any thoughts, feelings, or ideas that they had concerning AIDS. Fifty percent availed themselves of the opportunity to do so. The additional comments tended to reinforce or add to responses previously given but in addition reflected in very human terms the level of anger, fear, concern, compassion, and futility that this population experiences. The following are some excerpts from respondents' comments reflecting the above categories of concern.

"As a drug user, I know that satisfying my drug habit always came before the concern of getting AIDS, whether it meant using contaminated needles or not. I rationalized it when I thought about it by saying, 'I'm slowly killing myself anyways, so it doesn't matter if I get it.' A drug user is at a state of mind where they don't care and they are self destructive and irresponsible. If it is to be done by government and trying to provide them with the cleanest conditions for their drug use or set up more Methadone clinics to keep as many off the street as possible. I feel this is the most realistic way to deal with it."

"AIDS doesn't frighten me as much as it seems to frighten the public at large. I think the disease is being hyped by the media and I doubt that any one individual's chances of contracting the disease are as great as we are being led to believe."

"It's a very scary subject. I've gotten high with homosexuals, and I've used some nasty needles. And I'm glad I'm here at Spectrum House."

"I think the AIDS thing is real scary. To come down with it 5 or 6 years from now! And I also feel there is not enough being done about AIDS. They could test more people in Detox, clinics, etc. . . . They could even do it in jails, since most junkies visit there from time to time. I think the Federal Government should get involved in preventive measures!"

"AIDS to me is a scary problem that everyone should be aware of. I'm scared because I am homosexual and wonder because of the time it takes to show up if I could have it now, but I believe I don't, and having sex with someone now is scary and if I do I will use a condom."

"I gave this disease alot of thought, especially while recently incarcerated and in contact with a person afflicted with AIDS. When thinking clearly and logically, it is pretty frightening to think it's possible to have this disease inside of me and not knowing it for maybe years to come. This thinking didn't stop me, however, from getting high or make me take the time to find a sterilized needle. It is frightening because that is how unsafe I believe it to be. I believe it is also very sad that most IV drug abusers will suppress this fear of the disease and not take any precautions. There are IV drug abusers and IV drug users. With the drug users who are not totally into it 100%, I believe they can and do take some precautions. Personally, I need to be educated more on the disease."

"I don't know much about it, but I would like to know more. I also think it's very scary that I might have been exposed and don't know for sure."

"My knowledge of AIDS is limited. I would like to know more about this dreaded disease. I feel because of a lack of knowledge concerning AIDS, people inflicted with this ailment are treated improperly and cruelly. People tend to fear those with AIDS, and treat them as lepers."

"I don't know enough about it. Sometimes it seems someone invented it to wipe out junkies and faggots."

"I'm really scared to even learn about AIDS. Just the fact that it's a killer, and I feel people are not taking this seriously, and I don't know much about AIDS. But at this state, I'm willing to learn more about it. So I can help people who were like me."

"I'm really frightened by this epidemic and how it may even have effected me as a non-needle using cocaine abuser. Thank you for your concern and efforts."

"I think AIDS is the worst disease in the world, and the fact that two people I used to get high with a couple of years ago are now dying puts fear in me. But, I've talked about it honestly and openly, and realize worrying about getting sick won't do a thing to prevent it. All I can do is pray."

In summary, a survey of the perceptions of predominantly IV drug abusers concerning HIV/ARC/AIDS indicated that:

1. While most had some knowledge concerning how the disease was contracted, considerable confusion and/or lack of knowledge exists with respect to how to avoid HIV/ARC/AIDS.

2. Most felt that their IV drug use and/or sexual contacts made them prime candidates for contracting HIV.

3. Over one-half felt they had been exposed to HIV.

4. Eighty-percent felt that they could possibly contract AIDS.

5. Ninety percent wanted to be tested.

6. While most indicated that they should curtail sharing needles and sex with individuals suspected of being exposed to HIV, most felt that they would continue to associate with them even though at the time of "shooting dope" most could not control their activities.

7. Most felt that the greatest possibilities for prevention were in education and information, and a program of testing and screening.

8. The personal level of anxiety and hopelessness reflected by this population was quite high.

The suggestions for possible solutions to the containment of the AIDS problem put forth by those surveyed mirror the current thinking of public policy makers and those who work with potential and/or identified AIDS patients. The prevailing attitude which emerges in the proposed solutions is that there will always be drug addicts. The least-mentioned preventative approaches are related to research, so-called drug cures via maintenance, and drug treatment facilities. High priority is given to educational programming and making syringes available legally.

The data present a picture which is particularly not hopeful in terms of curtailing substance abuse when one considers that the survey was conducted in a long-term residential drug-free treatment program. However, what does emerge is a realistic understanding that one of the ways of preventing the spread of AIDS is by educating addicts in the importance of clean needles. In this regard and for this "at-risk" population, "safe" drug use may be more realistic than no drug use. More research needs to be done to determine how to best target risk reduction activities so that the impact will provide the greatest opportunity to limit the spread of AIDS.

References

Des Jarlais, D.C., S. Friedman, and M. Hopkins. 1985 Risk reduction for acquired immunodeficiency syndrome among intravenous drug users. *Ann. Intern. Med.* 103:775-59.

Eckholm, E. 1985. Women and AIDS: assessing the risks. *New York Times*, October 28, 8-9.

Ginzburg, H.M. 1984a. A survey of attitude concerning AIDS among clients in treatment. *Clinical Research Notes.* National Institute on Drug abuse, Rockville, Maryland.

Ginzburg, H.M. 1984b. Acquired immune deficiency syndrome (AIDS) and drug abuse. *Public Health Reports* 99(2):206-212.

Marmor, M., D. Des Jarlais, and S. Friedman. 1984. Lyden, M. El-sadr, W. The epidemic of acquired immunodeficiency syndrome (AIDS) and *Substance Abuse Treatment* 1:237-47.

17

Health Education and Knowledge Assessment of HIV Diseases among Intravenous Drug Users

Harold M. Ginzburg, MD, JD, MPH;
John French, MA; Joyce Jackson, MA;
Peter I. Hartsock, DrPH; Mhairi Graham
MacDonald, MBChB, FRCP(E), DCH;
and Stanley H. Weiss, MD.

The human immunodeficiency virus (HIV) (Gallo, Salahuddin, and Popovic 1984) is now recognized to be the causative agent of the endstage disease known as the acquired immunodeficiency syndrome (AIDS) (Wong-Staal and Gallo 1985). Between infection with the virus and endstage, AIDS is a spectrum of clinical conditions, each with a varying degree of symptomatology, clinical findings, and laboratory results (Sheretz 1985; Ho et al. 1985). Regardless of the clinical disease phase of the infective process, it appears that, once an individual is infected with the virus, the virus remains in the body indefinitely (Gallo, Salahuddin, and Popovic 1984). Thus, there is the need to decrease the rate at which individuals are exposed to and infected with HIV. Second, there is the need to decrease the rate at which infected individuals develop the more

Reprinted, with changes, from "Health Education and Knowledge Assessment of HTLV-III Diseases among Intravenous Drug Users," by Harold M. Ginzburg, John French, Joyce Jackson, Peter I Hartsock, Mhairi Graham MacDonald, and Stanley H. Weiss, *Health Education Quarterly* 13(4):373-82, 1986, by permission of John Wiley & Sons, Inc. (New York). Copyright 1986 by SOPHE.

severe clinical sequelae of HIV disease. This article focuses on the need to effectively intervene to decrease the rate of HIV transmission.

The majority of patients with AIDS are white male homosexuals, primarily living in Los Angeles, San Francisco, and the New York City areas (Centers for Disease Control 1985). Male homosexuals, independent of their history of intravenous drug use, represent 72% of all cases of AIDS (Centers for Disease Control 1985). (Eleven percent of these homosexuals have also used intravenous drugs.) Heterosexual intravenous drug users account for an additional 17% of the cases of AIDS (Centers for Disease Control 1985). Hemophiliacs, blood recipients, and infants of risk group members represent about 3% of AIDS cases (Centers for Disease Control 1985). These latter cases had no active role in acquiring an HIV infection.

The two largest risk groups for HIV infections, gay men and intravenous drug users, are able to minimize their risk of infection with HIV by choosing to alter certain aspects of their behavior. Thus, a significant issue in the development of preventive health strategies is to determine how to constructively influence these groups.

Peer group pressure can successfully influence change. The development of an effective peer intervention strategy requires organization, leadership, and funding. This structure exists in many gay communities; it generally does not exist within the intravenous drug-using community. Homosexuals are a major social and political force in several major cities, including Los Angeles, San Francisco, and New York; intravenous drug users have no organized social or political constituency.

Almost immediately after AIDS was recognized as being a disease that affected large numbers of homosexuals, the gay community mobilized, initiated education media campaigns, and was instrumental in helping to form health care facilities. There has been little mobilization within the intravenous drug-using community. Thus, the organization of public health education, prevention, and intervention programs for homosexuals may be far easier to accomplish than is development of a similar program designed to reach intravenous drug users and to change their behavior.

In this article, we will review the available data on public health strategies within the drug-using communities and present data that contradict the conventional wisdom that drug users are uneducable and are not concerned about HIV disease.

General Comments About Intravenous Drug Users

The intravenous drug-using community is a series of local clusters of those who voluntarily become involved with intravenous drugs. It is important to recognize that the word "community" refers only to a loose association of individuals whose common bond is obtaining and self-administering drugs as well as committing crimes together. Intravenous drug use is not synonymous with heroin self-administration, rather it also includes cocaine, amphetamines, and a host of other drugs which are commonly self-administered either by the intravenous or subcutaneous ("skin-popping") route.

The rates of admission to state or federally funded drug abuse treatment programs do not accurately reflect the nature and extent of drug use in any given community. While the national Client Oriented Data Acquisition Process (CODAP) collected data on nearly 200,000 admissions to drug abuse treatment during 1980 (Client-Oriented Data Acquisition Process 1981), there is no systematic data collection system for determining the number of admissions to private treatment clinics or the number of patients with drug-related problems being treated by individual practitioners.

By custom, tradition, or necessity, intravenous drug users share their needles, syringes (drug paraphernalia), and supply of drugs. The authors recently determined the extent of needle and syringe sharing for ten communities in New Jersey, and the cities of Washington, D.C. and New Orleans, Louisiana. The highest rate of needle and syringe sharing among intravenous drug users is in the northeastern portion to the United States. Among those in New Jersey who use their intravenous drugs on a daily basis, one-third share their drug paraphernalia with others on at least a daily basis. The rates of needle-sharing in Washington D.C. and New Orleans are significantly lower. These differences may reflect different law enforcement policies as well as different demographic characteristics of those sharing their drug paraphernalia. If a state has strong drug paraphernalia laws (with associated heavy penalties if convictions are obtained) drug users will be very reticent to carry their own drug paraphernalia. Under such circumstances they would prefer to "rent" what they need when they purchase their drugs. Similarly, if it is common practice for one member of a group to make the purchase and another to obtain the drug paraphernalia, then sharing will be more common. Sharing is more common among younger users and among those who use drugs several times a day.

The authors have noted an increased demand for sterile needles and syringes in both New York City and northern New Jersey. The federal government and various state and private organizations have developed pamphlets and other educational material to describe methods for sterilizing needles and syringes. These methods include boiling drug paraphernalia in water, or soaking them in either isopropyl alcohol or dilute (1:10) household bleach.

The National Cancer Institute, the National Institute on Drug Abuse, and the State Department of Health in New Jersey have conducted two knowledge assessment surveys during the past two years to determine whether intravenous drug users are aware of the nature of AIDS, its etiology, means of transmission, and clinical outcome.

The 1984 Knowledge Assessment Survey

The authors of this article had an opportunity to conduct a seroprevalence study among drug users in New Jersey during the fall of 1984. More than 1,000 drug abusers participated from ten drug treatment programs located throughout the state. This study was a cooperative venture between the treatment programs, the New Jersey State Department of Health, the National Cancer Institute (NCI), and the National Institute on Drug Abuse (NIDA). Unlike other studies among drug abusers, the authors found that there were essentially no refusals for this study. (Less than 5% of all clients approached refused to cooperate.)

In addition to the seroprevalence portion of the study, which determined the rates of HIV in the various communities, a detailed questionnaire was completed by the clients. They provided demographic data, information regarding specific sexual practices, and a detailed quantity-frequency drug use matrix, including routes of self-administration and needle-sharing patterns. The final component included a nine-item knowledge assessment questionnaire. The purpose of this questionnaire was to determine if there were any correlations between the prevalence of AIDS in a community and the knowledge about AIDS among intravenous drug users in that community. The assessment questionnaire was administered to and completed by a subsample of 175 drug abusers in four programs in communities with either a high, medium, or low prevalence of AIDS. The principal finding was that the amount of knowledge regarding AIDS did not correlate with the prevalence of AIDS in the community where the respondents resided. That is, independent of the seroprevalence of HIV antibodies in the community, or diagnosed and reported cases of AIDS to the New Jersey State Department of Health, the apparent knowledge level about AIDS was not statistically different among those drug abusers surveyed. The majority of the 175 drug abusers surveyed were men (57%). Fifty-eight percent were white, 34% were black, and the remaining 8% were Hispanic. The median age was 32 years. Approximately 60% had at least a high school education or GED certificate.

At the time of the knowledge assessment, there was active media coverage of the relatively large numbers of cases of AIDS in New Jersey. Also, whenever a known intravenous drug user was diagnosed as having AIDS, the word quickly travelled the streets. Individuals who had been sharing needles or having sexual relations with someone diagnosed as having AIDS approached treatment programs for knowledge, testing, and treatment for drug abuse related problems. At the time of this study, HIV antibody testing was only available as part of a research protocol, and thus research programs such as ours were the only source of antibody testing in New Jersey.

The results of this knowledge assessment survey were encouraging. Almost all those interviewed had heard of AIDS. A brief description of each of the nine items is presented in Exhibit 17-1.

Exhibit 17-1

The Nine Items from the 1984 New Jersey Health Survey
(single answer - multiple choice questions)

	percent correct
Recognition of what the initials AIDS stand for:	90
Geographic distribution of AIDS:	31
Knowledge about who are at highest risk for AIDS:	94
Means of transmissions of the AIDS virus:	95
Relative risk for men and women:	51
Means of reducing risk of becoming infected with the AIDS virus:	95
Identification of some of the symptoms associated with AIDS:	93
Means of avoiding AIDS:	93
Life expectancy of someone diagnosed as having AIDS:	76

More than 95% of those surveyed knew that intravenous drug users were at increased risk of becoming infected with HIV. Ninety percent were aware of the more severe symptoms of AIDS – severe pneumonias and the classic "purple spots" or lesions associated with Kaposi's sarcoma. Seventy-six percent knew that a great majority of those diagnosed with AIDS would die within two years after diagnosis, while an additional 9% indicated that they thought the disease could be adequately treated by physicians.

In order to determine whether this level of knowledge was the same for those in treatment as for those entering treatment, a similar study was conducted, in 1985, on new admissions to drug abuse treatment programs.

The 1985 Knowledge Assessment Survey

Approximately 1 year later, a similar knowledge assessment of intravenous drug users was conducted among 577 clients entering six similar drug abuse treatment programs in New Jersey. The sample, according to the New Jersey State Department of Health, was representative of all admissions to drug abuse treatment programs in the state with regard to age, sex, race, and ethnicity. The median age was 32.5 years. Approximately 50% were white, one-third were black, and the remaining one-sixth were Hispanic; approximately 30% were women.

The results of this survey indicated that there was a continued awareness of AIDS in the drug-using community. Intravenous drug users entering treatment were knowledgeable about what AIDS was, how it was spread, and the most common symptoms.

However, in New Jersey, individuals in treatment are only aware of some of the methods to sterilize drug paraphernalia. At the time of admission to treatment, only one-third of the clients were cognizant of the fact that a dilute household bleach solution would kill the AIDS virus. For those who continue to share their drug paraphernalia, knowledge about techniques for cleansing their "works" (drug paraphernalia) is critical. While an alternative method of cleansing drug paraphernalia includes boiling the needle and syringe, IV drug users in New Jersey believe that boiling a syringe or washing it repeatedly in hot water will "harden the plastic." (Repeated boiling will eventually remove the silicone-based lubricant used to permit the plunger to slide freely. Without lubricant, the plunger will become frozen in the barrel of the syringe.)

Having the knowledge is a first step to responsible action. The real issue, however, is not to what extent the intravenous drug user is knowledgeable about HIV diseases but rather, once they have become aware of the associated medical sequelae of infection with HIV, will they be willing to modify their behavior in order to decrease either their risk of initial exposure or their risk of subsequent repeated exposures? An educational survey, unfortunately, cannot answer this question. Behavioral studies are required to assess what an individual does with his or her newly acquired knowledge.

The distribution of the responses to a sample of the 1985 survey questions dealing with risk group identification, means of spread of the disease, and risk reduction activities are presented in exhibit 17-2. Approximately 90% of those interviewed identified homosexuals and intravenous drug users as the primary risk groups for AIDS. However, almost 11% thought that alcoholics were at risk. Only 57% of this sample were aware that infants of intravenous drug-using women were at risk for AIDS. Further education about the risk to offspring and sexual partners is necessary. Regardless of the route by which a sexually active intravenous drug user becomes infected, he or she can transmit the virus to others. However, the spread of the AIDS virus to nonintravenous drug users is most likely to occur during sexual intercourse. The intravenous drug user is aware that sexual relations and sharing needles with other people are the predominant means of spreading AIDS. More than 84% of those interviewed reflected this awareness in their responses.

More than one-third of those interviewed thought that once someone was exposed to the AIDS virus they would appear physically ill. This misinformation is extremely important if drug users believe they can safely share drug paraphernalia with those who do not appear to be clinically ill. Intravenous drug users have difficulty in understanding the concept of a carrier state. Historically, they have been able to determine if an individual had hepatitis by skin color changes. However, physical appearance is not a predictor of HIV infection; it is not possible to recognize those individuals infected with AIDS virus who have depressed T-cell ratios but who are otherwise healthy. Almost half of those entering treatment indicated that they were seeking treatment because they are afraid of AIDS

Exhibit 17-2

Representative Items from the 1985 New Jersey Health Survey
(multiple responses permitted for all questions)

Question:	Who does AIDS affect?	
Answers:	89.8%	Homosexual or bisexual men
	89.1	Intravenous drug users
	67.4	Women who have sex with men who are IV drug users
	64.3	Men who have sex with women who are IV drug users
	57.0	Babies born to women who use IV drugs or whose partners do
	56.7	Homosexual or bisexual women
	10.7	Alcoholics

Question:	AIDS is spread by:	
Answers:	28.2%	Contaminated drugs
	84.1	Sexual relations
	87.0	Sharing needles with other people
	16.3	Living in a home or working with a person who has AIDS

Question:	A drug user can reduce the risk of getting AIDS by:	
Answers:	7.8%	Always getting drugs from the same place
	81.8	Never sharing a set
	14.9	Wiping off a needle before use
	29.3	Soaking a set in a solution of 1 part bleach to 10 parts water for ½ hour and rinsing carefully

Question:	Once people are exposed to the AIDS virus, they:	
Answers:	34.0%	Will be visibly sick
	68.5	May not look sick but can pass the disease to others
	66.6	Will almost always die
	9.0	Have a good chance of remaining well

Question:	The reason I came into clinic today is: (multiple responses permitted)	
Answers:	30.3%	Family pressure
	67.9	Tired of running
	47.0	Afraid of AIDS and other diseases
	33.6	Afraid of getting arrested
	15.9	Legal pressure

Question:	I got my information about AIDS from: (multiple responses permitted)	
Answers:	77.8%	Television
	58.8	Radio
	69.0	Newspapers
	38.3	Leaflet or pamphlet
	33.1	At a drug program
	15.3	A drug program field worker in the street
	12.3	Other(s) (Specify)

and other diseases. This may be a significant motivational factor in prevention and treatment. Treatment promotes more than drug freeness; it promotes overall good health and longevity.

An apparent lack of recognition of the rapidly progressive fatal course of AIDS was detected in both the 1984 and 1985 surveys. The authors could not determine whether this was primarily deficient knowledge or denial on the part of the clients.

Educating the Intravenous Drug User

As a result of the 1984 findings (and prior to the availability of the 1985 findings) and the additional determination that needle-sharing patterns were essentially the same in all portions of the state, the New Jersey State Department of Health has initiated a series of innovative strategies for educating drug abusers about HIV diseases. One involves the use of indigenous health workers. These are former drug users who have completed a methadone maintenance treatment program; they are recruited and given an intensive training program on HIV diseases. They are also provided with written material to distribute. These indigenous health workers are specifically instructed to initiate conversations with drug users near "shooting galleries" (usually an abandoned building where drugs are sold and drug paraphernalia rented, so that a drug user neither has to carry his own drug supply or needle and syringe).

The core message communicated by the indigenous health workers is a description of what AIDS is and how it is transmitted. In addition, there is a more generic message to those using intravenous drugs: (1) if you are using intravenous drugs, you should consider treatment; (2) if you do not want to go into treatment, then cease sharing your drug paraphernalia; and (3) if you must share your needles and syringes, then attempt to sterilize them by boiling or soaking them in alcohol or dilute household bleach.

The positive impact of the indigenous worker program was actually noted several months before the second (1985) knowledge assessment survey. Nearly one in six drug users, in the 1985 survey, indicated that they had received some information about AIDS from the indigenous health workers assigned to their neighborhood. Of interest was the observation that the "street" price of needles and syringes increased as the demand for them increased. While this is an indirect measure of the effectiveness of the education program, it is not an insubstantial one.

Malaria and infectious hepatitis have been known for the past 3 decades to be transmitted among intravenous drug users through unsterile needles and syringes. However, there has never been a systematic effort to educate drug abusers about the hazards of needle-sharing or the means of attempting to keep their drug paraphernalia clean. In the past, there has only been one message—if you use drugs you should enter treatment; if you do not go into treatment, then whatever ill befalls you will be your own fault. Continued research is needed to measure the impact of the indigenous health care workers on decreasing the morbidity associated with other diseases frequently found among intravenous drug users.

Indigenous workers are one source of information. According to the 1985 survey, television and radio are also able to reach intravenous drug users and provide them with useful information; 78% of those surveyed reported that they obtained information about AIDS by watching television, while another 59% indicated that they had learned about various aspects of AIDS on the radio. Thus, media campaigns can be of value in reaching intravenous drug users. However, an assessment of peak viewing and listening times is required for this population, since prime time television and radio are also the prime times for hustling and purchasing drugs. Late night television and radio and afternoon "soap operas" may be the most productive times for television public service messages designed to reach intravenous drug users.

The value of a newspaper is limited to those who can read the language in which it is published. Overall, more than two-thirds of all those surveyed in 1985 indicated that they had obtained information about AIDS from newspapers. It is worth noting that whites gave positive responses most frequently and Hispanics less frequently to the statement concerning newspapers as a source of information. Hispanic newspapers are readily available in New Jersey. Literacy is the critical issue which must be considered in directing printed media campaigns to foreign language-speaking populations or to populations who did not receive their primary education in this country. Thus, the intravenous drug users are educable; however, community efforts are required to educate them.

Discussion

How realistic is the use of indigenous workers in minority communities? The Report of the Secretary of Health and Human Services' Task Force on Black and Minority Health was issued on 16 October 1985. The report documents the disparity in key health indicators among certain racial and ethnic groups in this country. Most importantly, the Task Force Report made a series of recommendations, which, although generic in nature, are applicable to the needs of intravenous drug users and have specific relevance to the problems of HIV diseases. The Task Force's recommendations serve to strengthen the conclusions which may be drawn from the two New Jersey knowledge surveys presented earlier. There is a need for outreach campaigns specifically designed for minority programs to disseminate targeted health information. Additionally, increased patient education must be accompanied by an improvement in health care provider awareness of minority cultural values, mores, and languages.

This Task Force also recommends the development of strategies to improve the availability and accessibility of health professionals to minority communities through the coordination of nonfederal and federal agencies. Technical assistance, from existing government and community agencies, must be provided so that minority health needs are met. The cooperation of federal, state, and local authorities has proved possible in developing and implementing the two knowledge assessment surveys and in implementing the indigenous health worker program.

The final recommendation of the Task Force related to the need to improve the quality, availability, and use of health care data pertaining to minority populations. Acquisition of health care data is only one building block in providing adequate medical care. These two surveys have demonstrated that drug users are educable. What is required is a means of ensuring that what is learned is put into practice.

In addition to the need for education and behavioral changes, adequate treatment resources need to be made available. A proper mixture of risk-factor identification, educational interventions, and prevention and treatment services needs to be shown to be cost-effective, even among intravenous drug users.

One potential limitation in the application of a volunteer-based model is the availability of educated, motivated, and concerned community members. When the high-risk group is a socially stigmatized and neglected group, such as intravenous drug users, the community may be unwilling to extend itself. Therefore, the use of indigenous health workers in New Jersey may be a substantive initial move forward, creating a community-based program to improve the overall health and well-being of inner city communities. This could be achieved by using the overwhelming public concern regarding HIV diseases to force an integrated community and state action plan to improve the availability of health care delivery to a population which has substantively been ignored by the mainstream of medical care and social concern.

Future Directions

More comprehensive and continuous educational programs are required to meet the specific needs of intravenous drug users, regardless of whether or not they are in treatment, or even interested in receiving treatment. These educational programs should also be targeted at the families and friends of intravenous drug users. Peer and family pressure may be necessary to persuade a drug user to modify his or her lifestyle, even if no formal clinical treatment for drug dependency is desired.

There are a number of public health prevention models that have been used during the past decade. Their success has varied. However, the common themes of persistence, identification of appropriate media and appropriate message, and the need for community involvement have been documented. The medical and social services alone cannot provide sufficient resources to educate and change behavior patterns. They are, however, able to provide leadership. A united community action is required to decrease the rate at which individuals are infected with HIV.

References

Centers for Disease Control. 1985. Acquired immunodeficiency syndrome (AIDS). *Weekly Surveillance Report*, 10 March.

Client-Oriented Data Acquisition Process. 1981. SMSA Statistics 1980, series E, number 23. NIDA, ADAMHA, PHS, Rockville, Maryland.

Gallo, R.C., S. Salahuddin, and M. Popovic, 1984. Frequent detection and isolation of cytopathic retroviruses (HIV) from patients with AIDS and at risk for AIDS. *Science* 224:500-3.

Ho, D.D., T. Rota, R. Schooley, and J. Kaplan. 1985. Isolation of HIV from cerebrospinal fluid and neural tissues of patients with neurologic syndromes related to the acquired immunodeficiency syndrome. *N. Engl. J. Med.* 313:1493-97.

Sheretz, R.J. 1985. Acquired immunodeficiency syndrome: a perspective for the medical practitioner. *Med. Clin. N. Am.* 69:637-55.

Wong-Staal, F., and R. Gallo. 1985. Human T-lymphotropic retroviruses. *Nature* 317:395-403.

18
AIDS Health Education for Intravenous Drug Users

Samuel R. Friedman, PhD; Don C. Des Jarlais, PhD;
and Jo L. Sotheran, MA.

Intravenous (IV) drug users are the second largest risk group for acquired immunodeficiency syndrome (AIDS) and the main source of infection for heterosexual partner and pediatric AIDS cases. IV drug users have an addiction and a subculture that make risk reduction difficult; for example, to refuse to share needles can endanger personal relationships, and carrying clean works (rather than renting them in a shooting gallery) risks arrest. In New York City, at least, knowledge about AIDS transmission is widespread among IV drug users, and most drug injectors report having changed their drug use practices to reduce their risks. The main functions of health education in areas where IV drug users have this level of knowledge are to disseminate news of new discoveries, reach those drug users who have not yet learned AIDS basics, reinforce what is already known, and provide information about new programs to help drug users deal with AIDS-related problems. To encourage behavior change requires going beyond simple education, however; it entails trying to

Reprinted, with changes, from "AIDS Health Education for Intravenous Drug Users," by Samuel R. Friedman, Don C. Des Jarlais, and Jo L. Sotheran, *Health Education Quarterly* 13(4):383-93, 1986, by permission of John Wiley & Sons, Inc. (New York). Copyright 1986 by SOPHE.

change IV drug users subculture. Drug user groups in the Netherlands and in New York City are attempting to do this from within
the subculture. Outside intervention requires repeated messages
from multiple sources: face-to-face, interactive communication and
perhaps the use of ex-addicts as health educators.

Introduction

IV drug users are the second largest risk group for AIDS. As of
10 February 1986, 17% of AIDS cases in the United States were
heterosexual IV drug users, and another 8% were IV drug users who
are homosexual or bisexual males.

In addition to being the second largest group at increased risk
for AIDS, IV drug users are the primary link to two other increased
risk groups – heterosexual partners and children. Of the 199 cases of
AIDS in heterosexual partners, 146 involve apparent transmission of
human immunodeficiency virus ([HIV] which is also referred to as
human T-lymphotropic virus type III [HTLV-III] and as lymphadenopathy-associated virus [LAV]) from an IV drug user to a
heterosexual partner. All but 24 of these IV-related heterosexual
transmission cases have been from males to females; the possibility
and efficiency of female to male sexual transmission of HIV is currently a matter of intense scientific debate (Eckholm 1985).

Children of IV drug users are also at increased risk for developing AIDS as a result of infection before or at birth. One hundred
and thirty-two of the 246 children with AIDS in the United States
have an IV drug user as a parent. The potential spread of HIV from
IV drug users to their sexual partners and their children thus inten-
sifies the already great need for control of the AIDS epidemic
among IV drug users.

Although vaccines and treatments for AIDS are currently being
developed, the need to test their safety and efficacy means that
years of effort will be required before they are ready for widespread
use (Altman 1986). In their absence, control of the epidemic will
depend upon changing behavior.

IV Drug Users and AIDS Prevention

The common image of IV drug users is one of persons whose lives are completely controlled by their drug habits. They are often viewed as people who cannot change their behavior even when they want to change. The high frequency at which IV drug users return to some level of drug injection after treatment supports the general idea that drug injection is very difficult to eliminate completely (Simpson, Savage, and Sells 1978). Current data on the response of IV drug users to the AIDS epidemic, however, indicate that many of them are nonetheless attempting to reduce their risks by reducing IV drug use or by trying to use safer injection practices. Before discussing these data, it will first be useful to review some characteristics of AIDS as a disease and of the social organization of IV drug use that affect AIDS prevention efforts.

AIDS as a Disease

There are two characteristics of AIDS as a disease that inhibit effective prevention efforts among IV drug users. First, AIDS has a long "latency" period between viral exposure and development of the disease. This is currently estimated to average 5 years (Lawrence et al. 1985). Thus, there may be considerable spread of the virus in a risk group in a city before AIDS cases serve as a warning notice. In New York City, for example, historically collected blood samples show high (30%) rates of HIV seropositivity among IV drug users 2 years before the discovery of the first cases of IV AIDS (Novick, in press).

Furthermore, the perceived time lag between exposure and noticeable disease is increased by the similarity between early AIDS-related symptoms (weight loss, fatigue, unexplained fevers, and night sweats) and the symptoms of intensive IV drug use. In one study we conducted, we found that 60% of seronegative IV drug users had experienced one or more symptoms consistent with AIDS in the five years prior to the interview (Des Jarlais, Friedman, and Spira, in press).

Social Organization of IV Drug Use and Its Implications for Health Education

IV drug use is not simply a matter of isolated individual behavior. IV drug users interact with each other in many ways that affect how often they shoot up and the ways in which they shoot up. Thus, attempts to change IV drug use behavior have to take account of the social organization of IV drug use.

In contrast to views that see IV drug use as simply a matter of individual pathology, it is more fruitful to describe IV drug users as constituting a "subculture," as this term has been used within sociological and anthropological research (Agar 1973; Coombs, Fry, and Lewis 1976; DuToit 1977; Weppner 1977; Johnson 1980). This calls our attention to the structured sets of values, roles, and status allocations that exist among IV drug users (Johnson 1973; Des Jarlais and Hopkins 1985). From the perspective of its members, participating in the subculture is a meaningful activity that provides desired rewards, rather than a psychopathology, an "escape from reality," or an "illness" (Preble and Casey 1969). Although there are regional and ethnic variations, it is nonetheless possible to analyze those who inject cocaine and/or heroine in the United States as constituting a single subculture in this sense (Agar 1973).

In the United States, the IV drug use subculture has been shaped in many ways by its relationship to the rest of society. Possession and sale of drugs are violations of the law, as are many of the activities undertaken to obtain money for purchasing the drugs. IV drug users are stigmatized, feared, mistrusted, disliked, scorned, and in some instances pitied. IV drug users, in turn, have similar negative feelings towards members of conventional society.

IV drug users maintain an uneasy balance between trust and mistrust among themselves. They need enough interpersonal trust to let them obtain drugs and the equipment and locations for injecting, and to maintain the sociocultural values and viewpoints that underpin the worth of "getting high." However, IV drug users also have a deep mistrust of other IV drug users. This mistrust stems from many experiences and interests: IV drug users compete for scarce goods (drugs and the money to buy them), hustle each other as well as "straights," and use violence to settle their disputes. Furthermore, their mistrust is heightened by the fact that law enforcement agencies make use of informers and undercover police officers.

Communication among IV drug users is oral rather than written or printed. Much of what they do is illegal, and written documents would be incriminating; many of them have difficulties in reading and writing. This oral subculture develops folklore belief systems that often interpret events in ways that minimize the disruption of IV drug users' activities and values (Goldsmith et al. 1984).

The sharing of works (the needles and syringes used for injecting illicit drugs) is deeply embedded in the IV drug use subculture. Such sharing serves both social bonding and economic functions. Sharing among "running partners" can symbolize their cooperative efforts to obtain drugs. Thus, efforts to reduce sharing works may encounter strong opposition from partners who feel their strongest friendships are under attack or who may need to share works to avoid withdrawal symptoms. The limited supply of needles and syringes for injection also encourages multiple users for the same works. (See Des Jarlais, Friedman, and Strug, in press, for a more complete discussion of the roles of needle sharing within the pre-AIDS IV drug use subculture.)

The risk of death was a part of IV drug user subculture long before AIDS. The annual pre-AIDS death rate among IV drug users who were not in treatment has been estimated as between 3.5% and 8% (Des Jarlais 1984). Thus, even though AIDS usually causes a slower and more painful death than does an overdose, IV drug users' fatalistic acceptance of the risk of death as part of their lifestyle has a tendency to reduce the deterrent effect of AIDS.

Public health efforts to prevent AIDS are made more difficult by the characteristics of the IV drug use subculture. The differences and hostility between the subculture and conventional society make public health authorities' efforts suspect in the eyes of many IV drug uses, and the contempt in which IV drug users are held makes it difficult for health educators to gain support for programs. Language and literacy problems reduce the potential effectiveness of written communications. IV drug users' generalized mistrust of each other makes it more difficult for them to organize a collective response to the AIDS epidemic.

IV Drug Users: Knowledge and Behavior Change in New York City

In spite of these difficulties stemming from the characteristics of AIDS and the social organization of IV drug use, IV drug users (at least in New York City) seem to have considerable knowledge about AIDS; and many have taken steps to protect themselves against the disease.

In the summer of 1984, as part of a larger study of exposure to HIV and its relationship to drug injection and needle-sharing, we conducted interviews with 59 patients in Manhattan methadone maintenance programs. We found considerable knowledge of AIDS in spite of all the forces already discussed. Thus, all the patients knew of AIDS; 55 (93%) knew that IV drug use was a way to get the disease, and 52 (88%) were able to name two or more ways one could get AIDS, with homosexual sex and IV drug use the most common means mentioned. Furthermore, 61% (36) were able to name at least one AIDS symptom correctly. The most frequent answers were weight loss (36%) and fatigue (31%).

Similarly, Selwyn et al. (1985) report that 97% of each of their samples (146 methadone maintenance patients and 115 incarcerated drug users) interviewed in New York City in 1985 knew that you can get AIDS from sharing needles. They also found, however, that false beliefs are widespread. For example, a majority of each sample believed that you can get AIDS by drinking from a shared cup (Selwyn et al. 1985).

IV drug users in New York City thus seem to have considerable knowledge about AIDS, as well as some false information. Given the common stereotype of drug users as incapable of change, we should consider whether their knowledge leads them to protective behavior changes. Our own and Selwyn's data indicate considerable reported individual behavior change. Most (59%) of the IV drug users we interviewed reported having made behavioral changes to avoid AIDS. Their modal changes were increasing the use of clean needles and/or the cleaning of needles (18/59 = 31%) and reduction of needle-sharing (17/59 = 29%). As a measure of protection against self-report biases, we also asked about whether their friends had made changes; 51% reported that their friends had changed their behavior. The extent of behavior change was not related to the educational level of the respondent.

Selwyn et al. report that over 60% of their respondents said they had made one of the following changes in order to avoid AIDS: stopping sharing needles while continuing IV drug injection, decreasing needle-sharing, stopping IV drug use altogether, or attempting to sterilize needles. In addition, many had attempted to use safer sex practices, with 48% decreasing their number of sex partners, using condoms, or taking other hygienic measures (Selwyn et al. 1985).

Furthermore preliminary analyses of a follow-up study indicate the possibility that increasing the consciousness of AIDS among drug users in methadone maintenance programs may lead them to cut down on drug injection. In 1984, we interviewed 314 methadone maintenance and drug detoxification patients about their drug injection patterns (in the context of AIDS); we also took blood samples to assess whether they had been exposed to HIV and to determine the state of their immune system. In 1985, approximately 9 months later, we attempted to reinterview them all. Among the 173 methadone patients, we achieved a 69% follow-up rate. Of these 119 reinterviewed methadone maintenance program patients, there were 84 who at the time of the first interview were active drug injectors who had already been in methadone maintenance programs for over 2 years. Their reported drug injection frequencies dropped significantly ($p < 0.05$) from an average of 16 times per month in the 2 years prior to the first interview to 6 injections per month during the period between interviews; 25 subjects quit injection totally. Further research, however, is needed before any definite conclusions can be reached about why their reported drug injections decreased.

Ethnographic information confirms the evidence that many drug users have been trying to protect themselves. For example, our ethnographic studies indicate that the illicit market in New York City for sterile needles has increased greatly since the AIDS epidemic began and that there has been some distribution of "free" sterile needles and syringes by drug dealers, as well as some fraudulent sale of used needles as new ones (Des Jarlais and Hopkins 1985; Des Jarlais, Friedman, and Hopkins 1985). Thus, based on both ethnographic and questionnaire data, it is clear that many New York City IV drug users have attempted to protect themselves against AIDS.

Health Education for IV Drug Users: Content

Since it appears that IV drug users can and do respond to information about AIDS, we should consider the content of health education directed at them. In doing this, it is necessary to start with the realization that knowledge about AIDS is changing rapidly, as is public policy. Thus, any program will need to change as new discoveries are made or as new policies are implemented.

Furthermore, we should consider the implication of the evidence that IV drug users already know a great deal about AIDS. Much of the basic information that health education programs convey is already known to most IV drug users (at least in New York City). Thus, the main function of education programs will be as follows: (1) disseminating news of new discoveries; (2) reaching those drug users who have not yet learned the basic facts about AIDS (who are an unknown proportion in most areas, although a minority in New York City); (3) reinforcing what is already "known" so that IV drug users are more likely to continue to engage in risk reduction continuously; and (4) providing information about new programs to help drug users deal with their AIDS-related problems, including information about groups that offer services to people with AIDS and efforts to deal with AIDS-related discrimination against drug users.

For IV drug users who are not going to quit using drugs, information should be distributed about the risks of sharing works and about how to clean needles in order to kill HIV. Printed materials containing this information are being used now in several states. There have been instances where such information has not been distributed to IV drug users under the belief that it might "encourage" IV drug use either by implying that it can be made safe from the risk of HIV infection or by suggesting that drug use is legitimate. The general trend across the country, however, has been to include specific information on the dangers of sharing works and how to sterilize them.

IV drug users also need information about HIV antibody testing, including how to get it, its limitations, its potential social risks, and its potential benefits. The limitations are important: first, the antibody tests have a small percentage of false positives and false negatives. These were estimated for any enzyme-linked immunosorbent assay (ELISA) test as being less than 2% false positives among blood donor and health care and laboratory control groups, and about 2% false negatives among AIDS patients, with 6% of the blood donor controls, 3% of the health care and laboratory controls, and 16% of the AIDS patients being borderline (and thus unclassifiable) on this test (Weiss, Goedert, and Sarngadharan 1985). Current technology in many testing centers is more demanding than this – as indeed it should be, given the potential consequences of errors – and uses an additional test to confirm or contradict the results of ELISA.

A second limitation is that some persons will correctly be measured as seronegative, but will already have been exposed to HIV and not yet had time to develop the antibody.

The antibody tests pose a potential risk to those who take them. This risk comes from the possibility that confidential test results will become known, whether through improper divulgence or by the subject telling them to other people. Such breaches of confidentiality could lead to problems, including possible loss of jobs or housing, family problems, or eventually, becoming the subject of any governmental restrictions that are instituted.

Benefits from being tested include stress reduction if one is seronegative, and the chance to reduce possible transmission to others if one is seropositive. Preliminary evidence suggests that continued injection after initial exposure to HIV increases immunosuppression (Des Jarlais, Friedman, and Marmor, in press), so seropositives may also be in a position to modify their behavior to reduce the chances of developing clinical AIDS.

Prevention of Transmission from IV Drug Users to Others

Information should also be disseminated about how IV drug users can protect their lovers and about the risks that potential children will be infected. Both the heterosexual partners and children are relatively large groups. A study of sexual relationships of male IV drug users found that almost 80% of them had their primary sexual relationship with women who did not inject drugs themselves. The size of the female heterosexual partner population was estimated to be at least half the size of the IV drug user population (Des Jarlais, Chamberlain, and Yankovitz 1984). IV drug users also have considerable numbers of children. A recently completed study of the children of methadone maintenance patients found an average of almost two children per patient, and a quarter of the patients indicated that they expected to have additional children (Deren 1985). The incidence of surveillance definition AIDS in both heterosexual partners and children has been low compared to the numbers of partners and children at risk—which suggests that these modes of transmission may be less likely to lead to AIDS than drug injection—but the incidence follows the same exponential increase as the cases in IV drug users (Des Jarlais, Thomas, and Deren, unpublished data).

Preventing AIDS among the sexual partners and unborn children of IV drug users will clearly be a necessary part of overall public health control of the epidemic. The previously mentioned finding by Selwyn et al., that 48% of the IV drug users they studied had attempted to use safer sex practices, indicates that many IV drug users are motivated to reduce the risk of infecting their lovers or future children (Selwyn et al. 1985).

The behavior changes needed to prevent heterosexual and in utero transmission are at least as complex and difficult as those associated with drug injection transmission. Disruption of ongoing sexual relationships and foregoing having children both involve considerable psychological costs. Until more is known about the probabilities of heterosexual and in utero transmission, it is difficult to provide full guidelines for the trade-offs of risk reduction and psychological costs. The same "safer sex" guidelines used for homosexual transmission (avoidance of anal sex and transfer of bodily fluids—particularly semen and blood; use of condoms), and, for women who are HIV antibody-positive, postponing voluntary pregnancies until more is known about transmission to children would seem to be minimal recommendations for prevention of AIDS among heterosexual partners and as yet unborn children.

From Knowledge to Behavior Change

As has already been discussed, IV drug users have considerable knowledge about AIDS, and many have engaged in risk-reduction behavior. However, maintaining safe injection practices is difficult. Social forces can lead an IV drug user to share works, as can difficulty in getting new works at a time when withdrawal threatens. Here, one role of public health interventions—including health education—should be to help IV drug users change selected aspects of their subculture and its environment. In particular, it has to become legitimate for an IV drug user to refuse to share works. Changing the subculture, in turn, depends upon an internal mobilization of IV drug users to change their practices and values, upon external support for these efforts, and perhaps upon legal and policy changes in the way the wider society approaches specific IV drug use practices. These issues are the focus of the remainder of this article.

Encouraging Subcultural Change

Reaching current and past IV drug users with information, and having the message accepted as accurate and as an appropriate basis for action, seems to be easier than one might expect from the estrangement between IV subculture and the larger society. This is evidenced by IV drug users' wide knowledge about AIDS that has been accepted from the mass media and by the extent to which IV drug users have changed their behaviors based upon this knowledge. However, outside support of the needed adjustments in IV subculture is likely to be more difficult. As discussed earlier, IV drug users communicate mainly by word of mouth, and so pamphlets and other printed materials are less useful than among other risk groups. Mass media (particularly radio and television) reach many drug users; however, the fact that most members of radio and TV audiences are not IV drug users – and, indeed, are hostile to drug users – means that acceptable messages may have to be too nonspecific to have the desired effects. Many IV drug users can be reached through programs at drug treatment centers, jails, or prisons; however, in some of these institutions, the social distance between staff and drug users is so great as to render information suspect.

Efforts to encourage subcultural change are more likely to be effective if they are carried out by an organization within the subculture rather than by isolated individuals or by outside agencies. Here, the response of the gay community to AIDS is a useful model. Gays have been able to mount a public response to the epidemic. They have created AIDS-related service and lobbying organizations such as the Gay Men's Health Crisis Center in New York City. There is a gay press that carries on extensive educational campaigns for readers as well as serving as a place to discuss the political and social implications of AIDS. The gay community also has been the base for the writing and production of plays about homosexuality and AIDS like *As is* and *The Normal Heart*. Collective organization and discussion of this sort are necessary in order to change deeply held subcultural values, such as those gays hold about sexual activity or those IV drug users hold about getting high.

IV drug users have not yet done anything comparable. IV users' responses to the AIDS crisis have primarily taken the forms of individual attempts at self-protection and market responses to the greater demand for new needles and syringes. Also, some drug dealers in New York are passing out pamphlets on how to avoid AIDS. However, rather than the self-organization that gays have engaged in to provide information, services, and a political voice during the health crisis, IV drug users have so far primarily relied on drug treatment centers and their related public agencies to do things for them.

On the basis of the gay public response to the epidemic, it appears that helping current and past IV drug users (and their lovers) set up similar projects to make information available and to represent their interests during the AIDS crisis might be a valuable health education measure. Such efforts will not be easy. IV drug users do not usually spend much time or energy in organizing activities, and their attempts to organize will meet hostility in some quarters. In these respects, they are "unorganizable"—just as Southern rural blacks were thought to be in the early 1950s or industrial workers in the early 1930s. However, given the importance of finding ways to provide IV drug users with knowledge about AIDS, such efforts should be attempted.

There are two examples that suggest that efforts at collective organization or drug users might be successful. First, although in a considerably different setting, drug users in the Netherlands have set up "Junkybond" organizations in Amsterdam, Rotterdam, and other cities (van de Wijngaart 1984; Buning 1986; Coutinho 1986). These groups were begun in 1980 as an attempt to resist changes in public policy towards drug use. The Junkybond was active in a campaign to reduce the spread of hepatitis among Dutch drug users; in Amsterdam, it was the essential organizational vehicle by which the Public Health Department was able to establish a program for the exchange of old syringes for new.

Second, an attempt to emulate the gay community's organizing efforts has recently been begun in New York by ex-users who are employed in drug programs (Friedman and Des Jarlais in press). They have set up the Association for Drug Abuse Prevention and Treatment (ADAPT) to provide support services for IV drug users who come down with AIDS, to educate past and present drug users about the risks of AIDS and how they can be minimized or avoided, to participate in public debates about drug use and AIDS, and generally to do what they can to help IV drug users change their behavior and subculture in ways that will reduce transmission of the disease. Although it is still too early to tell whether ADAPT will prosper, it has weathered some early difficulties in getting organized. Its concrete achievements include the production and distribution of pamphlets for drug users in the streets and in jail, and of several graphic posters as well as presentations at a number of conferences and public forums.

Techniques for Outside Intervention

Up to this point, we have discussed the different target groups for AIDS IV drug use prevention, evidence that IV drug users do change their behavior in order to reduce the risk of AIDS, specific information needed for risk reduction, and the value of encouraging self-organization in behalf of subcultural change. Little has been said about the techniques to use when providing information to IV drug users or their sexual partners. While there has been very little research in this area, several recommendations are appropriate.

First, one should think in terms of repeated messages from multiple sources. Education about AIDS should not be thought of in terms of a single packet of information to be delivered to the appropriate recipients, but in terms of maintaining behavior change over an indefinite time period. The strategies used in commercial advertising—of varied messages with a consistent theme repeated through as many sources of information as possible—are applicable to AIDS risk reduction.

There is also a need for face-to-face education to IV drug users about AIDS. The mass media and pamphlets/posters can reach many IV drug users at relatively low cost. Although language and literacy problems do restrict the effectiveness of these means of communications with IV drug users, a more important restriction comes from the impersonal nature of these means. AIDS and how it is transmitted are complex subjects, and communication will be much improved if the intended recipients have the opportunity to ask clarifying questions. It will be equally necessary to respond to the level of emotion aroused by information about AIDS. Too low a level may lead to the information being ignored, while too high a level may lead to psychological denial and lack of risk reduction. Only in a face-to-face situation will it be possible to gauge the level of emotional response and judge what additional information is needed to increase/decrease emotional response to the range where positive action is most likely. This argument assumes that the person providing the information is capable of assessing the emotional response of the IV drug users, or sexual partner of an IV drug user, through such cues as voice tone and body language. Making such assessments includes the ability to develop rapport with the person receiving the information and would be facilitated by knowledge of the IV drug use subculture. This ability should be seen as learned skill, requiring training and practice, rather than as an innate characteristic.

Earlier considerations suggest the value of using ex-addicts as health educators for providing AIDS information to current IV drug users. While training is clearly required, they have considerable advantages in developing rapport and credibility with current IV drug users based on their understanding of life as a drug user, their ability to sympathize with the difficulties involved in seemingly simple behavioral changes like refusing to share works with a friend who is confronting withdrawal, and their knowledge of street lore and language. Ex-addicts also serve as role models for stopping IV drug use among those they are educating. On the negative side, ex-addict health educators are faced daily with the lure and opportunity of reverting to drug use, so programs have to be structured so as to give them maximum support in resisting these pressures. Ex-addicts are currently being successfully used as AIDS educators in New Jersey, and a large-scale project utilizing ex-addicts is planned for New York.

Summary

Preventing the further spread of AIDS among IV drug users and from them to their sex partners and future children is a vital part of the fight against the disease. Although efforts in this direction will not be easy, there are many signs that they can have an impact.

Most notably, IV drug users have already begun to reduce their risks by changing their needle-use patterns and, to a limited extent, by reducing drug injecting.

Traditional approaches like posters, pamphlets, leaflets, and mass media campaigns will have a limited (but useful) effect in disseminating information and reinforcing its impact. However, in order to counteract the forces that lead IV drug users to ignore what they know about risk reduction, changes in the IV subculture and its environment need to be encouraged. Such subcultural changes are most likely to be encouraged to the extent to which they come out of organized efforts by current and former IV drug users; outsiders' attempts to intervene to facilitate change may be more likely to succeed if they are face-to-face interventions that draw upon the energies of present and former IV drug users.

References

Agar, M.H. 1973. *Ripping and running: a formal ethnography of urban heroin addicts.* New York: Seminar Press.

Altman, L.K. 1986. Who will volunteer for an AIDS vaccine? *New York Times*, C1, C7, 15 April.

Buning, E. 1986. The Amsterdam Helping System for Drug Addicts: a summary. Paper presented at the Conference on AIDS in the Drug Abuse Community and Heterosexual Transmission, 1 April, Newark, New Jersey.

Coombs, R.H., L. Fry, and P. Lewis, eds. 1976. *Socialization in drug abuse.* Cambridge, England: Schenkman.

Coutinho. R. 1986. Prevention of AIDS among drug users in Amsterdam. Paper presented at the Conference on AIDS in the Drub Abuse Community and Heterosexual Transmission, 1 April, Newark, New Jersey.

Deren, S. 1985. *A description of methadone maintenance patients and their children.* New York: New York State Division of Substance Abuse Services.

Des Jarlais, D.C. 1984. Research design, drug use and deaths: cross study comparisons. In *Social and medical aspects of drug abuse*, ed. G. Serban. New York: SP Scientific.

Des Jarlais, D.C., M. Chamberland, and S. Yancovitz. 1984. Heterosexual partners:

a large risk group for AIDS. *Lancet* 2:1345-47.

Des Jarlais, D.C. and W. Hopkins. 1985. Free needles for intravenous drug users at risk for AIDS: current developments in New York City. *N. Engl. J. Med.* 313:23.

Des Jarlais, D.C., S. Friedman, and W. Hopkins. 1985. Risk reduction for AIDS among intravenous drug users. *Ann Intern. Med.* 103:755-59.

Des Jarlais, D.C., S. Friedman, and M. Marmor. Continued injection as a co-factor for T4 cell loss among IV drug users exposed to HTLV-III/LAV. In press.

Des Jarlais, D.C., S. Friedman, and T. Spira. A stage model of HTLV-III/LAV infection in intravenous drug users. In press.

Des Jarlais, D.C., S. Friedman, and D. Strug. AIDS and needle sharing within the intravenous drug use subculture. In *The social dimensions of AIDS: methods and theory*, eds. D. Feldman and T. Johnson. New York: Praeger. In press.

Des Jarlais, D.C., P. Thomas, S. Deren. Intravenous Drug Users and Their Children (in preparation).

DuToit, B.M., ed. 1977. *Drugs, rituals and altered states of consciousness:* Rotterdam: A.A. Balkema.

Eckholm, E. 1985. Prostitutes' impact on spread of AIDS debated. *New York Times*, C1, 5 November.

Friedman, S.R. and D. Des Jarlais. Knowledge of AIDS, behavioral change, and organization among intravenous drug users. Stichting Drug Symposium. In press.

Goldsmith, D., D. Hunt, D. Strug, and D. Lipton. 1984. Methadone folklore: beliefs about side effects and their impact on treatment. *Human Organization* 43:330-40.

Johnson, B.D. 1973. *Marijuana users and drug subcultures.* New York: John Wiley.

Johnson, B.D. 1980. Toward a theory of drug subcultures. In *Theories on Drug Abuse,* NIDA Research Monograph 30, ed. D.J. Lettiere. Rockville, Maryland: National Institute on Drug Abuse, 110-19.

Lawrence, D.N., K. Lui, D. Bregman, T. Peterman, and W. Morgan. 1985. A model-based estimate of the average incubation and latency period for transfusion-associated AIDS. Paper presented at the International Conference on Acquired Immunodeficiency Syndrome (AIDS), 14 April, Atlanta, Georgia.

Novick, D., M. Kreek, and D. Des Jarlais. Antibody to LAV in parenteral drug abusers and methadone maintained patients: therapeutic, historical and ethical aspects. In press.

Preble, E., and J.H. Casey. 1969. Taking care of business: the heroin user's life on the street. *Int. J. Addictions* 4:1-24.

Selwyn, P.A., C. Cox, C. Feiner, C. Lipshutz, and R. Cohen. 1985. Knowledge about AIDS and high-risk behavior among intravenous drug abusers in New York City. Paper presented at the Annual Meeting of the American Public Health Association, 18 November, Washington, D.C.

Simpson, D.D., J. Savage, and S. Sells. 1978. *Data book on drug treatment outcomes.* Fort Worth, Texas: Institute of Behavioral Research.

Weiss, S.H., J. Goedert, and M. Sarngadharan. 1985. Screening test for HTLV-III (AIDS agent) antibodies: specificity, sensitivity, and application. *J.A.M.A.* 253:221-25.

Weppner, R.S., eds. 1977. *Street ethnography.* Beverly Hills, California: Sage.

van de Wijngaart, G.F. 1984. The "Junkie League" promoting the interests of the Dutch hard-drug user. Paper presented at The 14th International Institute of the Prevention and Treatment of Drug Dependence, May, Athens, Greece.

19
Knowledge about AIDS and High-Risk Behavior among Intravenous Drug Users in New York City

Peter A. Selwyn, MD; Cheryl Feiner, MPH; Charles P. Cox, MA; Carl Lipshutz, MA; and Robert L. Cohen, MD.

Introduction

After gay or bisexual men, intravenous (IV) drug users (IVDUs) currently form the second largest risk group for the acquired immunodeficiency syndrome (AIDS) in the United States (Curran et al. 1985). Sharing of contaminated needles has been implicated as the likely means of transmission among IVDUs of the virus believed to cause AIDS, human immunodeficiency virus (HIV), also referred to as human T-lymphotropic virus type III/lymphadenopathy-associated virus (Weiss et al. 1985; Friedland et al. 1985). Of the approximately 40,000 adult AIDS cases reported to the Centers for Disease Control through August 1987, 16% have occurred in heterosexual IVDUs, and 8% have occurred in gay or bisexual men who also used IV drugs (Centers for Disease Control 1987). In New York City and New Jersey, where IV drug-related AIDS is concentrated, IV drug users account for 35 and 51 percent, respectively, of total cases (New York City Department of Health 1987, New Jer-

Reprinted with permission of Gower Academic Journals, London, England. This chapter first appeared as an article in the November 1987 issue of *AIDS*.

sey State Department of Health 1987). The risk group of IVDUs also forms an important potential route for the spread of HIV infection to segments of the larger population, primarily through heterosexual and perinatal transmission (Centers for Disease Control 1985a, 1985b). There are an estimated 200,000 IVDUs in the New York metropolitan area, with most current seroepidemiologic reports estimating the prevalence of exposure to HIV at 50% or greater within this population (Ginzburg 1984a, 1984b; Des Jarlais, Friedman, and Hopkins 1985; Landesman, Ginzburg, and Weiss 1985; Spira et al. 1985).

The above data suggest that IVDUs occupy a pivotal position in the developing AIDS epidemic and that preventive interventions must focus at least in part on this key risk group. Public health education has been suggested as a means of reducing the spread of HIV infection and has been credited by some with already having had an impact on high-risk sexual activity among gay and bisexual men. Surveillance data have indicated a decline in incidence rates of rectal and pharyngeal gonorrhea among males in both New York City and San Francisco since the onset of the AIDS epidemic, and several studies have provided evidence of a concurrent decrease in high-risk sexual practices among gay men in both those cities (Centers for Disease Control 1984; Curran et al. 1985; McKusick Horstman, and Coates 1985; Centers for Disease Control 1985c; Martin 1986; Echenberg et al. 1986). Among IVDUs, however, comparable data on risk reduction are relatively lacking, and the development of educational campaigns has been problematic, perhaps due both to the elusive nature of this population and stereotyped image of IVDUs as incorrigible social outcasts.

Several studies have in fact suggested a high level of awareness about AIDS among certain groups of IVDUs, with perceived reductions in needle-sharing and the increased street demand for sterile needles noted as evidence of the impact of AIDS on drug-using behavior (Ginzburg 1984a, 1984b: Des Jarlais, Friedman, and Hopkins 1985; Friedman, Des Jarlais, and Sotheran 1986). Much of this information is anecdotal, however, involving small numbers of respondents; important questions remain concerning the extent to which the larger population of IVDUs has become aware of the risks of AIDS, the relationship of such knowledge of risk-taking behavior, and the persistence or decline of high-risk activities in this critical but not easily accessible group.

In an attempt to address some of these issues, we undertook a study with the following objectives: (1) to assess baseline levels of knowledge about AIDS among a large group of IVDUs, (2) to evaluate whether knowledge or concerns about AIDS had affected needle-sharing practices among IVDUs, (3) to determine reasons for continued needle-sharing and obstacles to risk reduction, and (4) to identify appropriate areas for intervention in an AIDS education program.

Methods

The study was conducted in May and June 1985, at two sites: a methadone maintenance treatment program located in the Bronx and the narcotic detoxification unit of a major detention facility in New York City. The methadone program provides long-term out-patient treatment for heroin addiction; at the detention facility site, narcotics addicts are identified immediately following arrest and undergo short-term detoxification with methadone after being assessed by prison medical staff for symptoms and signs of opiate withdrawal. Our intention in choosing these two sites was to be able to compare one group of current and former drug users already engaged in the treatment system with another group more closely approximating the world of the street addict.

Interviews of subjects were conducted by two interviewers (C. C. and C. L.). At the methadone program, interviewers were stationed each day in clinic waiting rooms where patients were awaiting daily medication and would periodically invite small groups of patients to participate in a confidential 10 to 15-minute survey about AIDS. Interviewers were not members of the treatment program staff, and patients were advised that no information concerning their participation in the survey would be communicated to treatment staff in any way. Patients volunteering to participate in the study were interviewed individually in a private room. At the detention facility, the interviewers visited the narcotic detoxification housing areas each day during the study period, making a similar presentation to that described above. Subjects who volunteered to participate were interviewed privately in a room adjacent to the housing area.

The interview instrument was a 42-item, interviewer-administered questionnaire, consisting of 21 questions designed to test subjects' general factual knowledge about AIDS and associated risk factors, with the remaining questions pertaining to basic demographic variables, subjects' IV drug and needle use practices, and sources of information about AIDS. The general knowledge items were posed as simple statements, with possible responses of true/false/don't know. In the analysis of the data, "don't know" recorded as incorrect. The questions on drug needle use were asked in a nonleading, open-ended fashion, with subjects' answers recorded verbatim and subsequently categorized into the most frequently occurring responses.

Statistical Considerations

Categorical data for independent sample groups were analyzed via the chi-square test and where appropriate by Fisher's exact test. Overall scores on the 21-item questionnaire were analyzed via the Wilcoxon rank-sum two-sample test, a nonparametric test, as they did not meet for this reason. Total percent correct for each individual test was calculated as the sum of the number of correct answers divided by the total number of questions, multiplied by 100.

Multivariate analyses were performed to examine the relationship between AIDS knowledge questionnaire scores, persistent needle-sharing behavior, and other variables. For questionnaire scores, a multiple regression analysis was used to describe the association between knowledge about AIDS and sociodemographic variables, including age, gender, race, marital status, and education, as well as study site. For persistent needle-sharing, stepwise multiple logistics regression was used to determine which factors were associated with persistent needle-sharing after adjustment for the presence of other variables. The predictor variables considered for the model included all those noted above as well as AIDS knowledge questionnaire scores and acquaintance with someone with AIDS. For the regression models, dummy variables were created when appropriate for the analysis of categorical data. Results of all regression analyses are presented by listing the significant variables (including intercept) and their associated regression coefficients and p values.

Statistical analysis was performed using the software package SAS from the SAS Institute, Inc., Cary, North Carolina.

Results

During the study period, there was a total of 876 patients enrolled in the methadone program, and 1,767 narcotics addicts were processed through the detention facility detoxification site. One hundred and forty-six patients volunteered to be interviewed at the methadone site, and 115 at the detention facility, for a total of 261.

Overall, subjects tended to be in their early 30s, nonwhite, poorly educated, and unemployed; there were slightly more men than women in the total sample. When analyzed by site of interview, respondents at the methadone clinic tended to be older, married, and somewhat better educated, with a greater percentage of females and whites. The inmates at the detention facility tended conversely to be younger, unemployed, black, single males. Study subjects did not vary significantly from the overall populations at each site with respect to age and race/ethnic group. There were, however, proportionally more women in the samples than in the general population at each site; 53% vs. 41% for the methadone program ($p < 001$), and 38% vs. 22% for the detention facility ($p < .001$). Subjects at the methadone program had been in continuous treatment for a median of 28 months (range: 1 to 153); as noted previously, inmates at the detention facility were all narcotics addicts interviewed within one week of arrest from the street.

Baseline Knowledge About AIDS

Subjects at both sites showed a great deal of personal concern about AIDS, with 77% indicating that they were worried about getting AIDS. Thirty-six percent of all respondents reported knowing one or more people with AIDS. Sixty-one percent indicated newspapers or magazines as a major source of information about AIDS, with 40% indicating the same for TV/radio. Inmate respondents were more likely to have received information from friends (32% vs. 14%, $p < .001$), and "the street," (28% vs. 11%, $p < 0.001$), and less likely to have gotten information from doctors and other health professionals (10% vs. 41%, $p < 0.001$).

Subjects at both sites did well on basic knowledge questions and had a virtually universal recognition of the AIDS risks associated with needle-sharing. There were also high percentages of correct answers on sexual transmission questions. Errors were more common on questions regarding certain risk-reduction techniques (e.g., the effectiveness of condom use) and were most frequent in the areas of popular misconceptions about AIDS and fears of casual contact. The methadone clinic group scored slightly better overall than did the detention center group, with a median percent correct of 71% vs. 67%, respectively ($p < .001$). (See table 19-1.)

The results of the multiple regression analysis with questionnaire score as the dependent variable indicated that increasing years of education (b=2.05, $p < .0005$) and the methadone program study site (b=-7.07, 1=detention center, o=methadone program site, $p < .002$) were both predictive of higher test scores, after controlling for the other variables.

Knowledge and Behavior Change

Subjects were asked whether knowing about AIDS had changed their IV drug use or needle-sharing practices. For this analysis, all those who had either stopped IV drug use or needle-sharing before learning of AIDS ($N = 68$), or who currently denied knowing about AIDS ($N = 12$), were excluded from consideration. The results indicate that of the remaining sample ($N = 181$), 63% had either stopped IV drug use entirely or stopped needle-sharing due to concerns about AIDS, based on self-report. Twenty percent of subjects reported persistent and undiminished needle-sharing, and 17% indicated ongoing but decreased needle-sharing. Those who had stopped IV drug use altogether due to fear of AIDS were concentrated at the methadone clinic, whereas persistent needle-sharers were more predominant among the inmate group.

Obstacles to Risk Reduction

All subjects were asked about current and past IV drug use and needle-sharing practices. Thirty-two percent (47/146) at the methadone clinic and 70% (80/115) at the detention facility reported needle-sharing within the prior year ($p < .001$). Among those reporting needle-sharing over the past year, however, 20/47 (55%) at the methadone program and 50/80 (63%) at the detention facility reported such behavior within the two months prior to the date of interview, which represented an approximate 40% decrease in needle-sharing for each of the two groups.

Table 19-1 Questionnaire Scores: Knowledge about AIDS (Selected Questions)*

	Methadone Clinic (n = 146)	Detention Center (n = 115)	P
	%	%	
AIDS attacks the body's immune system so it can't fight infections.	82	93	NS
Most people with AIDS will die from it.	88	72	.01
You can get AIDS by getting blood transfusions.	91	91	NS
Only homosexuals get AIDS.	92	82	.01
AIDS is caused by a virus.	85	58	.001
Women can pass AIDS on to their babies when they give birth.	90	83	NS
You can get AIDS from sharing needles.	97	97	NS
Women can get AIDS through sex with a man who has AIDS.	92	99	NS
Wiping off your needles with alcohol or putting them under a flame will prevent AIDS.	67	40	.001
Using a condom during sex may help prevent AIDS.	52	63	.02
You can get AIDS from giving blood.	64	32	.001
There is a blood test that will tell you if you have AIDS.	16	23	NS
There is a vaccine to prevent AIDS.	66	58	NS
You can tell by looking at a person if they have AIDS.	73	42	.001
You can get AIDS by drinking from the same cup as someone with AIDS.	40	16	.001
You can get AIDS by living in the same house as someone with AIDS.	60	39	.01

*Percent answering correctly to true/false questions.

Of the subgroup of 76 subjects reporting continued needle-sharing over the past two months, 67 (88%) indicated an awareness that by so doing they were increasing their risk for AIDS, with the remaining nine subjects (12%) stating that they were either unaware or dubious of such a risk. The reason most commonly given for continued needle-sharing, among those aware of the AIDS risks who still continued to share needles, was characterized as the need to inject drugs with no clean needle being available. This answer was indicated by 46% of all respondents and 71% of the methadone program group. The second most common reason, offered by 45% of the total and 52% of the detention facility inmates, was that needle-sharing was done only with a close friend or relative. Other less frequent responses indicated the habitual or social nature of needle-sharing practices. (See table 19-2.)

Univariate analysis of needle-sharers (N = 76) vs. nonneedle-sharers (N = 185) showed no association between needle-sharing and age, gender, marital status, and race/ethnic group. Needle-sharers were more likely to have less than a high school education (74% vs. 59%, p < .02), to have scored more poorly on the AIDS

Table 19-2 Self-Reported Reasons for Continued Needle Sharing*

	Methadone Program (n=21)	Detention Facility (n=46)	Total (n=67)**	P
	%	%	%	
Need to inject drugs/ no clean needle available	71	35	46	.01
Only share with close friend or relative	29	52	45	(.07)
Needle-sharing habitual, difficult to stop	10	17	15	NS
Enjoy social aspects of needle-sharing	0	11	7	NS

*Subjects allowed up to three responses to open-ended question regarding reasons for persistent needle sharing.
**Excludes nine of 76 persistent needle-sharers who stated that they were unaware that sharing needles increased AIDS risk.

knowledge questionnaire (median percent correct: 62% vs. 71%, *p* < .001), and to be from the detention center site (66% vs. 35%, *p* < .001). Acquaintance with someone with AIDS was not reported any less frequently among needle-sharers than non-needle-sharers (39% vs. 35%, *p* < .05).

The stepwise multiple logistics regression with persistent needle-sharing as the dependent variable showed that only study site (*p* < .0005) and AIDS knowledge questionnaire score (*p* < .0003) were significant predictors after adjusting for the other variables. The likelihood of needle-sharing was greater at the detention facility site and increased with lower questionnaire scores.

Discussion

Our results indicate that study subjects demonstrated both personal concern and factual understanding about AIDS, and that of those still engaging in needle-sharing after becoming aware of AIDS, over 60% had adopted some form of risk-reduction behavior by mid-1985.

As with any study based on self-reporting of behavior, this study runs the risks of recall and reporting biases. One might question the reliability of reports of drug and needle use at the two sites. As noted above, however, respondents were explicitly assured of confidentiality by interviewers who were not affiliated in any way with treatment program or detention facility staff, which may have enhanced the likelihood of accurate reporting. Patients were advised repeatedly that no information would be revealed to treatment staff; interviewers were trained to pose questions in an open-ended and nonjudgmental way.

Regarding the inclusiveness of the sample, it is not possible to calculate the number of participating patients as a true percentage of all patients at the two study sites, since the circumstances of the study did not permit an approach in which all eligible patients were approached individually and asked to participate. Rather, study volunteers were drawn from the available group of those patients present at the sites on the days and times that the interviewers were stationed there. Calculating the number of participating patients as a percentage of the total number of patients enrolled at either site would substantially underestimate the level of participation among those patients actually approached for the study.

Concerning the representativeness of the samples, the study groups did not differ significantly from the larger populations at each site by age or race/ethnic group, although as noted a greater percentage of female subjects was included in the study group at each location. At the methadone program site, this may have reflected the fact that female patients in the program are less likely to be employed than males, and therefore more likely to have the time to be interviewed (working patients tend in general to be medicated early in the day and not to spend additional time in clinic waiting rooms). At the detention facility site, females were over-represented because of certain institutional arrangements which made the female housing areas somewhat more accessible to the interviewers than the male areas. Notwithstanding the disproportionate number of female subjects, it is of note that, for the major measures of interest in the study (AIDS knowledge questionnaire scores and needle-sharing practices), there were no significant differences observed between male and female respondents at either site, either by univariate or multivariate analyses.

In anticipating the impact of potential selection and reporting biases on our data, we hypothesized that such biases, if present, would tend to operate toward the underreporting of high-risk behavior and the selection of a study group perhaps better informed and less involved in risk-taking behavior than the IV drug-using population as a whole. Even if such biases were operating, however, our data still indicate significant gaps in knowledge about AIDS, (especially concerning risk-reduction measures and fears of casual contact), with the persistence of risk-taking behaviors in over one-third of respondents despite knowledge of AIDS.

Our findings parallel those of other studies conducted in 1983 and 1984, with smaller groups of IVDUs, which found that the majority of respondents both expressed some concern about getting AIDS and were able to identify one or more facts about the disease (Ginzburg 1984a, 1984b; Des Jarlais, Friedman, and Hopkins 1985; Friedman, Des Jarlais, and Sotheran 1986). Our results support the view that drug users have in fact responded to the threat of AIDS through a reduction in needle-sharing, and would complement recent observations of the increased street level demand for sterile needles among IVDUs in New York (Des Jarlais, Friedman, and Hopkins 1985). The decreased prevalence of needle-sharing among methadone patients, and the not infrequent report in this group of having ceased IV drug use due to fear of AIDS, both suggest the potential importance of drug treatment in helping to interrupt the spread of AIDS in IVDUs.

The most frequent reason given for continued needle-sharing, even in the majority of cases where subjects were fully aware of the associated AIDS risks, was the need to inject drugs with no clean needle being available. This would support the hypothesis that, in certain situations at least, needle-sharing may not be the result of IVDUs being uneducated about the risks, but rather a simple calculus of the acute sickness of drug withdrawal vs. the more theoretical danger of some future disease in a setting where the only available needle is a used one. Des Jarlais, Friedman, and Hopkins have suggested that IV drug-using behavior involves such strong aversive conditioning that it may be virtually impossible to intervene rationally in the hurried steps between obtaining to preparing to injecting drugs among addicts seeking to avoid acute withdrawal symptoms (Des Jarlais, Friedman, and Hopkins 1985). Indeed, our finding that a substantial percentage of needle-sharers report doing so more out of expediency and the need to inject than out of ignorance is perhaps relevant to the current debate on the merits of increasing the availability of sterile needles to IVDUs as a means of reducing the transmission of HIV infection.

Our data also suggest, however, that needle-sharing may not always be due merely to the scarcity of sterile injection equipment, with 52% of needle-sharers in the inmate group responding that they only shared with close friends or relatives, and 11% alluding to the social aspects of this practice as explanation for their continued needle-sharing. This may reflect the ethnographic observations that needle-sharing serves a powerful social function in street addicts who lack many other social supports, and that the refusal to share needles with one's "running buddy" is akin to a sexual refusal between lovers. It may also be evidence of the common misconception, revealed in the AIDS knowledge questionnaire scores especially among the inmate group, that "you can tell by looking at a person if they have AIDS": the belief that only ill-appearing people are potential sources of infection may lead to a mistaken sense of security about needle-sharing partners. These findings would indicate that effective interventions among street addicts must address both the social networks and the factual misinformation which may promote persistent high-risk needle use.

Logistic regression analysis indicated that persistent needle-sharing was associated with lower scores on the AIDS knowledge questionnaire; this may suggest that even though knowledge is not sufficient to deter such behavior in the setting of acute drug withdrawal, perhaps in the long run knowledge and effective education may help reduce high-risk IV drug use practices. The analysis also indicated that the detention facility study site was in itself predictive of persistent needle-sharing, which would imply that prison settings may be particularly important locations for targeting AIDS education for drug users. Preliminary pre- and post-test data generated from an AIDS education program which was implemented at the same detention facility site following completion of the present study do in fact suggest post-test improvement for inmates' scores on an AIDS knowledge questionnaire similar to the one described here. Whether knowledge leads directly to changes in risk behavior clearly remains to be seen; nevertheless, such knowledge is at least an important prerequisite for change.

It has been suggested that, because of the illicit nature of IV drug use in our society, IVDUs are a hidden population, only becoming visible when they seek treatment, are hospitalized, or are arrested (Ginzburg 1984a). This phenomenon underscores the importance of drug treatment programs, medical institutions, and, as noted, correctional facilities as ideal sites for interventions to reduce the risks of AIDS among IVDUs. As for the large reservoir of IVDUs not in treatment or in the correctional system, more imaginative outreach and education campaigns may be needed. Education is only one part of the process, however, and the obvious next step would be to try to go beyond effecting changes in knowledge to affecting changes in behavior. Whatever strategies are adopted, they must of necessity include expanded drug treatment facilities, at present oversubscribed with long waiting lists and an estimated 6:1 ratio of IVDUs to available treatment slots in New York City. Bringing more IVDUs into contact with the treatment system would increase the possibility for AIDS education as well as provide an accessible alternative to ongoing uncontrolled needle use.

Finally, a truly comprehensive approach to the crisis of AIDS among IVDUs may need to include not only broad-based and innovative educational campaigns, nor only increased drug treatment facilities, but also perhaps, in the short term, strategies addressing the availability of sterile needles and syringes. Our data do not imply that merely increasing the supply of sterile injection equipment would eradicate needle-sharing in certain subgroups of IVDUs with deeply ingrained patterns of behavior. Nevertheless, our findings do suggest that it may be important to examine the issue of access to sterile needles and syringes in settings where the scarcity of such equipment may be a key factor in encouraging ongoing high-risk practices.

References

Centers for Disease Control. 1984. Declining rates of rectal and pharyngeal gonorrhea among males—New York City. M.M.W.R. 33:295-97.

———. 1985a. Heterosexual transmission of HTLV III/LAV. M.M.W.R. 34:561-63.

———. 1985b. Recommendations for assisting in the prevention of perinatal transmission of HTLV-III/LAV and AIDS. M.M.W.R. 34:721-32.

———. 1985c. Self-reported behavioral change among gay and bisexual men—San Francisco. M.M.W.R. 34:613-15.

———. 1987. AIDS program. *Weekly Surveillance Report*, 26 August.

Curran, J. W., W. Morgan, A. Hardy, H. Jaffe. 1985. The epidemiology of AIDS: current status and future prospects. *Science* 229:1352-57.

Des Jarlais, D. C., S. Friedman, and W. Hopkins. 1985. Risk reduction for the acquired immunodeficiency syndrome among intravenous drug users. *Ann. Intern. Med.* 103:755-59.

Echenberg, D. F. and G. Rutherford. 1986. The incidence and prevalence of LAV/HTLV-III infection in the San Francisco city clinic cohort 1985. Paper presented at the International Conference on AIDS, 23-26 June, Paris, France.

Friedland, G. H., C. Harris, and C. Small. 1985. Intravenous drug abusers and the acquired immunodeficiency syndrome (AIDS): demographic, drug use and needle sharing patterns. *Arch. Intern. Med.* 145:1413-17.

Friedman, S. R., D. Des Jarlais, and J. Sotheran. 1986. AIDS health education for intravenous drug users. *Health Education Quarterly* 13:383-93.

Ginzburg, H.M. 1984a. Intravenous drug users and the acquired immune deficiency syndrome. *Public Health Report* 99:206-12.

———. 1984b. A survey of attitudes concerning AIDS among clients in treatment. *Clinical Research Notes*, January. Rockville, Maryland: National Institute on Drug Abuse.

Landesman, S.H., H. Ginzburg, and S. Weiss. 1985. Special report: the AIDS epidemic. *N. Engl. J. Med.* 312:521-25.

Martin, J.L. 1986. Sexual behavior patterns, behavior change, and occurrence of antibody to LAW/HTLV-III among New York City gay men. Paper presented at the International Conference on AIDS, 23-26 June, Paris, France.

McKusick, L., W. Horstman, and T. Coates. 1985. AIDS and sexual behavior reported by gay men in San Francisco. *Am. J. Public Health* 75:493-96.

New Jersey State Department of Health. *Monthly AIDS Surveillance Report*, September 1, 1987.

New York City Department of Health, Surveillance Office. 1987. *AIDS Surveillance Update*, 26 August.

Spira. T.J. et al. 1985. HTLV-III/LAV antibodies in intravenous drug abusers: comparison on high-and-low-risk areas for AIDS. Paper presented at the International Conference on Acquired Immune Deficiency Syndrome (AIDS), 14-17 April, Atlanta, Georgia.

Weiss, S.H. 1985. Risks for HTLV-III/LAV exposure and AIDS among parenteral drug users in New Jersey. Paper presented at the International Conference on Acquired Immune Deficiency Syndrome (AIDS), 14-17 April, Atlanta, Georgia.

PART V

Social and Ethical Implications of AIDS

Acquired immunodeficiency syndrome (AIDS) is a disease surrounded by ethical questions as challenging as the medical uncertainties that still remain unanswered. Because of the prejudice that often accompanies an AIDS diagnosis—the prejudice of being labeled a member of a high-risk group, such as homosexual/bisexual or intravenous drug user, as well as the societal fears attached to the transmission of human immunodeficiency virus (HIV)—patients with this disease are often denied legal and social rights.

In Part V, authors from the fields of social work, medicine, and law examine some of the social and ethical issues associated with AIDS, especially in the case of the intravenous drug abuser. In Chapter 20, "AIDS: The Social Dimension," Siegel looks at AIDS as a disease of morally prohibited behaviors and the resultant difficulties faced by the AIDS patient in the realm of housing, jobs, and obtaining medical treatment. She notes that the medical uncertainty still surrounding some aspects of AIDS transmission contributes in large degree to the prejudices of society toward AIDS patients. The consequences may be the isolation of these patients, at a time when they most need the help and care of their friends and family.

Legal and ethical issues involved in the AIDS diagnosis or HIV seropositive status are the focus of Ginzburg (and Gostin) in Chapter 21. The author(s) note that many ethical questions will continue to call upon the judgment of treatment professionals: who should be informed of a patient's HIV exposure? What are the rights of the spouse, lover, or family of the HIV seropositive patient? Can or should physicians be required to report individuals with AIDS to governmental agencies? Should HIV testing sites be provided in order to prevent high-risk individuals from donating blood to assess

229

their own seropositivity? The privacy of medical records of AIDS patients, the duty to warn, and the risk of discrimination are all important legal issues that attend a diagnosis with AIDS.

20
AIDS: The Social Dimension

Karolynn Siegel, PhD.

Illness is a social state as well as a physical condition. Becoming ill has not only personal consequences, but also far reaching interpersonal implications as well. The assignment of a diagnosis affects both the behavior of the individual labeled as sick and the actions of others toward the patient (Freidson 1984). An understanding of how the responses of others influence the adaptation of the individual with the acquired immunodeficiency syndrome (AIDS) to his/her disease can help elucidate the psychiatric sequelae of the illness. This article describes several aspects of the public's reaction to AIDS and how these responses have become sources of significant psychological distress for both people with AIDS (PWAs) as well as others at substantial risk for infection with the causative viral agent, the human immunodeficiency virus (HIV).

AIDS and Scientific Uncertainty

From the outset of the AIDS epidemic, the disease has repeatedly been referred to as a "medical mystery." The scientific uncertainty that continues to surround a number of issues related to

Reprinted, with changes, from "AIDS: The Social Dimension," by Karolynn Siegel, *Psychiatric Annals* 16(3):168-72, by permission of Slack, Inc.

modes of transmission of the disease, and the relative infectivity of different groups of individuals exposed to HIV have contributed to the public impression that little is understood about AIDS and other HIV-related diseases. In reality, AIDS has been well characterized, both epidemiologically and clinically, in a relatively short period of time. Nevertheless, the public's perception of the scientific community's perplexity about these matters has led to the conclusion that it is wisest in matters of policy regarding infected individuals to err on the side of extreme precaution, even if such a position compromises the civil rights of certain groups.

The September 1985 controversy over whether New York City school children with AIDS should be permitted to attend classes with their peers highlighted the differences of opinion that exist even within the medical community concerning the relative risks of various types of nonintimate contact. Each side was able to present medical specialists who supported their position. When disagreement exists among the experts, the opportunity is created for nonexperts to assert their views and for these opinions to be accorded greater legitimacy than could occur under less controversial circumstances. Lay opinion, however, is often influenced more by fear, and by personal and moral values, than by the available scientific evidence.

The inability of the scientific community to develop an efficacious treatment for HIV diseases, and especially AIDS, or to rapidly develop a vaccine to contain the spread of the virus, has been a source of great consternation to the general public. Concomitantly, these perceived "failures" have heightened the public's feelings of being exposed and defenseless in the face of a terrifying illness. We live in a society in which knowledge is equated with power and mastery; conversely, lack of understanding is associated with weakness and a lack of control. This epidemic has caused much of the public to lose sight of the fact that a good deal of uncertainty characterizes many areas of medical practice, completely unrelated to AIDS.

Another source of ambiguity for the lay public concerns the number of clinical conditions, other than AIDS, which have been associated with HIV. AIDS-related complex (ARC), is an ill-defined constellation of different symptoms, usually associated with generalized lymphadenopathy and the presence of antibodies to HIV. There are also vast numbers of individuals who have been found to have antibodies to HIV, but who remain asymptomatic. Estimates of the prevalence of HIV infection among intravenous drug users range from 10% to more than 50% in various United States cities (MacDonald 1986) and between 17% and 68% (Curran et al. 1985) for homosexual men. A final group, perhaps numbering well into the millions, are defined by the Centers for Disease Control as being "at high risk" for HIV diseases, by virtue of either their lifestyle (sexually active male homosexuals, bisexuals, or intravenous drug users) or their receipt of contaminated blood or blood products (transfusion recipients, hemophiliacs, and neonates).

At the present time, there is considerable debate concerning the relative risks of developing AIDS once an individual has been infected with HIV or even after an individual has developed ARC. Cofactors or host susceptibility factors that may determine who will go on to develop HIV-related diseases remain incompletely unidentified. This incomplete scientific understanding on this and other points has permitted much public speculation on three issues: (1) the relative efficiency of different modes of transmission, (2) the ultimate number of individuals who will be infected with HIV who will develop and die of AIDS, and (3) the degree of risk experienced by the heterosexual portion of the population.

The first issue, the relative efficiency of various modes of transmission remains an area of some ambiguity. While it is generally recognized that unprotected anal intercourse is the riskiest sexual practice, the degree of risk inherent in deep kissing and oral intercourse, for example, remains uncertain. Casual (nonsexual) contact is also widely agreed to present no threat. Nevertheless, available poll data indicate that despite concerted efforts to educate the public that AIDS cannot be spread by casual contact, a significant percentage of the population is still misinformed.

When 1,500 adults were asked in a national survey if they thought it was safe or unsafe to associate with someone who had AIDS, assuming there is not physical contact, 36% said they thought it was unsafe and 7% were undecided (ABC News 1985).

Furthermore, there is little differentiation made by the many among those who are in risk groups, those who are seropositive, those with ARC, and those who have endstate HIV disease – AIDS. Fear seems to override the ability to maintain such distinctions. Thus, many more people are treated "as if" they had the disease than is warranted. This inclusive social definition of people with

AIDS has intensified with the public's sense of threat from the epidemic. It has also caused a great deal of personal anguish for risk group members, seropositive individuals, and those with ARC who, although not meeting the Centers for Disease Control surveillance criteria for a diagnosis of the disease, are treated by many as people with AIDS. These individuals have difficulties in managing their own fears and anxieties about their uncertain future when many respond to them as if they already have the fatal disease. Inevitably, the reactions of others become incorporated into the individual's self-perception, making it increasingly difficult for him/her to maintain a sense of psychological and physical well-being.

Evidence of the tendency of a substantial proportion of the population to exaggerate the prevalence of AIDS cases is available from a poll which surveyed 1,500 adults (ABC News 1985). Respondents were asked, "To the best of your knowledge, is the number of AIDS cases in the U.S. closer to a million or 10,000?" A full 29% incorrectly answered a million; another 8% said they didn't know.

The second issue, the ultimate number of individuals who will be infected with HIV and who will develop and die of AIDS, is the more frightening one. Public perceptions tend to largely discount the available scientific evidence that progress has been made in stemming the transmission of this disease. The present capacity to screen blood for the presence of HIV antibodies has minimized the risk of transfusion-associated AIDS. The new heat treatment procedure in the manufacture of factor VIII will minimize future cases of pediatric AIDS.

There is also considerable research evidence that a large proportion of homosexual and bisexual men have modified their sexual practices in an effort to prevent becoming infected or infecting others (Joseph et al. 1985; McKusick, Hortsman, and Coates 1985; Siegel and Bauman 1986).

Data also exist which indicate that many intravenous drug users are also making changes in their behavior in response to the threat of AIDS. One study of patients in methadone treatment found that over 90% knew AIDS was transmitted through sharing works and that 59% reported having adopted changes in their behavior to reduce their risk of AIDS (Des Jarlais and Friedman 1986). Another study of methadone patients and intravenous drug users under arrest found that 97% of the respondents were aware that AIDS was transmitted through needle-sharing, and over 60% said they had changed their behavior to reduce their chances of getting AIDS (Selwyn et al. 1985). The Institute of Medicine Report (1986) notes that these self-reports are supported by studies of the illicit market in sterile needles in New York City, which indicate that this market has increased greatly since the start of the epidemic.

A final issue on which there remains considerable uncertainty is the extent to which AIDS represents a significant health threat to nonhigh-risk group individuals. While there has been intermittent discussion in the mass media of the potential danger of the growing spread of AIDS beyond the established risk groups into the wider heterosexual community, there have also been periodic reassurances that the proportion of AIDS cases accounted for by nonrisk group members has remained relatively stable over time. Such seemingly conflicting messages have resulted in a sense of confusion among many regarding the actual magnitude of the risk of infection to most heterosexuals.

The proportion of PWAs among the various high-risk groups has remained relatively constant over the past several years (Fauci 1985). However, media coverage concerning the high prevalence of AIDS among heterosexual Africans and reports of United States cases of bidirectional heterosexual transmission continue to nurture the fear of the spread of the disease beyond the established high-risk groups in the United States. Regardless of the objective reality, much of the public has responded to the threat of AIDS and PWAs in terms of their subjective perception of events. Because of the fatal nature of AIDS and the odium ascribed to it, the sense of peril evoked by AIDS has been exceptional. In an effort to attenuate the public's sense of danger, social constructions (interpretations) of HIV-related disease have emerged that foster the ostracism of individuals infected with the virus.

AIDS As a Stigmatized Disease

AIDS was first identified in a small number of homosexual men in 1981 (Curran et al. 1985). Initial case-control studies revealed an association between a diagnosis of AIDS, and the number of sexual partners and certain sexual practices (Marmor et al. 1982; Jaffe et al. 1983). These findings contributed to an early popular stereotype that all PWAs engaged in a lifestyle characterized by a preoccupation with sexual gratification as reflected in a large number of anonymous furtive contacts (the so-called "fast lane sex"). Although subsequent research has revealed significant within- and between-group diversity in the sexual behavior of gay individuals with AIDS, ARC, and those infected with HIV although currently asymptomatic, this initial public image has persisted.

Initially, the syndrome was labeled by some as "GRID," Gay Related Immune Deficiency Syndrome. This perception has been perpetuated by the media, especially by their frequent use of the terms "gay plague" to refer broadly to AIDS and the reference to "gay cancer" when they refer to Kaposi's sarcoma.

The gay community quickly mobilized to respond to the AIDS crisis. Gay organizations were founded to meet the social support needs of PWAs. These groups received substantial media coverage and therefore buttressed the public's perception that AIDS was essentially a gay disease.

Once the association between AIDS and homosexuality was stated by the media, community reactions to AIDS were inextricably linked with attitudes toward homosexuality. While there has been greater societal tolerance of homosexuality as an alternative lifestyle in recent years, a 1982 opinion poll indicated that only one-third of the adult population of this country felt that homosexuality was an acceptable alternative lifestyle (Newsweek 1983). It is important to recognize that at the time there was still relatively little public awareness of AIDS. There is some evidence for assuming that the base of acceptance of homosexuality as an acceptable alternative lifestyle has been considerably eroded during the past 3 years. In a 1985 poll of 1,000 adults, 37% said their "opinion about homosexuals" had changed "for the worse" as a result of the AIDS epidemic (Gallup Organization Poll 1985). Furthermore, the growing social and political influences of the Moral Majority and other fundamentalist groups that denounce homosexuality have served as a countervailing force to the trend toward greater tolerance for homosexuality.

The fundamentalist groups have charged homosexuals with violating the cherished values of family life, procreation, and the lasting commitment with another individual through the institution of marriage. They have sought to emphasize the association of AIDS with homosexuality, even suggesting, in some instances, that the epidemic represents an act of divine retribution for the practice of unnatural sexual acts.

Intravenous drug abusers are a similarly stigmatized group. They are stereotypically viewed as antisocial deviants who are out of control of their lives and driven by their habit (Institute of Medicine 1986). This group is also typically viewed as being socially isolated and segregated from most of society. In reality, of course, intravenous drug abusers are represented in all social strata. Still, at the present time, because it is more widely recognized that gay individuals are well integrated into all social classes and occupations in American society and therefore that most of us are likely to have daily contact with them, they are perceived by more of the public as a more immediate threat. This is especially true for those who continue to hold the belief that the disease can be spread through casual contact.

Because intravenous drug users and homosexual men account for the overwhelming proportion of AIDS cases, an attitude held by a substantial segment of society is that AIDS is a self-inflicted disease: gay men have their own licentious behavior to blame for their plight, just as drug abusers have their needling sharing behavior to blame. A consequence of this interpretation is that many individuals with AIDS have been denied the privileges associated with being physically ill. Patients with AIDS do not receive empathy, sympathy, support, and assistance normally afforded the ill in our society.

AIDS and Morality

HIV diseases also are sexually transmitted diseases. They are sexually transmitted independent of the sexual preference of either partner. This is a significant factor in the public's response to this illness. Sexually transmitted diseases are widely regarded as the outcome of sexual excess and low moral character. Because of the traditionally strong association between sexual behavior and morality in American society, those who suffer from sexually transmitted diseases have commonly been viewed as depraved. Once the patient is so judged, his suffering is met with much less concern or compassion.

The image of wanton sexual behavior provokes primitive alarm. Every society has felt the necessity to establish customs to regulate sexual behavior. The universality of such mores suggests they perform a function essential to the preservation of society. On some collective preconscious or unconscious plane, gay men might be perceived as undermining the social order through their transgression of sexual customs. The resulting sense of danger may account for some of the seemingly unreasoned reactions toward gay men. Calls for quarantining gay men, regardless of whether they have been infected with HIV, are clearly inappropriate. Intravenous drug users are also considered social "pariahs." Drug abuse and homosexuality have been variously defined, throughout history, as sinful, criminal, and as evidence of mental illness.

Many segments of society wish to physically and socially distance themselves from the "defiled" PWAs. These sentiments have led to the growing social isolation of PWAs as well as high-risk group members. A principal social function of the labeling of some behaviors as deviant and applying social sanctions to those who practice these deviant acts is to reaffirm the existing norms and social barriers. Social labeling serves to provide definitional boundaries between the "upright" and the "normal" on the one hand, and the "corrupt" and "deviant" on the other.

The Social Consequences

Social support systems can effectively buffer many illness-related stresses and mitigate their potentially deleterious effects (Shumaker and Brownell 1985). However, PWAs are frequently denied the support physically ill individuals receive because of prevalent fears of contagion through casual contact and the social devaluation of those afflicted.

Not infrequently, the gay male diagnosed with AIDS has never informed his family of his sexual orientation. Thus, he is simultaneously confronted with the task of revealing both his gay lifestyle and his fatal illness. Most families can adjust to these revelations; some cannot. The sense of loss and abandonment, generated by family rejection, is profound. Some gay men are so fearful of rejection that they never disclose their lifestyle or their diagnosis to their family. They prefer to tell those who ask that they have "cancer."

Finally, the lovers and gay friends of some PWAs have dissolved relationships when the diagnosis of AIDS is revealed. While PWAs frequently state that they understand their ex-partner's and friends fear and panic, the sense of abandonment and loss that result do cause extraordinary distress. Gay men expect rejection from heterosexuals; they have generally assumed the acceptance and succor of their own homosexual community. A strong sense of betrayal often results when such support is not forthcoming.

In interviewing gay men today, one often discerns a certain self-doubt about their personal worth. Among those who had not achieved self-acceptance of their lifestyle prior to the AIDS epidemic, self-reproach is quite common. While many do not blame their choice of a homosexual lifestyle for this disease, an undercurrent of guilt and shame is still detectable in a substantial proportion of gay men. It is difficult to assess the role society's disparagement of homosexuals plays in promoting these feelings. Some PWAs manifest what has been termed "internalized homophobia." They have incorporated society's prejudicial judgments about their lifestyle into their own self-image (Christ and Wiener 1985).

Intravenous drug users with AIDS are also unlikely to obtain adequate support. Their sexual partners may flee when they learn of the PWAs illness. When they enter the medical care system they are likely to feel that the health professionals they encounter are unresponsive to their needs. These professionals tend to be ethnically, culturally, and socioeconomically dissimilar from the intravenous drug users and as a result feel uncomfortable with these patients. Their discomfort and lack of understanding of the drug users lifestyle often causes the health professional to interact with the patient in a distant, perfunctory manner. A mutual distrust of one another further exacerbates these problems.

Social Isolation

PWAs, people with ARC, seropositive individuals, and even risk group members frequently feel the need to conceal their diagnosis or lifestyle from their neighbors, landlords, and employers. They fear eviction and termination of employment. Loss of job often means a loss of medical insurance as well.

The necessary sexual and personal precautions PWAs are advised to follow to avoid infecting others, as well as to protect themselves, enhance their sense of isolation. Proscriptions against certain familiar forms of intimacy and relatedness create a feeling of separateness.

The medical community is changing its assertions about the range of uses the HIV serum antibody tests will have. While there is the potential for misuse — e.g., attempting to use the antibody tests

as a surrogate for determining whether an individual is homosexual—there is also a clinical utility in determining whether an individual is infected with HIV. Because health and life insurance
companies are considering the use of the antibody test in screening
applicants, it is important to state emphatically that the antibody
test is not capable of determining whether an infected individual will
develop either AIDS or ARC.

In most states, AIDS is a reportable disease to the state department of health. In Colorado, the presence of HIV antibodies is a
reportable condition to that state's health department. Thus, issues
of confidentiality and how the information will be used become critical issues. Mandatory testing is only required of those individuals
donating blood and military recruits. What policies will health and
life insurances attempt to adopt? Gay men fear mandatory testing.
They may be denied potential benefits or access to services. They
may be labeled, stigmatized, and ostracized from their social communities. These fears are especially poignant for the gay whose
sexual orientation is known to only a few.

At present, it is possible to avoid being tested for the presence
of HIV antibodies. Fears among intravenous drug users that they
may be tested if they enter treatment programs may serve as a barrier to their receiving help with their addiction. Many drug abusers
are suspicious and distrustful of large organizations or official agencies. This too, serves to reinforce their sense of isolation and alienation. Additionally, because drug users do not constitute an organized community, they have little political power with which to
oppose violations of their rights.

Thus, the spector of the loss of fundamental opportunities and
protections produces extraordinary stress for PWAs and high-risk
group members. This stress may be clinically manifested as diffuse
anxiety, reactive depression, and somatic complaints.

Conclusions

The medical uncertainties that still accompany HIV disease, the
fatal nature of AIDS, and the opprobrium that accompanies the illness, have resulted in constant public attention. A January 1986 poll
revealed that 76% of adults believe that AIDS already represents a
threat to the "general public" (Singer and Rogers 1986). Another

11% believe AIDS will come to represent such a threat in the next several years.

One collective response has been to socially and physically distance those who are perceived to represent a danger to the larger society. The social and psychological costs to those shunned has been enormous. Mental health professionals who are committed to the alleviation of emotional anguish must assume a public leadership role in addressing HIV and AIDS-associated social problems. They should seek not only to alleviate distress, but also to combat the prejudice and social discrimination that produce such suffering.

References

ABC News/Washington Post Poll. September 1985.

Christ, G.H., and L. Wiener. 1985. Psychosocial issues in AIDS. In *AIDS: etiology, diagnosis, treatment and prevention*, eds. V.T. Devita, S. Hellman, and S. Rosenburg. New York: Lippincott.

Curran, J.W., W. Morgan, and A. Hardy. 1985. The epidemiology of AIDS: current status and future prospects. *Science* 229:1352-57.

Des Jarlais, D.C., and S. Friedman. 1986. AIDS among intravenous drug users: current research in epidemiology, natural history and prevention strategies. Paper prepared for Committee on a National Strategy for AIDS. Institute of Medicine, National Academy of Sciences, Washington, D.C.

Fauci, A.S. 1985. Acquired immunodeficiency syndrome: an update. *Ann. Intern. Med.* 102:800-13.

Freidson, E. 1984. *The profession of medicine.* New York: Dodd Mead.

Gallup Organization Poll. November 1985.

Institute of Medicine. 1986. *Confronting AIDS: directions for public health, health care and research.* Washington D.C.: National Academy Press.

Jaffe, H.W., K. Choi, and P. Thomas. 1983. National case-control study of Kaposi's sarcoma and *pneumocystis carinii* pneumonia in homosexual men. Part I. Epidemiological results. *Ann. Intern. Med.* 99:145-51.

Joseph, J.G., C. Emmons, and R. Kessler. 1985. Changes in sexual behavior of gay men: relationships to perceived stress and psychological symptomatology.

Paper presented at the International Conference on the Acquired Immunodeficiency Syndrome (AIDS), 14-17 April, Atlanta, Georgia.

MacDonald, D.I. 1986. Coolfont report: a PHS plan for prevention and control of AIDS and AIDS virus. *Public Health Reports* 101:34-348.

Marmor, M., A. Friedman-Kein, and L. Laubenstein. 1982. Risk factors for Kaposi's sarcoma in homosexual men. *Lancet* 1:1083=87.

McKusick, L., W. Hortsman, and T. Coates. 1985. AIDS and sexual behavior reported by gay men in San Francisco. *Am. J. Public Health* 75:493-96.

Newsweek. 1983. Poll on homosexuality. *Newsweek.* 8 August, p. 33.

Selwyn, P.A., C. Cox, C. Feiner, C. Lipshutz, and R. Cohen. 1985. Knowledge about AIDS and high risk behavior among intravenous drug abusers in New York City. Paper presented at the Annual Meetings of the American Public Health Association, November, Washington, D.C..

Shumaker, S.A., and A. Brownell. 1985. Toward a theory of social support. *Social Forces* 40:11-33.

Siegel, K., and L. Bauman. 1986. Patterns of change in sexual practices among gay men in New York City. Paper presented at the Annual Meetings of the American Sociological Association, August, New York.

Singer, E., and T. Rogers. 1986. Public opinion and AIDS. *AIDS and Public Policy* 1:8-13.

21
Legal and Ethical Issues Associated with HIV Diseases

Harold M. Ginzburg, MD, JD, MPH; and
Larry Gostin, JD.

Human immunodeficiency virus (HIV)-associated diseases have been primarily reported among groups that are considered separate from the mainstream of society—male homosexuals and intravenous drug users (Curran, Morgan, and Hardy 1985; Centers for Disease Control 1985a, 1985b). Both homosexuality and intravenous drug use are often associated with status offenses. That is, homosexual activity between consenting adults is considered to be a felony in many jurisdictions; the United States Supreme Court is to examine the constitutionality of these statutes this term. Possession of narcotics, or drug paraphernalia, regardless of any intent to distribute the drug, is also punishable by incarceration in most jurisdictions. Medical conditions associated with either of these proscribed behaviors have negative or pejorative social value. However, it would be a mistake for public health officials or health care personnel to be influenced by these punitive or "popular" social attitudes toward primary risk groups.

There are a great number of legal and ethical issues concerning those at risk of, or actually infected with, HIV; we discuss only a few

Reprinted with changes, from "Legal and Ethical Issues Associated with HTLV-III Diseases," by Harold M. Ginzburg and Larry Gostin, *Psychiatric Annals* 16(3):180-85, by permission of Slack, Inc.

of the more important issues here. Patients with acquired immunodeficiency syndrome (AIDS) have similar legal expectations to
those of other patients: the right to provide informed consent to
testing procedures, such as the diagnostic tests for infections with
HIV, treatment, and participation in research protocols; confidentiality of medical records; and the right to make a will for the dis-
position of their property, as they wish. For AIDS patients, these
basic expectations can be complicated by the fact that many will
have neurological damage caused by HIV infection, and their competency may be under question (Snider, Simpson, and Nielson 1983;
Navia and Price 1986).

Those infected with HIV suffer the stigma of having an infectious and potentially lethal virus and are often members of risk
groups with histories of unequal access to treatment. Private discrimination in areas of employment, housing, and insurance have
long been experienced by high-risk group members; disclosure of
their HIV antibody status can trigger further discrimination. Public
officials are pursuing methods for slowing the spread of the virus
and are under pressure to initiate protective measures: quarantine,
segregation in prison facilities, expulsion from treatment facilities
and from certain occupations such as school teaching, food handling,
the armed forces, and health care. These measures can interfere
with the liberty, autonomy, or privacy of risk group members. Even
public meeting places such as bathhouses and gay clubs are being
targeted for closure or strict regulation, thus affecting freedom of
association of those who frequent these establishments.

Other generic issues that may need to be addressed when dealing with patients with HIV-related diseases include the rights and
responsibilities of surviving partners in homosexual couples to
determine funeral arrangements and to safeguard property rights
after death; similar problems, including child custody matters, must
also be dealt with by heterosexual couples, especially if they are not
married.

In this article, the legal and ethical issues associated with HIV
disease will be identified, discussed, and described. However, an initial caveat is necessary. The law is reactive. Laws are passed to meet
the perceived needs of the community. Interpretation of a law occurs when the court attempts to apply that law or legal principle to
the controversies before it. Thus, if there is the potential for avoid-
ing litigation by the preparation of proper informed consent docu-

ments, living wills, interviews transfers, and health and antidiscrimination regulations, then such actions should be initiated. Anticipatory legal planning often prevents needless, time-consuming, and expensive litigation.

Confidentiality of a person's HIV antibody status is particularly important because of the potential personal, social, and economic harms that may result from disclosure of this information. Thus, blood banks, health care personnel, and researchers have all sought to scrupulously ensure the confidentiality of records. Federal regulations exist to protect the confidentiality of drug and alcohol records (Confidentiality of alcohol and drug abuse patient records 1985). Federal regulations also exist to protect the identity of research subjects (Protection of identity of research subjects 1979). There are no equivalent federal protections for doctor-patient communications. However, patients' confidences are protected at common law and by statute in a number of states (*Matter of Application quash subpoena duces tecum in grand jury proceedings* 1981). There is a common law doctor-patient privilege that protects the confidentiality of records even against judicial process unless overridden by a compelling state interest (AIDS Legal Guide 1984). The purpose of the physician-patient privilege is to promote an honest, therapeutic relationship with full communication (AIDS Legal Guide 1984). Confidentiality is to be maintained, but information can be shared with other clinicians on a "need to know" basis; there is also a reporting requirement for some infectious diseases in all states.

Privacy and Reporting Requirements

Information concerning an individual's health status belongs to that individual, unless it is required to be shared with a government agency. State laws require the reporting of specific infectious diseases for case identification, case finding, and treatment. Each state establishes which diseases are reportable to its state health department. Centers for Disease Control-defined AIDS is a reportable disease in most states. Colorado and Minnesota are the only states that require the reporting of those who have antibodies to HIV. The Centers for Disease Control have developed a definition of adult and pediatric AIDS, and maintain a semianonymous registry of such cases (Centers for Disease Control 1985a, 1985b). A soundex coding system is used to report AIDS cases from New York and other jurisdictions. This system was initiated to provide reassurance to physicians that patient identity will be protected.

A person with HIV infection has the right to keep this information private under some state laws and constitutional provisions. The United States Constitution has been determined to protect in matters relating to personal sexual conduct and the use and selection of contraceptives (Griswold 1965; Eisenstat 1972).

Privileged communication is information that is private and not subject to disclosure. A privilege is usually recognized between priest and penant, doctor and patient, lawyer and client, and husband and wife. Insurance records are only privileged in ten states; medical records are not privileged in Nebraska, New Mexico, and South Carolina (Sourcebook of Criminal Justice Statistics 1984); states do not have privileged communication statutes (Sourcebook of Criminal Justice Statistics 1984). Patients, therefore, have a right to be concerned about their ability to control the dissemination of their sensitive and potentially damaging medical information. Special protections for HIV-related medical data may need to be provided in those jurisdictions that currently lack the appropriate medical records and privileged communication statutes if AIDS patients and others who may be actively infective are to seek medical care and treatment.

The Duty to Warn

Individuals with antibodies to HIV, including AIDS patients, have a right to confidentiality of their medical records. But is there a duty to warn those in foreseeable danger of contracting HIV from the patient with AIDS? Recent litigation wherein one adult sexual partner sues the other because of the failure to warn of the potential exposure to herpes suggests that analogous law suits involving HIV may be filed in due course (Kathleen 1984). Must married partners, who find that they have been infected with HIV, as determined by the ELISA test and confirmed by the Western blot test, inform their spouses? These tests indicate that there are antibodies to the virus. They do not indicate, with certainty, that the individuals were infective at the time the tests were conducted. If the female partner has not been notified that her male consort has been found to demonstrate the presence of antibodies, and becomes pregnant and delivers an infant with AIDS or early evidence of HIV related diseases, is there liability? If there is liability, to whom and for what? By analogy, there have been instances of wrongful birth suits. Who is legally and ethically responsible for providing medical care of an infant with AIDS or other evidence of HIV-related diseases? Does the ultimate responsibility rest with the public hospital, or with the local, state, or federal government? AIDS assistance acts, such as the one passed by the New Jersey legislature in 1984, provide some economic relief.

Mental Competency

Reports by Navia (1986) and Snider, Simpson, and Nielson (1983) that HIV is neurotropic present a series of medical and legal conundrums. Initially, all of the neurological symptoms observed in AIDS patients were thought to be due to secondary infections that resulted from a compromised immune system. However, more recent research has demonstrated that HIV directly attacks neuronal tissue. The resultant clinical picture resembles Alzheimer's disease, but with a much more rapid clinical progression of the dementia (Snider, Simpson, and Nielson 1983). In a short span of time, individuals become demented. They are unable to care for themselves. Family (or significant others) need to be informed of the patient's condition and take necessary actions if the dementia has already progressed to a stage in which judgment is substantively impaired. Patients and their "significant others" need to anticipate the degenerative process and arrange for a power of attorney or a court-appointed guardian to deal with financial matters and funeral arrangements. If an AIDS patient agrees to participate in a research protocol and becomes incompetent to withdraw his or her consent, who will protect the patient? Consent of a patient who subsequently becomes incompetent is ineffective. Must research protocols stop when a patient becomes demented unless prior arrangements have been made? Clearly, these issues must be resolved in the near future or many research studies analyzing the endstages of the neurological aspects of AIDS will never be initiated and completed. Protection of the human rights of these patients must be ensured by courts and institutional review boards consistent with the importance of continuing research endeavors.

The incompetency of patients that may result from AIDS dementia is also a major problem in areas such as treatment and disposal of property. Many patients suffering from a fatal disease have personal choices to make about the level to which they wish to have continued life thrust on them by extraordinary means. Further, when they die, some may wish to make provisions for close relationships that were not bound by marriage and which are not recognized by the state. Once the diagnosis of AIDS is made and confirmed, the prognosis is poor and the possibility of dementia foreseeable. In those circumstances, state legislatures must devise procedures for allowing the patient to plan while competent, e.g., by making a durable power of attorney, a living will, or by making his or her wishes known in guardianship proceedings.

Public Health Powers

HIV-related diseases have generated a primitive community response based on a mixture of irrational prejudice and understandable fear. Historically, American communities have periodically introduced public health powers such as quarantine on those with infectious disease, particularly those who are considered socially unacceptable (Brandt 1985). The quarantine programs for prostitutes, during both World War I and II, were ineffective in controlling venereal diseases (Brandt 1985). Communities must be made to understand that any coercive public health measures must be based upon "public health necessity." Such powers can only be justified where there is clear medical and epidemiologic evidence to demonstrate their effectiveness, and where the rights of individuals are not simply set aside. Expulsion of AIDS patients from society does not protect the community. Curran, Morgan, and Hardy (1985) have estimated that, for every AIDS case reported, there are at least 50 to 100 asymptomatic infectious carriers of the AIDS virus in both the intravenous drug-using community and the sexually active homosexual and bisexual communities. Thus, removing the symptomatic without identifying and removing the asymptomatic does not protect a community. Rather, it gives that community a false sense of security until the next asymptomatic carrier becomes ill.

Discrimination

There has also been a great deal of pressure to exclude AIDS patients from various occupations, housing, and medical resources.

School boards, for example, have refused admission to children with AIDS in New York City. This discriminatory activity has occurred in the face of evidence that the spread of HIV among children through saliva and social contact is minimal (Current Trends 1985). The Centers for Disease Control has promulgated guidelines for addressing the needs of school children who are symptomatic (Current Trends 1985). These guidelines have met with significant opposition. In the final analysis, some school boards are asking Centers for Disease Control for a legal guarantee that if they follow Centers for Disease Control guidelines their children will be protected. The Centers for Disease Control cannot give a legal guarantee that some child, infected with HIV, will not bite a classmate and infect him with the virus. There are very few scientific certainties, and few scientists are willing to give unqualified statements about the certainty of an infectious disease not spreading between two individuals who will have some contact with each other.

Some jurisdictions, such as Los Angeles, have passed city ordinances that designate AIDS as a handicap. This designation precludes patients with AIDS from being discriminated against by employers. Patients with AIDS are thus "entitled" to continue to be employed as health care workers, even if they are known to be actively infected with HIV and other secondary infections. What are the rights of those they will come in contact with? Health care workers are concerned about becoming infected with HIV by an accidental needlestick; patients have the same rational fears about their service providers. What is the responsibility and liability of a viremic and infective health care professional to his or her patients? Health care workers with infectious hepatitis, type B, can be prevented from providing direct medical care until they are serum antigen-negative. When does alleged discrimination become redefined as reasonable practice?

Availability of Alternative Test Sites for HIV Antibody Testing

Preliminary estimates suggest that 8% to 10%, per year, of HIV seropositive individuals will develop AIDS; an equal or higher rate is associated with the development of AIDS-related conditions, including generalized lymphadenopathy, neurological complications, diverse malignancies, and other carcinomas (Curran, Morgan, and

Hardy 1985; Wong-Staal and Gallo 1985). For those who do not become acutely ill, chronic degenerative diseases may evolve (Wong-Staal and Gallo 1985). Thus, it is understandable that those members of high-risk groups may want to know their antibody status. This is especially important when Wong-Staal and Gallo state that their coworkers can isolate HIV from peripheral blood of more than 80% of people with serum antibodies to the virus, and that this is a conservative estimate because of technical difficulties with some of the blood specimens (Wong-Staal and Gallo 1985).

The Food and Drug Administration has licensed commercial assays that can determine the presence of HIV antibodies in blood and blood products. The approved indications for the use of this product is in the testing of blood and blood products by blood banks. In some areas, patient and physician access to these tests have been limited. In New York City, where more than one-third of all cases of AIDS have been reported, the Commissioner of Health, on 8 February 1985, issued an emergency order restricting the use of the HIV antibody test to blood bank screening and research purposes only and making it illegal for commercial laboratories to perform the test for private physicians (Caiazza 1985). Therefore, it is not surprising to have individual clinicians report that their high-risk patients are donating blood so that they may find out whether or not they are carrying antibodies to HIV (Caiazza 1985).

The value of alternative test sites is obvious and has been documented; at an alternative test site in Massachusetts, 13% of high-risk group members were positive (Forstein, Page, and Carwell 1985). Not only is an emotional strain being placed on those who wish to know their status, but in their quest for their antibody status they may be threatening potential recipients of their blood products. While the antibody test is sensitive and specific, it does not determine whether or not an individual is viremic. A recently infected individual may be viremic (virus positive) and antibody negative (Wong-Staal and Gallo 1985).

Blood banks voluntarily screen all donated blood and blood products for the presence of antibodies to HIV. Blood that has been determined to have antibodies to HIV is not used for human purposes. The blood banks request that members of high-risk groups not donate blood; they also ask donors to indicate if their blood should only be used for research purposes. This provides an opportunity for someone who gives blood during a "blood drive" to divert his or her blood from use without having to explain to friends or colleagues why they have not donated blood. However, there is no guarantee that someone who wants to know their antibody status, and elects to donate blood to obtain their test results, will indicate to the blood bank staff that their blood should not be used. Therefore, both to further protect his country's blood supply, and to provide clinically useful results to patients, it might be advisable to either expand the alternative test site program or permit commercial laboratories to conduct HIV antibody testing.

Conclusions

The entire range of HIV infection poses a host of legal and ethical issues that require careful thought. Central to the resolution of these issues are the rights of privacy and confidentiality of patients to avoid disclosure of their disease status, except to clinicians, researchers, and public health officials. Patients with HIV infection also retain their ordinary right to provide informed consent in relation to research, testing, and treatment. The increasing number of such patients whose competency is in question raises issues that society has already considered in depth in the context of mental health, aging, and dying. Finally, individuals should retain their freedom of movement in the face of increased pressure on public health officials to exercise compulsory powers.

These rights of liberty, autonomy, and privacy apply to patients infected with HIV, as they do to any other patients. But, these rights are not absolute. They may yield to a compelling state interest, but only where there is clear scientific evidence that they are necessary for public health. As yet, no such evidence exists to justify deprivation of the rights of HIV-infected patients.

References

AIDS Legal Guide: A Professional Resource on AIDS-Related Legal Issues and Discrimination. 1984. New York: Lambda Legal Defense and Education Fund, Inc., 18-23.

Brandt, A.M. 1985. *No magic bullet: a social history of venereal disease in the United States since 1880.* New York: Oxford University Press.

Caiazza, S.S. 1985. Letter to the editor. *N.*

Engl. J. Med. 313:1158.

Centers for Disease Control. 1985a. Revision of the case definition of acquired immunodeficiency syndrome for national reporting—United States. 1985. *Ann. Intern. Med.* 103:402-3.

———. 1985b. Acquired immunodeficiency syndrome (AIDS). *Weekly Surveillance Report.* 18 December.

Confidentiality of alcohol and drug abuse patient records. 1985. *40 FED. REG. 27802-21.*

Curran, J.W., W. Morgan, and A. Hardy. 1985. The epidemiology of AIDS: current status and future prospects. *Science* 229:1352-57.

Current trends. 1985. Education and foster care of children infected with human T-lymphotropic virus type III/lymphadenopathy associated virus. *M.M.W.R.* 34:517-21.

Eisenstat v. Baird, 405 U.S. 438 (1972).

Forstein, M., P. Page, and R. Carwell. 1985. Letter to the editor. *N. Engl. J. Med.* 313:1158.

Griswold v. Connecticut, 381 U.S. 479 (1965).

Kathleen v. Robert, 150 Cal.Apped 992, 198 Cal Rptr 273 (1984).

Matter of Application quash subpoena duces tecum in grand jury proceedings, 56 N.Y. 2d 348, 452 N.Y.S.2d 361, 437 N.E.2d 1118 (1981).

Navia, B.A., and R.W. Price. 1986. Dementia complicating AIDS. *Psych. Ann.* 16:158-66.

Protection of identity of research subjects. 1979. 44 FED.REG. 20382-87. (1979).

Snider, W.D., D. Simpson, and S. Nielson. 1983. Neurological complications of acquired immune deficiency syndrome: analysis of 50 patients. *Ann. Neurol.* 14:403-18.

Sourcebook of Criminal Justice Statistics 1984. 1985. Washington, D.C.: General Printing Office, p. 629.

Wong-Staal, F., and R. Gallo. 1985. Human T-lymphotropic retroviruses. *Nature* 317:395-403.

22
Drug-Dependent Populations: Legal and Public Policy Options

Larry Gostin, JD.

Intravenous (IV) drug users are a major risk group for human immunodeficiency virus infection in the population. They comprise approximately 17% of cases of acquired immunodeficiency syndrome (AIDS) reported to the Centers for Disease Control (1987). More important, they are probably the population in which HIV infection is spreading most rapidly. New York City has an estimated 250,000 heroin addicts; fully 37% of the city's 9,709 reported cases involve present or past IV drug users as a risk factor (Centers for Disease Control 1987).

HIV infection among IV drug users is also probably the single most important reason for the spread of the infection to nonrisk groups, including heterosexuals and children. Some two-thirds of all heterosexual cases of AIDS involve present or past IV drug users, their sexual partners, or their children (Centers for Disease Control 1987).

Preventing the continued spread of HIV infection within drug-dependent populations is one of the major contemporary public health objectives. But the task is also one of the most difficult. HIV infection among IV drug users is caused primarily by the sharing of

The author expresses his appreciation to Michael Witt, Warner & Stackpole, for his able assistance with this chapter.

253

contaminated needles. This behavior is extremely resistant to change. First, IV drug users are usually physically and mentally dependent on the drug. It is unrealistic to expect them to give up their habit easily. Second, the population tends to be less educated and responsive to traditional modes of public education. IV drug users are an insular minority immersed in their own culture. As a result, modification of their behavior using public health education techniques is a formidable task. There are, however, some signs that the population is beginning to understand the danger from HIV infection (Craddock, Bray, and Hubbard 1983; Des Jarlais, Friedman, and Hopkins 1985). Third, obtaining sterile (infection-free) needles is extremely difficult and usually unlawful (Ginzburg et al. 1986). Even if this population consciously chose to use their drugs more safely, they would have difficulty finding sterile equipment. The legalism and moralism attached to illicit drug use stands as a formidable obstacle to controlling the epidemic among drug users.

Given the difficulty of developing a public health strategy to cope with the spread of HIV infection in drug-dependent populations, what is the appropriate course? In this chapter, I propose a voluntary, well-funded system comprising the following elements: (1) identify drug users who are HIV positive; (2) provide a program of education, counseling, and treatment, using traditional clinics as well as innovative outreach programs; and (3) provide a legal milieu to encourage voluntarism and cooperation through confidentiality and antidiscrimination statutes.

It may be argued that if the disease is so devastating, and if the foregoing voluntary programs provide a useful strategy, why not impose compulsory measures? I will also seek to state the case against the introduction of compulsory screening, reporting, and personal control measures. A more complete statement of this case has been published elsewhere (Gostin and Curran 1987a, 1987b; Gostin, Curran, and Clark 1987).

Identification of HIV Infection: Screening and Reporting

IV drug users already have a dependency which seriously threatens their life and well being. The threat of HIV infection adds to the health risks. The additional threat of HIV infection can be a motivator for change of behavior. While drug-dependent people may not stop taking drugs entirely, they have a strong incentive for using sterile needles to prevent HIV infection.

One of the foundations for voluntary alteration of behavior is knowledge about serologic status. Individuals can make the best decisions about the health of themselves and others if they are tested for HIV antibodies. Knowledge of HIV seropositivity can allow a person to take precautions in the future with respect to needle-sharing and sexual contacts. It may also serve as an incentive for seeking early treatment.

Testing for HIV should be widely available to IV drug users. Facilities for testing should be located in centers for the treatment of drug dependency. Outreach programs should be designed to inform drug-dependent people of the importance of testing, and where they can go for cost-free and confidential testing. Test sites should be in convenient urban locations. Alternative test sites often have long waiting times, inconvenient locations, and uncertain confidentiality protection. The Centers for Disease Control (1986) has recommended wide-scale testing among high-risk populations. At the time of this writing, however, there has been no development of a strategic plan or allocation of adequate resources (McAuliffe, 1987).

Screening for HIV infection among IV drug users comprises one element of a comprehensive program to alter high-risk behavior. Should such screening programs be mandatory? one proposal would be to require screening as a condition of entry into treatment centers for drug dependency.

There are strong reasons against a compulsory screening program (Gostin and Curran 1987a; Gostin, Curran, and Clark 1987). The objective of collecting information about seropositivity is to educate and counsel the individual to willingly alter his or her behavior. There is no evidence for the proposition that compulsory testing for HIV infection will produce voluntary changes in behavior. Individuals who are willing and able to change their behavior could voluntarily submit to testing.

It could be argued, of course, that the force of law could be used if individuals did not change their behavior. But the consequence of using compulsory screening and control measures would be to deter cooperation by the IV drug population. IV drug users would be concerned about the use of the test information to impose restrictions on their freedoms and to trace their intimate contacts. One possible consequence, then, of requiring a compulsory test as a precondition for entry into a treatment program is that participation in that program might be discouraged. IV drug treatment programs have a vital public health function which could be undermined by introducing compulsory measures. Thus, even if a marginal individual benefit from compulsory screening could be demonstrated, the benefit would be outweighed by the potential damage to important public health programs. Proponents of compulsory screening at IV drug treatment centers have the burden of demonstrating a public health benefit from the test information which overrides the negative consequences.

Education, Counseling, Treatment, and Rehabilitative Services

Testing for HIV antibodies will indicate whether a person is infected. But that information is of little benefit unless it is accompanied by clear and focused information about the meaning of the test. High-risk groups must receive information on how to live in a way which promotes health and strengthens the immune system. They must also receive clear and explicit information on how to avoid catching or transmitting the infection (Friedman et al. 1986; Ginzburg et al. 1986).

Public education and counseling are important for any group at risk for AIDS, but IV drug users present special challenges. Many consider it a useless endeavor to try to educate this population. No comprehensive educational campaigns have been directed towards IV drug users to try to promote safer needle-using behavior. The federal government and many state governments have taken a legalistic-moralistic view which presents an obstacle to effective education. IV drug use, it is asserted, is unlawful. For those wishing to change this unlawful behavior, there are clinics. The idea that people should be taught to use illegal drugs more safely has barely reached the attention of policymakers. This attitude is beginning to change, and some education programs are now being instituted (Craddock, Bray, and Hubbard 1983; Des Jarlais, Friedman, and Hopkins 1985).

The resistance of IV drug users to behavior change means that the public education message must "reach out" into the communities where they live. Innovative projects are being implemented in those areas where drug abuse is endemic, such as in New York City and northern New Jersey. These programs utilize people who were formerly a part of the drug use community to inform people in graphic terms about the dangers of using unsterilized needles, the methods of sterilizing needles, and the importance of testing and treatment. Well-funded outreach programs are essential to ensure that IV drug users receive the education and support needed to impede the spread of HIV infection.

Programs of education are beginning to have some impact among IV drug users. Studies from New York and New Jersey have shown that IV drug users are educable. In two New Jersey surveys, IV drug users entering treatment were able to identify the signs and symptoms of HIV disease, and were knowledgeable about means of transmission. They understood that behaviors such as sharing needles are dangerous. Apparently, the powerful health risk of HIV infection, when presented in clear terms, is a message which can be understood (Craddock, Bray, and Hubbard 1983; Des Jarlais, Friedman, and Hopkins 1985).

Policymakers must contend with the fact that many IV drug users are not going to quit their habit by simple education or even treatment. Given the fact that they will continue using drugs, it is essential that they receive clear information on the safer forms of needle use. They should be informed not to share needles; if they continue to share, then needles should be sterilized.

Treatment and rehabilitation of persons with drug dependency are an indispensable part of the public health function. At present, there are long waiting lists for treatment centers in many American cities with high rates of HIV infection. It is estimated that 750,000 people use IV drugs at least once a week; a similar number inject drugs less often (Ginzburg 1986). The vast majority of these people are not in treatment, and those who are spend an average of only six months as drug-free individuals. It simply makes no sense to face an epidemic spread in large part by shared use of needles without adequate drug treatment facilities. The law already proscribes IV drug abuse. But, short of preventive confinement, IV drug users will continue to spread the infection, unless they are given public support to help free them from physical dependency. Publicly provided treatment and financial support are necessary public health measures in this context.

Clean Needle Program

Harold Ginzberg (1986) explained the method of transmission of HIV through needle-sharing in a recent symposium issue on AIDS in *Law, Medicine and Health Care*:

> "Drug abusers self-administer heroin and cocaine parenterally in a non-sterile manner. The 'dose' is diluted with reagents (ranging from baking soda to strychnine) and injected, usually into a vein, through unsterile needles and syringes ('works') that, in many cases, have been used by other drug abusers."

Drug-dependent people, then, can inject themselves with HIV by the common practice of sharing drug paraphernalia. This can occur in private or in "shooting galleries" where there is a custom and camaraderie connected with sharing. Thus, one reason for the dangerous practice of sharing needles is purely social. This social aspect can only be broken by getting clear public health information to people in their communities and galleries. Stricter law enforcement for the purpose of preventing drug use and closing shooting galleries are unlikely to dissuade those who are physically dependent.

The most important reason for unsafe needle-sharing is not social, but legal and financial. The possession of drug paraphernalia is illegal across the country (Witt, 1986, personal communication). Most states do allow the purchase of insulin needles and syringes. However, many states in the Northeast, where IV drug use and IV infection are most prevalent, require a medical prescription for the purchase of hypodermic needles. In these states, the possession and use of needles is strictly limited. In Massachusetts, for example, only specified health care professionals can be in possession of hypodermic syringes, needles, or any instrument adapted for the administration of controlled substances by injection. A physician may write a written prescription for a patient under his or her immediate charge for the administration of controlled substances. A wholesale druggist or surgical supplier must keep careful records of the sale of syringes and needles. Failure to comply with this law is punishable by fine and imprisonment. If a person is charged with illegally possessing hypodermic syringes or needles, he or she has the burden of proving that he or she has sufficient authority or licenses to possess them.

The "legitimate medical purposes" doctrine is intended to hold a prescription invalid unless it was prescribed in good faith for a therapeutic purpose. On its face, this would prohibit a physician from prescribing for the purposes of injection of illicit drugs. An argument could be made that a physician can validly prescribe for the purpose of preventing transmission of HIV. This would not, however, seem to comport with the current consensus on what constitutes proper medical practice.

Perhaps the greatest public health challenge is to devise policies which encourage safer patterns of behavior among drug-dependent people, without appearing to condone use of illicit drugs. It is necessary to take a bold step to help drug-dependent people to behave in a safer manner. The prospects for such a bold change in policy look grim in the face of government insistence that drug abuse is a crime that will be dealt with strictly. A comprehensive public health program should include the following:

1. Easier access to cost-free, sterile needles.

2. Use of intensive individual and group counselling, treatment, and rehabilitation services as an integral part of any needle distribution program.

3. Public education on the health risks of HIV, the use of non-sterile needles and how to obtain treatment and sterile needles.

This is a politically difficult proposal because it appears both to condone and to encourage criminal behavior. However, a properly devised public health program would not promote illicit drug use. The objective is not simply to distribute sterile needles but to ensure safer needle use, as well as education, treatment, and rehabilitation.

Any needle distribution system would have to carefully control distribution of the needles. If a "needle exchange" program were adopted, dependent persons could exchange dirty needles for clean ones. If distribution centers were utilized rather than pharmacies, they could provide a focal point for intensive education, counseling, and encouragement to seek treatment.

Another alternative would be to loosen the legal regulations of prescriptions for sterile needles. Physicians could prescribe a sterile needle, expressly for the purpose of preventing transmission of disease through dirty equipment. Such prescriptions could be filled at specially licensed pharmacies or distribution centers, where HIV education programs could occur. Clearly, there are practical problems with this approach. Physicians who generally do not practice in the drug-dependency area would be faced with hard choices. Physicians and pharmacists could feel discomfort with such a legal responsibility; such discomfiture could be addressed through separately licensing the practitioners or pharmacies, while educational programs at the state licensure board level could address the scope of the practitioners' duties and constraints in this area. Unfortunately, looser regulation also has the potential for abuse by practitioners. Nevertheless, people who are physically dependent on drugs will find ways to get needles if we do not provide them. It is further unlikely that a physician-operated system would promote the use of illicit drugs.

It may be wise to establish one of these programs on a trial basis in a designated area. As part of this trial, we could test the needle-sharing patterns of those outside the experimental areas, with several different experimental programs. Experimental programs might test the utility of authorizing only certain facilities, with special controls for distribution of needles and individual and professional accountability.

One difficulty with an experimental program is that it might lead to stockpiling of needles which will be sold or even reused after the experimental program is over. Temporary programs could well exacerbate the problem. Longer term "clean needle" programs, therefore, would be a better alternative. This problem could be obviated also by careful controls, perhaps through a needle exchange program.

Whatever method is adopted, it is clear that some kind of "clean needle" program is essential. Public health officials cannot ignore the rapid spread of disease among people who have little meaningful control over their behavior. As an adjunct to education, counseling, and treatment, public health officials are well advised to adopt a clean needle program.

Confidentiality and the Duty to Warn

Confidentiality is of major importance in the areas of drug dependence and AIDS. Such information can include, for example, medical and social histories of sexual practices, or the extent and frequency of illicit drug usage. These data are universally regarded as confidential, and HIV-infected people are predominantly members of risk groups subject to persistent prejudice and discrimination.

There are already special statutes at the federal and state levels which provide for confidentiality of information about treatment for IV drug dependency (Pascal 1987). Most state statutes classify AIDS as a communicable, as opposed to a venereal, disease. Under these statutes, AIDS patients are afforded inadequate or nonexistent confidentiality protection. A few states, such as California and Massachusetts, have enacted specific legislation or regulations to protect the confidentiality of HIV antibody test results. Adequate statutory protection of confidentiality is essential because enlisting the cooperation of risk groups with public health objectives is largely dependent upon their expectations of privacy.

Balanced against the duty of confidentiality is the obligation to protect others from transmission of HIV. Courts have held that health care professionals must disclose confidential patient information to those who are in foreseeable danger of serious harm from their patients. The benchmark case is *Tarasoff* v. *The Regents of California*, 551 P.2d 340 (1976), which found a psychologist liable for failure to warn a third party of his patient's intention to murder her. The duty to protect third parties from contracting an infectious disease predates *Tarasoff* (Gostin, Curran, and Clark 1987). Early courts have held that a physician owes a duty to warn specific individuals in foreseeable danger of contracting an infection from his patient (*Wojcik* v. *Aluminum Co. of America*, 18 Misc.2d 740 [1959]; *Hoffmann* v. *Blackman*, 241 So.2d 752 [Fla. App. 1970]).

In a recent United States Court of Appeals case, it was held that there was no legal obligation to warn the general public of hepatitis B in the community; before a duty to warn exists, a physician must be aware of specific risks to specific persons (*Gammill* v. *U.S.*, 727 F.2d 950 [1984]). Thus, a reasonably specific and high degree of potential harm is required before the courts will find an affirmative duty to disclose confidential information.

The duty to protect third parties from transmission of HIV arises in relation to specific persons who the physician knows are likely to have an intimate exchange of bodily fluids with the patient. The steps the physician must take to fulfill this "duty to protect" are unclear though. But they at least include a threshold obligation to advise the patient of his responsibility to warn close contacts of his infection and to behave safely.

Those who test for the presence of HIV antibodies take on duties owed both to the patient to keep test results confidential and to third parties to protect them from foreseeable danger of contracting the infection. Physicians and public health officials, particularly in states with strict HIV confidentiality protection, face potential liability either way they decide. There are already strict statutory protection of confidentiality in relation to treatment for drug dependency. But the applicability of these statutes or general confidentiality statutes to AIDS is unclear. Strong confidentiality statutes, which make an explicit exception for foreseeable risks to specific persons, such as a spouse, are required.

In the absence of such a statute, physicians should consider maintaining confidentiality by counseling patients to inform their sexual contacts. When there are strong clinical grounds for believing that a specific contact has not been informed who is in serious danger from exposure to HIV, then the prudent course for the physician is to notify the contact of the positive serological status of the patient. Such a determination must be made, of course, in light of the specific state statutes and case law relating to confidentiality of medical information and testing results, and the duty to warn.

Antidiscrimination

Drug-dependent people with HIV infection are a minority which are virtual outcasts in society. There is a potential for significant discrimination against this group. Discrimination can occur in relation to jobs, insurance, and housing.

The Federal Rehabilitation Act of 1973 prohibits discrimination against the handicapped. There are similar "handicap discrimination" statutes in most states. Two questions arise from these statutes. First, do they protect IV drug users; and second, do they protect people with infectious diseases, including HIV infection or AIDS?

The Federal Rehabilitation Act was amended to exclude alcohol and drug-dependent people whose current abuse prevents the proper performance of their jobs. However, prior abuse or a condition in remission may still qualify as a handicap under that Act. Under state law in many jurisdictions, alcohol and drug dependency do qualify as handicaps. In *Hazlett* v. *Martin Chevrolet* (496 N.E.2d 478 [1986]) the Ohio Supreme Court held that dismissal of an employee who requested a leave of absence to obtain treatment for his dependency was unlawful discrimination on the basis of his handicap.

The Federal Rehabilitation Act has recently been held by the U.S. Supreme Court to cover infectious diseases. In *School Board of Nassau County* v. *Arline* (55 U.S.L.W 4245 [1987]) Justice Brennan wrote:

"Society's accumulated myths and fears about disability and disease are as handicapping as are the physical limitations that flow from actual impairment. Few aspects give rise to the same level of public fear and misapprehension as contagiousness . . . . The Act is carefully structured to replace such reflexive reactions with actual or perceived handicaps with actions based upon reasoned and medically sound judgments."

In a footnote, the U.S. Supreme Court explicitly refused to decide whether the 1983 Act protects carriers of HIV. Nonetheless, the *Arline* decision will give IV drug users with HIV infection a large measure of protection against discrimination.

In order to clarify some of these issues, some states have passed statutes explicitly giving protection against discrimination based upon real or perceived HIV infection or AIDS. These statutes, together with those protecting confidentiality, provide a milieu to encourage voluntarism and cooperation among IV drug users.

Summary and Conclusions

I have sought to identify briefly a cogent public health strategy for impeding the alarming spread of HIV among IV drug users. Federal and state governments urgently need to allocate substantial financial and personnel resources to provide:

1. Widespread testing and counseling in treatment centers and urban areas where IV drug users live.

2. Education focused on IV drug users, including innovative outreach programs. Such educational programs should include clear and explicit information on how to obtain clean needles, and how to sterilize needles.

3. Treatment and rehabilitation centers of sufficient number and quality to help reduce the incidence of IV drug use.

4. Devise "clean needle" programs to help drug-dependent people to remain free of HIV infection. Bold and innovative programs need to be developed. Alternatives include free distribution of sterile needles, needle exchange, and prescription programs.

5. Provide a legal milieu to encourage voluntarism and cooperation through strict statutory protection of confidentiality and against invidious discrimination.

Only through a comprehensive, well-coordinated, and well-funded program, as briefly examined herein, can we expect to significantly reduce HIV infection and mortality within a highly vulnerable and dependent population.

References

Centers for Disease Control. 1986. Additional recommendations to reduce sexual and drug abuse-related transmission of HTLV-III/LAV. *M.M.W.R.* 35:152-55.

———. 1987. Acquired immunodeficiency syndrome (AIDS). *Weekly Surveillance Report.*

Craddock, S. G., R. M. Bray, and R. L. Hubbard. 1983. *Drug use before and during drug abuse treatment: 1979-1981 TOPS admission cohorts.* Research Triangle Park, North Carolina: Research Triangle Institute.

Des Jarlais, D. C., S. R. Friedman, and W. Hopkins. 1985. Risk reduction of acquired immunodeficiency syndrome among intravenous drug users. *Ann. Intern. Med.* 103:755-59.

Freidman, S. R. 1986. Health education for intravenous drug users. *Health Education Quarterly* 12:383-94.

Ginzburg, H. M. 1986. Intravenous drug abusers and HIV infections: consequence of their actions. *Law, Medicine and Health Care* 14:268-72.

Ginzburg, H. M. 1986. Health education and knowledge assessment of HTLV-III diseases among intravenous drug users. *Health Education Quarterly* 13:373-82.

Gostin, L. and W. J. Curran. 1987a. Legal control measures of AIDS: reporting requirements, surveillance, quarantine, and regulation of public meeting places. *Am. J. Public Health* 77:214-18.

———. 1987b. AIDS screening, confidentiality, and the duty to warn. *Am. J. Public Health* 77:361-65.

Gostin, L., W. J. Curran, and M. Clark. 1987. The case against compulsory case finding in controlling AIDS—Testing, screening, and reporting. *Am. J. Law Med.* 12:1-47.

McAuliffe, W. E. 1987. *Intravenous drug use and the spread of AIDS.* Governance, Massachusetts: Harvard Journal of Public Policy.

Pascal, C. B. 1987. Selected legal issues about AIDS for drug abuse treatment programs. *J. Psychoactive Drugs* 19:1-12.

Afterword

Acquired Immuno-
deficiency Syndrome:
Current and Future Trends

W. Meade Morgan, PhD; and
James W. Curran, MD, MPH.

The first cases of acquired immunodeficiency syndrome (AIDS) were reported in 1981 in five young homosexual men from Los Angeles diagnosed with *Pneumocystic carinii* pneumonia (Centers for Disease Control 1981). Since that time, the number of cases in the United States has continued to increase, resulting in considerable morbidity and mortality (Centers for Disease Control 1986a). The cost of medical care and social services has been high, and medical practitioners and public health officials have expressed concerns about the adequacy and availability of personnel and facilities to meet future needs. Planning for the future requires accurate projections of the number of persons with AIDS and other medical and social problems related to human immunodeficiency virus (HIV) infection. (The designation human immunodeficiency virus [HIV] has recently been proposed by a subcommittee of the International Committee for the Taxonomy of Viruses as the appropriate name for the retrovirus that has been implicated as the causative agent of AIDS [Coffin 1986].) As a basis for planning, trends among AIDS cases reported to the Centers for Disease Control were analyzed, and empirical models were used to project the number and the distribution of AIDS cases through 1991. In this paper, we provide a detailed description of the demographic projections that serve as

Reprinted with permission from "Acquired Immunodeficiency Syndrome: Current and Future Trends," by W. Meade Morgan and James W. Curran. *Public Health Reports* 101 (5):459-64.

the basis for the "Public Health Service Plan for the Prevention and Control of AIDS and the AIDS Virus" (Coolfont Report 1986).

Trends in the numbers of AIDS cases in the United States meeting the surveillance definition and reported to the Centers for Disease Control were analyzed for the period beginning June 1981 through 16 May 1986. Surveillance for AIDS is conducted by health departments in every state, district, and United States territory. In many areas, public health officials routinely contact hospital personnel to assist in detecting and reporting cases and use record systems such as death certificates, tumor registries, and laboratory data to supplement and validate hospital-based surveillance. Confidential case reports are recorded on a standard form which includes data on patient demographics, opportunistic disease(s), risk factors, and laboratory tests. Information from the forms, without personal identifiers, is coded and computerized either at Centers for Disease Control or at health departments where it is then transmitted electronically to Centers for Disease Control.

The models used to project the number and the distribution of AIDS cases by patient group, geographic area of residence, gender, race, and age are empirical in the sense that they reflect observed trends in the distribution of reported cases and assume that these trends will continue unchanged over time (Curran 1985). The projections involve a two-stage process. First, the cases reported each month are adjusted to obtain estimates of the cases actually diagnosed during that month. Second, a quadratic polynomial is fitted using weighted linear regression to the adjusted case counts as transformed by a modified Box-Cox (1964) method, and the resulting model is projected to 1991. The transformation was used to obtain homoscedastic weighted residuals suitable for calculating confidence intervals. The 68% (one standard deviation) confidence bounds account for the usual residual variance in the model as well as the statistical error introduced by adjusting the case counts and applying the Box-Cox transformation. The bounds are valid under the assumption that the quadratic polynomial model, as fit under the Box-Cox transformation, will hold throughout the entire period.

To obtain estimates for the number of AIDS-associated deaths, survival times were calculated from surveillance data using the Kaplan-Meier (1958) method for life table analysis. The estimated median survival time was 12 months and the cumulative 3-year survival was estimated to be 28%. Because of a lack of follow-up information related to patients' deaths, surveillance data will considerably overestimate the true survival rates after the first year. To project AIDS-related mortality reasonably through the third year after diagnosis and beyond, it was assumed that the cumulative survival times follow a negative exponential distribution with 50% of patients living at most 1 year and only 12% surviving for more than 3 years (Moss 1984). The distribution was applied to the upper and lower bounds for projections on the incidence of AIDS to obtain a range for the number of AIDS-related deaths through 1991.

Changes in the distribution of diagnosed cases over time were tested using the chi square test for linear trends when testing proportions or the Spearman rank correlation when testing continuous variables. To project future trends in the distribution of cases, weighted linear regression on the logits of proportions was used. For each month from January 1983 until April 1986, the logit of the proportion of AIDS cases in each category was calculated:

$$(\text{logit}(p) = \log(p) - \log(1 - p)).$$

Weights were taken to be proportional to the inverse of the approximate variance of logit(p), that is $np(1 - p)$ where n is the number of AIDS patients diagnosed in the given month, and p is the proportion of patients in the particular category. The changes in the logit proportions were assumed to be linear over time. Quadratic effects were rarely statistically significant and were not considered further. Only cases diagnosed after 1982 were used to order to allow time of diagnosis and reporting to have stabilized. The parameter estimates were restricted so that the projected proportions of cases in both 1986 and 1991 would sum to 100%. For the 1991 estimates, 68% confidence bounds on the resulting proportions were calculated.

Results

Between 1 June 1981 and 19 May 1986, physicians and health departments in the United States reported 20,766 cases of AIDS. Of these, 20,473 (98.6%) were diagnosed in adults and 293 (1.4%) in children. The number of cases has increased steadily, but the doubling times continue to lengthen, indicating that the rate of increase is not exponential. For example, between July 1981 and February 1982, approximately 1,000 cases of AIDS had been diagnosed and reported. This number increased to 2,000 by July 1983, a 6-month doubling time. More recently, the number of cases has increased from 10,000 in May 1985 to 20,000 by April 1986, a doubling time of 11 mo.

Exhibit A-1 depicts the projected incidence of AIDS through 1991. The adjustment for reporting delays indicates that 25,000 cases will be reported that have already been diagnosed through April 1986, although only 20,076 cases had been reported as of that time. It is projected that 15,800 new AIDS cases will be diagnosed in 1986, increasing to 74,000 cases in 1991 (table A-1). The current number of cases is projected to double in 13 to 15 months, while the cumulative case total of 270,000 by the end of 1991 will represent a doubling over a 2-year period from the end of 1989.

Exhibit A-1

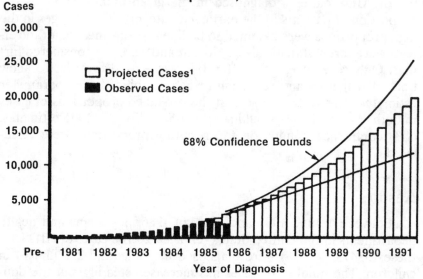

Incidence of AIDS in the United States
by Quarter of Diagnosis
Projected from Cases Reported as of
April 30, 1986

[1]Adjusted for reporting delays.

Table A-1 Incidence of AIDS and associated mortality, United States, May 19, 1986

Year	Number of cases diagnosed during year	Projected cases		Number of deaths during year	Projected deaths	
		Lower bounds	Upper (68 percent) bounds		Lower range	Upper range
1981 and before	321	...	...	146	...	...
1982	1,002	...	...	382	...	...
1983	2,736	...	...	1,225	...	...
1984	5,456	...	...	2,829	...	...
1985[1]	8,775	...	...	5,178	...	...
Projected						
1986	15,800	14,800	16,400	9,000	8,700	9,200
1987	23,000	21,000	25,000	14,000	13,000	15,000
1988	33,000	27,000	36,000	21,000	18,000	23,000
1989	45,000	33,000	51,000	30,000	24,000	33,000
1990	58,000	40,000	69,000	41,000	31,000	47,000
1991	74,000	46,000	92,000	54,000	37,000	64,000

[1]The numbers of diagnoses and deaths for 1985 are underestimated since reporting for this year is not yet complete.

The relative distribution of reported adult and pediatric cases has not changed significantly over time ($p < 0.15$). It is projected that 1.4% of 1986 cases (200) will occur in children under 13 years of age, decreasing slightly to 1.2% (1,000) of cases in 1991.

Trends by Patient Group

Ninety-four percent (18,879) of the total reported adult cases can be placed in patient groups that suggest a possible means of disease acquisition: heterosexual intravenous drug abusers (17%); homosexual or bisexual men with a history of intravenous drug abuse (8%); homosexual or bisexual men who are not known intravenous drug abusers (65%); persons with hemophilia (1%); heterosexual sex partners of persons with AIDS, HIV infection, or persons who are at increased risk for AIDS (1%); and recipients of transfused blood or blood components (2%). The remaining 6% of adult cases have not been classified by recognized risk factors, although 40% of these cases occurred in persons born in Haiti or in central African countries where heterosexual transmission is thought to account for a major share of the cases (Pape 1983; Castro 1985).

The relative proportion of reported cases among the patient groups with the largest numbers of cases has remained stable over time since 1982 (table A-2), while slight but statistically significant changes have occurred in the smaller patient groups. The most significant change is a decline in the proportion of AIDS patients born outside the United States, in Haiti, or central African countries ($p < 0.0001$). The number of reported cases among persons born outside the United States has doubled in the past 18 months compared with a doubling in 11 months for all other AIDS cases in adults. If current trends continue, this group will account for 1.3% of cases diagnosed in 1986 and only 0.3% of those diagnosed in 1991. The initially higher proportion of AIDS cases among Haitians may have been due to the migration to the United States during the period 1978 to 1981 of persons who were already infected (Hardy 1983; Castro 1985). Two other shifts in the distribution of cases are statistically significant. First, the proportion of diagnosed cases associated with blood transfusions and in hemophilia patients has increased slightly ($p < 0.01$) even though the proportion remains small (2.4% of the total adult cases). No cases of AIDS have been

Table A-2 Adult cases of AIDS with projections for 1991, by patient group, United States, May 19, 1986

Patient group	Reported cases, by year of diagnosis								Projected cases			
	1983 & before		1984		1985		1986		1986		1991		
	No.	Percent	No.	Percent	No.	Percent	No.	Percent	No.	Percent	Percent	Lower, Upper (68%) bounds	No.
Homosexual, bisexual men[1]	2,868	72.3	4,000	74.3	6,373	73.4	1,757	71.9	11,300	72.6	70.0	(67.3, 72.6)	51,100
Heterosexual IV drug users	687	17.3	907	16.8	1,479	17.0	451	18.5	2,700	17.3	16.4	(14.5, 18.5)	12,000
Hemophilia patients	19	0.5	43	0.8	86	1.0	12	0.5	200	1.0	1.4	(1.0, 2.0)	1,000
Transfusion recipients	45	1.1	77	1.4	164	1.9	46	1.9	300	2.0	2.5	(1.8, 3.5)	1,800
Other heterosexual cases:													
Heterosexual contacts	36	0.9	65	1.2	151	1.7	52	2.1	300	2.0	5.0	(3.6, 6.8)	3,700
Born outside United States[2]	174	4.4	126	2.3	128	1.5	35	1.4	200	1.3	0.3	(0.2, 0.4)	200
Other, none of the above	138	3.5	165	3.1	297	3.4	92	3.8	600	3.7	4.5	(3.5, 5.8)	3,200
Total	3,967	100.0	5,383	100.0	8,678	100.0	2,445	100.0	15,600	100.0	100.0	....	73,000

[1]12 percent of homosexual, bisexual men are also reported to have a history of IV drug use.

[2]Includes persons born in countries in which most AIDS cases have not been associated with known risk factors but where heterosexual transmission is believed to play a major role.

reported in persons who only received transfusions after routine HIV antibody testing of donors began in the spring of 1985, although one case of a seronegative donor transmitting infection has been reported (Centers for Disease Control 1986c). These continuing increases represent cases among persons infected prior to April 1985 as well as increased recognition of the disease among transfusion recipients, particularly elderly patients. The empirical model projects that 2.0% of adult AIDS cases in 1986 will be in persons whose only risk factor is the receipt of transfused blood or blood components and that this will increase to 2.5% in 1991.

The proportion of cases in the heterosexual contact risk group also has increased from 1983 to 1986 ($x < 0.0001$), although the total number of cases identified in this group is small (1.5%). If current trends continue, the proportion of heterosexual contact cases is projected to be 2.0% in 1986, increasing substantially to 5.0% in 1991. In addition to those cases reported as a result of heterosexual contacts, it is likely that a major portion of the cases without identified risk factors result from heterosexual transmission of the AIDS virus. An estimated 7% of cases diagnosed in 1986 will be among heterosexual contacts, persons born outside of the United States, and persons with no identified risk factor; the majority of cases in these three groups are thought to result from heterosexual transmission. The proportion in these groups is projected to increase to nearly 10%·in 1991.

Trends by Geographic Area

The geographic distribution of diagnosed adult AIDS cases has changed markedly from 1983 to 1986 (table A-3). The proportion of cases outside New York City is primarily due to an increasing proportion of United States cases among homosexual men from other areas. The proportion of homosexual cases from outside of New York City and San Francisco has increased from 50% of cases diagnosed before 1984 to 65% of those diagnosed after 1984. The number of reported AIDS cases doubled in the past 14 months in New York City, in 13 months in San Francisco, and in 10 months in the remainder of the United States. By 1991, only 12% of cases are projected to be diagnosed in the New York City and 8% in the San Francisco Standard Metropolitan Statistical Area (SMSAs) with

Table A-3

Adult cases of AIDS with projections for 1991,
by geographic area, United States, May 19, 1986

	Reported cases, by year of diagnosis							
	1983 & before		1984		1985		1986	
Geographic area	No.	Percent	No.	Percent	No.	Percent	No.	Percent
New York City SMSA	1,527	38.5	1,662	30.9	2,354	27.1	754	30.8
San Francisco SMSA	442	11.1	591	11.0	866	10.0	284	11.6
Florida	286	7.2	368	6.8	572	6.6	122	5.0
Remainder, United States	1,712	43.2	2,762	51.3	4,886	56.3	1,285	52.6
Total	3,967	100.0	5,383	100.0	8,678	100.0	2,445	100.0

	Projected cases					
	1986		1991			
Geographic area	Percent	No.	Percent	Lower, Upper (68 percent) bounds		No.
New York City SMSA	24.9	3,900	11.9	(10.8,	13.1)	8,700
San Francisco SMSA	10.1	1,600	8.1	(7.1,	9.3)	5,900
Florida	5.7	900	3.2	(2.7,	3.7)	2,300
Remainder, United States	59.2	9,200	76.9	(75.0,	78.8)	56,100
Total	100.0	15,600	100.0	....	....	73,000

Note: SMSA - Standard Metropolitan Statistical Area.

80% of the cases outside of these areas which had reported more than half of the cases from 1981 to 1983.

Trends by Race, Gender, and Age

The distribution of cases by race in adults did not change significantly from 1983 to 1986 (table A-4), and there has been a marginally significant increase in the proportion of persons with AIDS

Table A-4

Adult cases of AIDS with projections for 1991,
by race, United States, May 19, 1986

| | Reported cases, by year of diagnosis | | | | | | | |
| | 1983 & before | | 1984 | | 1985 | | 1986 | |
Race	No.	Percent	No.	Percent	No.	Percent	No.	Percent
White	2,294	57.8	3,270	60.7	5,256	60.6	1,452	59.4
Black	1,036	26.1	1,307	24.3	2,114	24.4	603	24.6
Hispanic	568	14.3	747	13.9	1,227	14.1	370	15.1
Other, unknown	69	1.7	59	1.1	81	0.9	20	0.8
Total	3,967	100.0	5,383	100.0	8,678	100.0	2,445	100.0

	Projected cases					
	1986		1991			
				Lower, Upper		
Race	Percent	No.	Percent	(68 percent) bounds		No.
White	61.0	9,500	64.2	(62.2,	66.2)	46,900
Black	23.8	3,700	20.8	(19.3,	22.5)	15,200
Hispanic	14.5	2,300	14.8	(13.3,	16.4)	10,800
Other, unknown	0.8	100	0.2	(0.1,	0.3)	100
Total	100.0	15,600	100.0	···	···	73,000

who are women (p = 0.09, table A-5). There has also been a small but significant increase in the age of patients (p = 0.02). The mean age among patients diagnosed before 1984 is 36.3 years compared with 37.8 years for those diagnosed after 1984. Ninety-three percent of the reported cases are men. Sixty percent are white, 25% are black, and 14% are Hispanic; less than 1% of adult cases are in persons between 13 and 19 years of age, 21% between 20 and 29 years of age, 48% between 30 and 39, 21% between 40 and 49, and 9% are over 49. The increase in age has occurred primarily among heterosexual intravenous drug users whose mean age has increased from 34.2 years for those diagnosed before 1983 and 35.1 for those diagnosed after, and among blood transfusion recipients whose mean ages increased from 50.0 to 55.2 years, respectively. The increase in age among adults is not significant if either heterosexual intravenous drug users or transfusion recipients are excluded (p > .15).

Table A-5

Adult cases of AIDS with projections for 1991,
by gender, United States, May 19, 1986

	Reported cases, by year of diagnosis							
	1983 & before		1984		1985		1986	
Gender	No.	Percent	No.	Percent	No.	Percent	No.	Percent
Male	3,707	93.4	5,045	93.7	8,097	93.3	2,254	92.2
Female	260	6.6	338	6.3	581	6.7	191	7.8
Total	3,967	100.0	5,383	100.0	8,678	100.0	2,445	100.0

	Projected cases						
	1986		1991				
Gender	Percent	No.	Percent	Lower, Upper (68 percent) bounds		No.	
Male	92.3	14,400	90.2	(88.4,	91.7)	65,800	
Female	7.7	1,200	9.8	(8.3,	11.6)	7,200	
Total	100.0	15,600	100.0			73,000	

Trends among Pediatric Cases

Fifty-four percent of 159 pediatric cases have been in children born to a parent with a history of intravenous drug abuse, an additional 10% (28) are among children of parents with AIDS or are at other risk for AIDS, and 13% (39) are in children born to Haitian parents. Fifteen percent (44) of pediatric AIDS cases are in children who have received blood transfusions, and 4% (12) have hemophilia. Risk factor information is incomplete or missing for the remaining 4% (11 cases).

The distribution of pediatric cases by the patient's age, race, and geographic region has not changed significantly from 1983 to 1986. However, the number of cases is relatively small so that there is less ability to detect trends. Forty-nine percent of the cases were diagnosed under 1 year of age. Sixty percent of the children are black, and 21% are Hispanic; 38% have been reported from New York City, 14% from New Jersey, and 14% from Florida. The distribution of pediatric cases by geographic area is similar to that of cases in women who use intravenous drugs or are born outside of the United States.

Discussion

AIDS will become an even more serious public health problem in the United States during the next 5 years, with a concurrent need for medical and social services for AIDS patients. The empirical model projects that 74,000 patients will be diagnosed in 1991 alone. An estimated 70,000 patients diagnosed during previous years will also require care during 1991.

These projections are conservative, since they are based only upon cases reported to Centers for Disease Control. A review of death certificates over a 3-month period in four different metropolitan areas in the United States suggests that an additional 10% of diagnosed cases of AIDS are not reported to the Centers for Disease Control (Hardy 1986). At least an additional 10% of patients may be seriously ill with other group IV HIV infections (Centers for Disease Control 1986b) which do not fit current surveillance criteria (such as severe constitutional disease of "wasting syndrome" without a specific opportunistic infection or tumor). Thus, the figures we present may underestimate by 20% or more the future morbidity and mortality due to HIV infection.

Because of the lengthy period between infection with HIV and the diagnosis of AIDS, most of the cases projected to occur in the next 5 years will be among persons already infected. Thus, the majority of cases in 1991 will be in intravenous drug abusers and homosexual and bisexual men. Cases in "other heterosexual men and women" are projected to increase to more than 7,000 (nearly 10%). Most of these will occur among those already infected. Future trends in the geographic distribution of cases also reflect the current distribution of AIDS virus infection.

The empirical models do not consider the availability of therapy, vaccine, preventable cofactors, or the effectiveness of primary prevention efforts. If effective therapeutic regimens soon become widely available, the course of disease could be altered for those already infected. However, effective primary prevention of future HIV infections through vaccines, counseling and testing, and education will have little impact on the number of cases occurring before 1990 due to the long incubation period and the large number of persons already infected. In some areas, prevention efforts have already been successfully implemented so that the empirical model may overestimate future cases, that is, among persons with hemophilia and recipients of transfusions.

Epidemiologic models for projecting the future incidence of AIDS will require additional information on the incidence, prevalence, and natural history of HIV infection and on the effectiveness of efforts to prevent virus transmission. Our current understanding of the severity of AIDS and projections for the future underscore the need for continued commitment to research for a vaccine and therapy. Primary prevention and education activities must be widely implemented now throughout the United States to curtail the further spread of infection and future AIDS cases.

References

Box, G. P., and D. Cox. 1964. An analysis of transformations. *J. R. Stat. Soc.* (series B) 26:211-52.

Castro, K. G. 1985. Risk factors for AIDS among Haitians in the United States. Paper presented at the International Conference on Acquired Immune Deficiency Syndrome (AIDS), 16 April, Atlanta, Georgia.

Centers for Disease Control. 1981. *Pneumocystis pneumonia* – Los Angeles. *M.M.W.R.* 30:250-52.

———. 1986a. Update: acquired immunodeficiency syndrome – United States. *M.M.W.R.* 35:17-21.

———. 1986b. Classification system for human T-lymphotropic virus type III/lymphadenopathy-associated virus infections. *M.M.W.R.* 35:334-49.

———. 1986c. Transfusion-associated human T-lymphotropic virus type III/lymphadenopathy-associated virus infection from a seronegative donor-Colorado. *M.M.W.R.* 35:389-91.

Coffin, J. 1986. Human immunodeficiency viruses (letter). *Science* 232:697.

Coolfont Report. 1986. A PHS plan for prevention and control of AIDS and the AIDS virus. *Public Health Report* 101:342-48.

Curran, J. W. 1985. The epidemiology of AIDS current status and future prospects. *Science* 229:1352-57.

Hardy, A. M. 1983. The incidence rate of acquired immunodeficiency syndrome in selected populations. *J.A.M.A.* 253:215-20.

Hardy, A. M. 1986. Using death certificates to determine the level of AIDS case reporting. Paper presented at the International Conference on Acquired Immune Deficiency Syndrome (AIDS), 23 June, Paris, France.

Kaplan, E. L. and P. Meier. 1958. Nonparametric estimation from incomplete observations. *J. Am. Stat. Assoc.* 53:457-81.

Moss, A. R. 1984. Mortality associated with mode of presentation in the acquired immune deficiency syndrome. *J. Natl. Cancer Inst.* 73:1281-84.

Pape, J. 1983. Characteristics of the acquired immunodeficiency syndrome (AIDS) in Haiti. *N. Engl. J. Med.* 309:945-90.

Epilogue

The rising incidence of acquired immunodeficiency syndrome (AIDS) among intravenous drug users poses a broad spectrum of questions for substance abuse treatment professionals and society. For no other high-risk group have methods of intervention in virus transmission become such a matter of legal and moral debate; and, by the same token, no other high-risk group poses a threat of similar magnitude to the nondrug-abusing heterosexual population. Intravenous drug users with AIDS are both a problem mainstream society would prefer to forget, and one that is most dangerously forgotten.

Because the use of intravenous drugs is illegal, there has been a subtle yet pervasive prejudice against the treatment and education of intravenous drug users. For what other risk group, for example, would an interventive measure—such as giving out sterile needles to reduce human immunodeficiency virus (HIV) transmission—be condemned as a matter of immorality rather than dealt with constructively in the interest of public health? The reluctance to pursue any and all means of intervention now will have a profound impact on the cost and availability of health care in the future if HIV transmission continues at its current rate.

The funding of health care for intravenous drug users with AIDS-related complex (ARC) and AIDS is another question that must be dealt with by the public health system. Many such drug users have neither jobs nor insurance.

For those who work directly with intravenous drug users in a substance abuse treatment setting, the questions posed by AIDS range from the theoretical to the very practical. Inevitably, more cases of ARC and AIDS among intravenous drug users will begin to be seen in ambulatory and residential substance abuse treatment programs as the spread of the virus progresses; this means that such programs will need to consider the implementation of policies for dealing with these cases, in addition to active educational efforts for all clients and staff. Should drug users with HIV infection, ARC, or AIDS be permitted to enter drug treatment programs? Is the addict with AIDS physically capable of undergoing substance abuse treatment? What precautions should be taken to protect not only the health of the HIV seropositive client, but also that of other clients and staff in a residential drug treatment program? Finally, can the arduous task of treatment for addiction be justified to a client who realizes his/her life may be shortened considerably by a diagnosis of AIDS?

Despite the fact that a cure for AIDS remains uncertain, the implications of the research presented in *AIDS and IV Drug Abusers: Current Perspectives* are hopeful. Far from indicating that intravenous drug users are unconcerned about their health and incapable of change, researchers working with this population both "on the street" and in treatment have found high levels of awareness and concern. This concern may take the form of attempts to purchase "clean" needles, reducing or even stopping drug use, or the development of better health habits. Whatever form it takes, the potential for change clearly exists, prodded, at least in part, by knowledge and anxiety about AIDS.

Among sexually active homosexual and bisexual men, who still comprise the largest percentage of cases of AIDS, educational efforts made by the homosexual community itself have demonstrated effectiveness in influencing behavior change. Within this population, men are reducing their high-risk sexual behaviors, with a concomitant reduction in the incidence of venereal disease. The impact of such behavior change, according to Morgan and Curran, will not have an effect on the spread of AIDS for some years in the future, because of the disease's long incubation period and the likelihood of HIV infection prior to intervention efforts. It is reasonable to expect the same to be true of intravenous drug users, among whom rates of HIV seropositivity, in some urban areas, mirror those found among homosexual men in 1981, at the start of the AIDS epidemic. Unlike homosexual and bisexual men, however, intravenous drug users do not have a structured community to facilitate the spread of information about AIDS. For that reason, active educational intervention with this population is critical now, since, as the research reflects, it may have a profound impact on the spread of AIDS to other, non-drug-using heterosexuals.

Many researchers and clinicians, including those whose work is featured in *AIDS and IV Drug Abusers: Current Perspectives*, have already begun investigating the potential for various types of AIDS education for intravenous drug abusers. A great deal of work still remains, however. Continuing efforts are needed to overcome the initial denial of intravenous drug users and to develop educational modules that will have maximum effectiveness. As the course of the AIDS epidemic continues, so will the development of better means of assessing the success or failure of such educational programs – for finding out whether lessons learned in treatment and while "straight" remain effective when drug users return to the community or, possibly, to their former lifestyle.

The challenges presented by AIDS will be ongoing ones for our society. Willingness to face the issues raised by this disease – and raised by researchers like those whose papers are collected in this volume – may ultimately be the most effective means of fighting its continued spread.

Glossary

Acquired Immune Deficiency Syndrome (AIDS): The endstage manifestation of infection with the Human Immunodeficiency Virus (HIV), which destroys important components of the human immune system. Persons with the disease develop infections that would not occur with normal immunity. The Centers for Disease Control have strict criteria for a diagnosis of AIDS. These include a positive test for exposure to HIV and certain abnormalities in T-cell ratios, as well as a number of infections and cancers, including the following: histoplasmosis, isoporiasis, candidiasis, various forms of pneumonia, especially *Pneumocystis carinii* pneumonia, enterocolitis, meningitis, esophagitis, encephalitis, chronic mucocutaneous herpes simplex, cytome-galovirus infection, chronic progressive multifocal leukoen-cephalopathy, Hodgkin's disease, non-Hodgkin's lymphoma, Burkitt's lymphoma, liver cancer, cancer of the oropharynx, chronic lymphocytic leukemia, lung cancer, and Kaposi's sarcoma in individuals under age 60. Also included in the Centers for Disease Control definition are central nervous system abnormalities caused by infection with the HIV itself.

AIDS-Related Complex (ARC): A variety of chronic symptoms that occur in persons who are infected with Human Immunodeficiency Virus, but whose conditions do not meet the Centers for Disease Control definition of AIDS. ARC symptoms may include unexplained swollen lymph glands, fever, weight loss, fatigue, and persistent diarrhea. Most doctors consider two of these symptoms and two laboratory findings, such as indication of opportunistic infection or some immune system abnormality, as indicative of ARC.

Antibody: A protein produced by blood B-lymphocytes to eliminate specific infectious agents.

Antigen: A substance that is foreign to the body and stimulates the formation of antibodies to combat its presence.

Asymptomatic carrier: A person who has an infectious organism within the body but feels or shows no outward symptoms.

B-lymphocyte: A kind of white blood cell that produces antibody in response to stimulation by an antigen.

Candida albicans: A yeast that causes whitish patches in the mouth and/or esophagus. The infection is called candidiasis or thrush.

Case-control study: An epidemiological study design in which individuals with a disease or health problem are matched on a variety of factors with others who do not have the disease or health problem for purposes of comparison. Some matching factors may be age, race, socioeconomic status, occupation, or area of residence.

Case fatality rate: The proportion of individuals with a disease, in this case AIDS, who have or are projected to die of that disease.

Casual contact: Day-to-day contact between Human Immunodeficiency Virus-infected persons and others at home, at work, or at school. This type of contact does not include sexual or needle-sharing interaction.

Cell-mediated immunity: A defense mechanism in which T-lymphocytes called helper T-cells and killer T-cells work together to stimulate immune response and eliminate cells that are infected with infectious agents.

Cofactor: Any factor, such as stress, malnutrition, or infection with another microorganism, that increases the likelihood of developing a particular disease.

Count: The most basic quantitative measure in epidemiology. The term refers to a notation that X people in a particular population have, for example, developed Human Immunodeficiency Virus infection.

Cytomegalovirus (CMV): A member of the herpesvirus group which infects most of us during our childhood or adult life. It can be associated with a congenital infection of infants and infections in bone marrow transplant patients and other patients who have undergone procedures that cause immune suppression. It causes pneumonia and inflammations of the retina, liver, kidneys, and colon in AIDS patients.

Cytopathic: Cellular destruction.

DNA (deoxyribonucleic acid): A nucleic acid found in the nucleus of cells that transmits hereditary characteristics.

ELISA: The "enzyme-linked immunosorbent assay," a rapid screening test used to detect antibody to Human Immunodeficiency Virus.

Endemic: The constant presence of a disease within a given community or area.

Epidemic: The occurrence of a group of illnesses in a community or region that is in excess of normal occurrence.

Epidemiology: The study of the distribution and causes of disease within populations.

Epstein-Barr virus: The virus that is the cause of infectious mononucleosis; it has also been linked with the development of Burkitt's lymphoma in Africa and nasopharyngeal carcinoma in China.

Etiology: The cause or origin of a disease.

False negative: A negative test result for a condition that actually is present.

False positive: A positive test result for a condition that is actually not present.

Helper-suppressor T-cell ratio: Ratio of the number of helper T-cells to the number of suppressor T-cells; the normal ratio of 2:1 is reversed in people suffering from AIDS.

Herpes simplex: Two types (I and II) of viruses which are members of the herpesvirus family, and are associated with cold sores of the mouth and lips and genital ulcers.

Herpesvirus group: A group of human viruses including the herpes simplex viruses, varicella zoster virus, cytomegalovirus, and Epstein-Barr virus.

Hepatitis B: An inflammation of the liver caused by a virus and commonly spread by needle-sharing among intravenous drug users.

HIV: The Human Immunodeficiency Virus, cause of AIDS.

HTLV-III: The human T-cell lymphotropic virus type III, the name once given by the National Cancer Institute to the virus now known as Human Immunodeficiency Virus.

Humoral immunity: A defense mechanism involving production of antibodies in body fluids, such as serum and lymph, which are directed against bacteria, viruses, and other foreign antigens.

Immune-system: The body's major mechanism for resisting disease-causing organisms, consisting of specialized cells and proteins in blood and other body fluids.

Immunodeficient: Having an impaired or nonfunctioning immune system.

Immunosuppressed: Abnormal functioning of the immune system, often as the result of drugs used in certain medical illnesses, i.e., cancer chemotherapy.

Incidence: The number of new cases of a disease in a population over a period of time.

Incubation period: Latency: the period of time between infection with a virus and the development of symptoms.

Interstitial pneumonitis: An acute inflammation of the lungs, which, if it persists for more than two months, is indicative of AIDS in children unless another cause is diagnosed.

Intravenous: Injected into a vein through a needle.

Kaposi's sarcoma: A cancer of the cells lining blood vessels. In the United States, it typically appeared only in men over 50 years of age until its appearance in young men with cases of AIDS appeared in the United States in 1978.

Latency: Period of time during which a virus remains inactive in the body.

LAV: Lymphadenopathy-associated virus, the name given by French researchers to the virus now known as Human Immunodeficiency Virus.

Lymphadenopathy: Swelling of the lymph glands principally in the neck, armpits, and groin, a symptom of AIDS-Related Complex.

Lymphocytes: White blood cells involved in immune response.

Macrophage: A white blood cell that destroys foreign particles in the blood stream.

Mutation: A change or deviation from inherited characteristics.

Mycobacterium avium-intracellulare: A rare form of bacteria, related to the bacteria that causes tuberculosis, that causes many infections in AIDS patients, although it normally does not infect people with healthy immune systems.

Needle-sharing: The most likely means of the transmission of Human Immunodeficiency Virus in intravenous drug use. The virus is transmitted through blood that remains in the needle or syringe after injection, not through the injected drug itself.

Opportunistic infection: An infection that would not normally affect a person with a healthy immune system.

Parenteral: Involving introduction or injection into the blood stream.

Pneumocystis carinii pneumonia: A life-threatening pneumonia commonly diagnosed in AIDS patients but rarely in others, caused by a parasite, *Pneumocystis carinii*.

Prevalence: The total incidence of a disease in a given population at a particular time.

Proportion: The ratio of infected individuals in a particular population or risk group; for example, 100 Human Immunodeficiency Virus-infected individuals would, in a particular city, comprise differing proportions if the number of intravenous drug users in that city were 2,500 or 7,500. Proportion is expressed as a percentage (i.e., 100/2,500 or 4%).

Rate: An expression of proportion in which time is taken into account. For example, the rate of AIDS cases in a specific risk group indicates the probability of the number of cases that will develop in the future.

Retrovirus: A class of virus having the ability to transform their own genetic material, RNA, into DNA, and thus incorporate themselves into the genetic structure of an infected cell.

Reverse transcriptase: The enzyme used by retroviruses to transform their RNA genetic material to DNA.

RNA (ribonucleic acid): A nucleic acid that regulates the production of proteins within a cell.

Seroconversion: The development of antibodies to a particular virus.

Serologic study: A comparison of the serum of individuals.

Seropositive: Producing a positive reaction to antibody tests for Human Immunodeficiency Virus.

Shooting gallery: A place where drug addicts gather to administer drugs, i.e., a vacant apartment, etc. Needle-sharing often occurs in such shooting galleries.

Syndrome: A particular pattern of symptoms and signs that serve to indicate the presence of a disease.

T4 (CD4) lymphocyte: The helper T-cell that is the primary target of Human Immunodeficiency Virus. It plays a key role in the human immune system.

Toxoplasma gondii: A parasite causing brain inflammation, called toxoplasmosis, in AIDS patients.

Western blot technique (or Immunoblot): A more exacting test for antibodies to Human Immunodeficiency Virus. Because the Western blot is more expensive to perform than the ELISA test, it is usually used only to confirm a positive result on the ELISA test.

"Works": Paraphernalia, such as hypodermic needles and syringes, used by intravenous drug users.

Bibliography

ABC News/Washington Post Poll. September 1985.

Agar, M. H. 1973. *Ripping and running: a formal ethnography of urban heroin addicts.* New York: Seminar Press.

AIDS Legal Guide: A Professional Resource on AIDS-Related Legal Issues and Discrimination. 1984. New York: Lambda Legal Defense and Education Fund, Inc., 18-23.

Allison, M., R. Hubbard, E. Cavanaugh, and J. Rachal. 1983. *Drug abuse treatment process: descriptions of TOPS methadone, residential, and outpatient drug free programs.* Research Triangle Park, North Carolina: Research Triangle Institute.

Altman, L. K. 1986. Who will volunteer for an AIDS vaccine? *New York Times,* C1, C7, 15 April.

Ammann, A. J. 1985. The acquired immunodeficiency syndrome in infants and children. *Ann. Intern. Med.* 103:734-37.

Ammann, A. J., D. Wara, and S. Dritz, 1983. Acquired immunodeficiency in an infant: possible transmission by means of blood products. *Lancet* 1:956-58.

Anderson, R. E., and J. Levy. 1985. Prevalence of antibodies to AIDS-associated retrovirus in single men in San Francisco. *Lancet* 1:217.

Angarano, G., G. Pastore, L. Monno, T. Santanio, N. Luchena, and O. Schiraldi. 1985. Rapid spread of HTLV-III infection among drug addicts in Italy. *Lancet* 2:1302.

Auerbach, D. M., W. Darrow, and H. Jaffe. 1984. Cluster of cases of the acquired immune deficiency syndrome: patients linked by sexual contact. *Am. J. Med.* 76:487-92.

Barre-Sinoussi, F., J. Chermann, and F. Rey. 1983. Isolation of a T-lymphotropic retrovirus from a patient at risk for acquired immune deficiency syndrome (AIDS). *Science* 220:868-71.

Battin, P. 1982. *Ethical issues in suicide.* Englewood Cliffs, New Jersey: Prentice-Hall.

Box, G. P., and D. Cox. 1964. An analysis of transformations. *J. R. Stat. Soc.* (series B) 26:211-52.

Brandt, A. M. 1985. *No magic bullet: a social history of venereal disease in the United States since 1880.* New York: Oxford University Press.

Bray, R. M. 1982. *Approaches to the assessment of drug use in the Treatment Outcome Prospective Study.* Research Triangle Park, North Carolina: Research Triangle Institute.

Britton, C. B., and J. Miller. 1984. Neurological complications in acquired immune deficiency syndrome (AIDS). *Neurol. Clin.* 2:315.

Brown, S. M., B. Stimmel, and R. Jaub. 1974. Immunologic dysfunction in heroin addicts. *Arch. Intern. Med.* 134:1001-6.

Buning, E. 1986. The Amsterdam Helping System for Drug Addicts: A Summary. Paper presented at the Conference on AIDS in the Drug Abuse Community and Heterosexual Transmission, 1 April, Newark, New Jersey.

Caiazza, S. S. 1985. Letter to the editor. *N. Engl. J. Med.* 313:1158.

Califano, J. A. 1982. *Report on drug abuse and alcoholism.* New York: Warner Press.

Carlson, J. R., M. Bryant, and S. Hinrich. 1984. AIDS serology in low- and high-risk groups. *J.A.M.A.* 253:3405-8.

Castro, K. G., M. Fischl, and S. Landesman. 1985. Risk factors for AIDS among Haitians in the United States. Paper presented at the International Conference on Acquired Immunodeficiency Syndrome (AIDS), session 11, Atlanta, Georgia.

Centers for Disease Control. 1981a. *Pneumocystis* pneumonia – Los Angeles. *M.M.W.R.* 30:250-2.

———. 1981b. Kaposi's sarcoma and *Pneumocystis* pneumonia among homosexual men – New York City and California. *M.M.W.R.* 30:305-8.

——. 1982a. Diffuse, undifferentiated non-Hodgkin's lymphoma among homosexual males. *M.M.W.R.* 31:277-79.

——. 1982b. *Pneumocystis carinii* pneumonia among persons with hemophilia A. *M.M.W.R.* 31:315-67.

——. 1982c. Opportunistic infections and Kaposi's sarcoma among Haitians in the United States. *M.M.W.R.* 31:353-54.

——. 1982d. Update on acquired immune deficiency syndrome (AIDS) United States.*M.M.W.R.* 31:507-14.

——. 1982e. Acquired immunodeficiency syndrome (AIDS): precautions for clinical and laboratory staffs. *M.M.W.R.* 31:577-80.

——. 1982f. Update on acquired immune deficiency syndrome (AIDS) among patients with hemophilia A. *M.M.W.R.* 31:644-52.

——. 1982g. Possible transfusion-associated acquired immune deficiency syndrome (AIDS) – California. *M.M.W.R.* 31:652-54.

——. 1983a. Prevention of acquired immunodeficiency syndrome (AIDS): report of inter-agency recommendations. *M.M.W.R.* 32:101-3.

——. 1983b. Update: acquired immunodeficiency syndrome (AIDS) United States. *M.M.W.R.* 32:688-91.

——. 1983c. Immunodeficiency among female sexual partners of males with acquired immunodeficiency syndrome (AIDS) – New York. *M.M.W.R.* 31:697-98.

——. 1984a. Prospective evaluation of health-care workers exposed via parenteral or mucous-membrane routes to blood and body fluids of patients with acquired immunodeficiency syndrome. *M.M.W.R.* 33:181-82.

——. 1984b. Declining rates of rectal and pharyngeal gonorrhea among males New York City.*M.M.W.R.* 33:295-97.

——. 1984c. Antibodies to a retrovirus etiologically associated with acquired immunodeficiency syndrome (AIDS) in populations with increased incidences of the syndrome. *M.M.W.R.* 33:377-79.

——. 1984d. Update: acquired immunodeficiency syndrome (AIDS) in persons with hemophilia. *M.M.W.R.* 33:589-91.

——. 1984e. Acquired immunodeficiency syndrome (AIDS) – United States. *M.M.W.R.* 33:661-64.

——. 1984f. Acquired immunodeficiency syndrome (AIDS). *Weekly Surveillance Report*, 31 December.

——. 1985a. Revision of the case definition of acquired immunodeficiency syndrome for national reporting United States. *Ann. Intern. Med.* 103:402-3.

——. 1985b. Provisional public health service inter-agency recommendations for screening donated blood and plasma for antibody to the virus causing acquired immunodeficiency syndrome. *M.M.W.R.* 34:1-5.

——. 1985c. Update: prospective evaluation of health-care workers exposed via the parenteral or mucous-membrane route to blood or body fluids of patients with acquired immunodeficiency syndrome United States.*M.M.W.R.* 34:101-3.

——. 1985d. Revision of the case definition of acquired immunodeficiency syndrome for national reporting – United States. *M.M.W.R.* 34:373-75.

——. 1985e. Results of human T-lymphotropic virus type III test kits reported from blood collection centers United States.*M.M.W.R.* 34:375-76.

——. 1985f. Heterosexual transmission of HTLV-III/LAV. *M.M.W.R.* 34:561-63.

——. 1985g. Update: evaluation of human T-lymphotropic virus type III/lymphadenopathy-associated virus infection in health-care personnel – United States. *M.M.W.R.* 34:575-78.

——. 1985h. Self-reported behavioral change among gay and bisexual men – San Francisco. *M.M.W.R.* 34:613-15.

——. 1985i. Recommendations for preventing transmission of infection with human T-lymphotropic virus type III/lymphadenopathy-associated virus in the workplace. *M.M.W.R.* 34:682-95.

——. 1985j. Recommendations for assisting in the prevention of perinatal transmission of HTLV-III/LAV and AIDS. *M.M.W.R.* 34:721-32.

———. 1985k. Acquired immunodeficiency syndrome (AIDS). *Weekly Surveillance Report*, 10 March.

———. 1985l. Acquired immunodeficiency syndrome (AIDS). *Weekly Surveillance Report*, 25 November.

———. 1985m. Acquired immunodeficiency syndrome (AIDS). *Weekly Surveillance Report*, 18 December.

———. 1986a. Update: acquired immunodeficiency syndrome United States. *M.M.W.R.* 35:17-21.

———. 1986b. Update: acquired immunodeficiency syndrome Europe. *M.M.W.R.* 34:35-45.

———. 1986c. Classification system for human T-lymphotropic virus type III/lymphadenopathy-associated virus infections. *M.M.W.R.* 35:334-49.

———. 1986d. Transfusion-associated human T-lymphotropic virus type III/lymphadenopathy-associated virus infection from a seronegative donor Colorado.*M.M.W.R.* 35:389-91.

———. 1987. AIDS program. *Weekly Surveillance Report*, 16 February.

Chaiken, J. M., and M. Chaiken. 1982. *Varieties of criminal behavior.* Santa Monica, California: Rand Corporation.

Chamberland, M. E., K. Castro, and H. Haverkos. 1984. Acquired immunodeficiency syndrome in the United States: an analysis of cases outside high-incidence groups. *Ann. Intern. Med.* 101:617-23.

Cheingsong-Popov, R., R. Weiss, and A. Dalgleish. 1984. Prevalence of antibody to human T-lymphotropic virus type III in AIDS and AIDS-risk patients in Britain. *Lancet* 2:476-80.

Christ, G. H., and L. Wiener. 1985. Psychosocial issues in AIDS. In *AIDS: etiology, diagnosis, treatment and prevention*, ed. V. T. De-Vita, S. Helman, and S. Rosenburg. New York: Lippincott.

Client-Oriented Data Acquisition Process. 1981. *SMSA statistics 1980*, series E, number 23. NIDA, ADAMHA, PHS, Rockville, Maryland.

Clumeck, N., F. Mascart-Lemone, and J. De Mauberge. 1984. Acquired immunodeficiency syndrome in African patients. *N. Engl. J. Med.* 310:492-97.

Cobb, S. 1976. Social support as a moderator of life stress. *Psychosom. Med.* 28:300-14.

Coffin, J. 1986. Human immonodeficiency viruses (letter). *Science* 232:697.

Cohen, H., M. Marmor, and D. Des Jarlais. 1985a. Behavioral risk factors for HTLV-III/LAV seropositivity among intravenous drug abusers. In *The International Conference on the Acquired Immunodeficiency Syndrome: Abstracts.* Philadelphia, Pennsylvania: American College of Physicians.

———. 1985b. Behavioral risk factors for HTLV-III/LAV seropositivity among intravenous drug abusers. Paper presented at the International Conference on Acquired Immune Deficiency Syndrome (AIDS), 14-17 April, Atlanta, Georgia.

Cohen, M. A., and J. P. Merlino. 1983. The suicidal patient on the surgical ward: a multidisciplinary case conference. *Gen. Hosp. Psychiat.* 5:65-71.

Confidentiality of alcohol and drug abuse patient records. 1985. 40 FED. REG. 27802-21 (1985).

Conte, J. E., Jr. 1983. Infection-control guidelines for patients with acquired immunodeficiency syndrome (AIDS). *N. Engl. J. Med.* 309:740-44.

Coolfont Report. 1986. A PHS plan for prevention and control of AIDS and the AIDS virus. *Public Health Report* 101:342-48.

Coombs, R. H., L. Fry, and P. Lewis, eds. 1976. *Socialization in drug abuse.* Cambridge, Massachusetts: Schenkman.

Cooper, D. A., J. Gold, and P. Maclean. 1984. Acute AIDS retrovirus infection: definition of a clinical illness associated with seroconversion. *Lancet* 1:537-40.

Coppola, V., and M. Zabarsky. 1983. Coming out of the closet. *Newsweek*, 8 August.

Coutinho, R. 1986. Prevention of AIDS among Drug Users in Amsterdam. Paper presented at the Conference on AIDS in the

Drug Abuse Community and Heterosexual Transmission, 1 April, Newark, New Jersey.

Craddock, S. G. November 1983. *Drug use before and during drug abuse treatment: 1979-81 TOPS admission cohorts.* Research Triangle Park, North Carolina: Research Triangle Institute.

Curran, J. W. 1985. The epidemiology of AIDS – Current status and future prospects. *Science* 229:1352-57.

Curran, J. W., D. Lawrence, and H. Jaffe. 1984. Immunodeficiency syndrome (AIDS) associated with transfusions. *N. Engl. J. Med.* 310:69-75.

Curran, J. W., et al. 1985. The epidemiology of AIDS: current status and future prospects. *Science* 229:1352-57.

Current Trends. 1982. Acquired immune deficiency syndrome (AIDS): precautions for clinical and laboratory staff. *M.M.W.R.* 31:577-80.

———. 1985. Education and foster care of children infected with human T-lymphotropic virus type III/lymphadenopathy-associated virus. *M.M.W.R.* 34:517-21.

Davis, K. C. 1983. Acquired immune deficiency syndrome in a patient with hemophilia. *Ann. Intern. Med.* 98:284-86.

Deren, S. 1985. *A description of methadone maintenance patients and their children.* New York: New York State Division of Substance Abuse Services.

Derogatis, L. R., G. Morros, and J. Frtting. 1983. The prevalence of psychiatric disorders among cancer patients. *J.A.M.A.* 249:751-57.

Desforges, J. F. 1983. AIDS and preventive treatment in hemophilia. *N. Engl. J. Med.* 308:94-95.

Des Jarlais, D. 1983. *Heroin influx update.* New York: New York State Division of Substance Abuse Services, Bureau of Research.

———. 1984. Research design, drug use and deaths: cross study comparisons. In *Social and medical aspects of drug abuse*, ed. G. Serban. New York: SP Scientific.

Des Jarlais, D., and G. Uppal. 1980. Heroin activity in New York City, 1970-1978. *Am. J. Drug Alcohol Abuse* 7:335-46.

Des Jarlais, D. C., M. Chamberland, and S. Yancovitz. 1984. Heterosexual partners: a large risk group for AIDS. *Lancet* 2:1346-47.

Des Jarlais, D. C., S. Friedman, and M. Hopkins. 1984. Risk reduction for the acquired immunodeficiency syndrome among intravenous drug users. *Ann. Intern. Med.* 103:755-59.

Des Jarlais, D. C., and W. Hopkins. 1985. Free needles for intravenous drug users at risk for AIDS: current developments in New York City. *New Engl. J. Med.* 313:23.

Des Jarlais, D. C., S. Friedman, and T. Spira. 1985. A stage model of HTLV-III/LAV in intravenous drug users. In *Problems of drug dependence*, ed. L. Harris. Rockville, Maryland: National Institute on Drug Abuse.

Des Jarlais, D. C., N. Jainchill, and S. Friedman. 1986. AIDS among IV drug users: epidemiology, natural history and therapeutic community experiences. *Proceedings of the 9th World Conference of Therapeutic Communities*, 69-73.

Des Jarlais, D. C., S. Friedman, and D. Strug. 0000. AIDS and needle sharing within the intravenous drug use subculture. In *The social dimensions of AIDS: methods and theory*, eds. D. Feldman and T. Johnson. New York: Praeger (in press).

Des Jarlais, D. C., S. Friedman, and M. Marmor. 0000. Continued injection as a co-factor for T4 cell loss among IV drug users exposed to HTLV-III/LAV (in press).

Deuchar, N. 1984. AIDS in New York City with particular reference to psychosocial aspects. *Br. J. Psychiat.* 145:612-19.

DeVita, V. T., S. Hellman, and S. Rosenberg, eds. 1985. *AIDS: etiology, diagnosis, treatment and prevention.* Philadelphia, Pennsylvania: J. B. Lippincott.

Dilley, J. W. 1984. Treatment interventions and approaches to care of patients with acquired immune deficiency syndrome. In *Psychiatric implications of acquired immune deficiency syndrome*, eds. S. E. Nichols and D. G. Ostrow. Washington, D.C.: American Psychiatric Press, 62-80.

Duncanson, F. P., D. Hewlett, and S. Maayan. 1985. Tuberculosis and the acquired immunodeficiency syndrome in non-Haitian intravenous drug abusers. In *The International Conference on the Acquired Immunodeficiency Syndrome: Abstracts.* Philadelphia, Pennsylvania: American College of Physicians.

Durack, D. T. 1981. Opportunistic infections and Kaposi's sarcoma in homosexual men. *N. Engl. J. Med.* 305:1465-67.

DuToit, B. M., ed. 1977. *Drugs, rituals and altered states of consciousness.* Rotterdam: A. A. Balkema.

Echenberg, D. F., and G. Rutherford. 1986. The incidence and prevalence of LAV/HTLV-III infection in the San Francisco city clinic cohort 1985. Paper presented at the International Conference on AIDS, 23-26 June, Paris, France.

Eckholm, E. 1985. Women and AIDS: assessing the risks. *New York Times*, 28 November, pp. 8-9.

——. 1985. Prostitutes' impact on spread of AIDS debated. *New York Times*, 5 November, C1.

Eisenstat v. Baird, 405 U.S. 438 (1972).

Emmons, C. 1986. Psychosocial predictors of reported behavior change in homosexual men at risk for AIDS. *Health Education Quarterly*, 3:331-45.

Engel, G. L. 1977. The need for a new medical model: a challenge for biomedicine. *Science* 196:129-36.

——. 1982. The biopsychosocial model and medical education: who are to be the teachers? *N. Engl. J. Med.* 306:802-5.

Evatt, B. L., R. Ramsey, and D. Lawrence. 1984. Acquired immunodeficiency syndrome in patients with hemophilia. *Ann Intern. Med.* 100:499-504.

Evatt, B. L., E. Gomperts, and S. McGougal. 1985. Coincidental appearance of LAV/HTLV-III antibodies in hemophiliacs and the onset of the AIDS epidemic. *N. Engl. J. Med.* 312:483-86.

Fauci, A. S. 1985. Acquired immunodeficiency syndrome: an update. *Ann. Intern. Med.* 102:800-13.

Fauci, A. S., M. Macher, and D. Longo. 1984. Acquired immunodeficiency syndrome: epidemiologic, clinical immunologic and therapeutic considerations. *Ann. Intern. Med.* 100:92-106.

Feorino, P. M., H. Jaffe, and E. Palmer. 1985. Transfusion-associated acquired immunodeficiency syndrome: evidence for persistent infection in blood donors. *N. Engl. J. Med.* 312:1293-96.

Forstein, M., P. Page, and R. Carwell. 1985. Letter to the editor. *N. Engl. J. Med.* 313:1158.

Francis, D. P., P. Feorino, and J. Broderson. 1984. Infection of chimpanzees with lymphadenopathy-associated virus (letter). *Lancet* 2:1276-77.

Freidson, E. 1984. *The profession of medicine.* New York: Dodd Mead.

Friedland, G. H., C. Harris, and C. Butkus-Small. 1985. Intravenous drug abusers and the acquired immunodeficiency syndrome: demographic, drug use, and needle-sharing patterns. *Arch. Intern. Med.* 145:1413-17.

Friedman, S., D. Des Jarlais, and J. Sotheran. 1986. AIDS health education for intravenous drug users. *Health Education Quarterly* 13:383-93.

Friedman, S. R., and D. Des Jarlais. Knowledge of AIDS, behavioral change, and organization among intravenous drug users. Presented at the Stichting Drug Symposium. In press.

Gallo, R. C., S. Salahuddin, and M. Popovic. 1984. Frequent detection and isolation of cytopathic retroviruses (HTLV-III) from patients with AIDS and at risk for AIDS. *Science* 224:500-3.

Gallup Organization Poll. November 1985.

Ginzburg, H. M. 1984a. A survey of attitudes concerning AIDS among clients in treatment. *Clinical Research Notes.* National Institute on Drug Abuse, Rockville, Maryland.

Ginzburg, H. M. 1984b. Intravenous drug users and the acquired immune deficiency syndrome. *Public Health Reports* 99(2):206-12.

Ginzburg, H. M. 1984c. Intravenous drug users and the acquired immune deficiency syndrome. *Public Health Reports* 99:206-12.

Goedert, J. J., M. Sarngadharan, and R. Biggar. 1984. Determinants of retrovirus (HTLV-III) antibody and immunodeficiency conditions in homosexual men. *Lancet* 2:711-16.

Goedert, J. J., and W. Blattner. 1985. The epidemiology of AIDS and related conditions. In *AIDS etiology, diagnosis, treatment and prevention*, ed. V. T. DeVita, S. Hellman, and S. A. Rosenberg. Philadelphia, Pennsylvania: J. B. Lippincott, 1-30.

Goldberg, R. J. 1981. Management of depression in the patient with advanced cancer. *J.A.M.A.* 246:373-76.

Goldsmith, D., D. Hunt, D. Strug, and D. Lipton. 1984. Methadone folklore: beliefs about side effects and their impact on treatment. *Human Organization* 43:330-40.

Gottlieb, M. S., R. Schroff, and H. Schanker. 1981. *Pneumocytis carinii* pneumonia and mucosal candidiasis in previously healthy homosexual men. *N. Engl. J. Med.* 305:1425-31.

Griswold v. Connecticut, 381 U.S. 479 (1965).

Groopman, J. E., S. Salahuddin, and M. Sarngadharan. 1984. HTLV-III in saliva of people with AIDS-related complex and healthy homosexual men at risk for AIDS. *Science* 226:447-49.

Grossman, R. J. 1984. Psychosocial support in AIDS: a practitioner's view. In *AIDS*, eds. A. Friedman-Kien and L. J. Lauberstein. New York: Masson, Inc.

Guinan, M., P. Thomas, and P. Pinsky. 1984. Heterosexual and homosexual patients with the acquired immunodeficiency syndrome. *Ann. Intern. Med.* 100:213-18.

Hackett, T. P., and N. Cassem. 1970. Psychological reactions to a life-threatening illness. In *Psychological aspects of stress*, ed. H. Abram. Springfield, Illinois: Charles C. Thomas, 29-43.

Hardy, A. M. 1986. Using death certificates to determine the level of AIDS case reporting. Paper presented at the International Conference on AIDS, 23 June, Paris, France.

Hardy, A. M., J. Allen, and W. Morgan. 1985. The incidence rate of acquired immunodeficiency syndrome in selected populations. *J.A.M.A.* 253:215-20.

Harris, C., C. Small, and R. Klein. 1983. Needle sharing as a route of transmission of the acquired immune deficiency syndrome. In *Twenty-Third Interscience Conference of Antimicrobial Agents and Chemotherapy*, Abstract 632A. Las Vegas, Nevada: American Society for Microbiology.

Harris, C. A., C. Cabradilla, and R. Klein. 1983. Immunodeficiency in female sexual partners of men with acquired immune deficiency syndrome. *N. Engl. J. Med.* 308:1181-84.

———. Antibodies to a core protein of lymphadenopathy-associated virus and immunodeficiency in heterosexual partners of AIDS patients. In *Twenty-Fourth Interscience Conference on Antimicrobial Agents and Chemotherapy*, Abstract 64. Washington, D.C.: American Society for Microbiology.

Haussman, K. 1983. Treating victims of AIDS poses challenge to psychiatrists. *Psychiatric News*, 5 Aug.

Heidegger, M. 1962. *Being and Time.* J. Macquarrie and E. Robinson, Translators. New York: Harper and Row.

Hirsch, M. S., G. Wormser, and R. Schooley. 1985. Risk of nosocomial infection with human T-cell lymphotropic virus III (HTLV-III). *N. Engl. J. Med.* 312:1-4.

Ho, D. D., R. Schooley, and T. Rota. 1984. HTLV-III in the semen and blood of a healthy homosexual man. *Science* 226:451-53.

Ho, D. D., T. Rota, R. Schooley, and J. Kaplan. 1985. Isolation of HIV from cerebrospinal fluid and neural tissues of patients with neurologic syndromes related to the acquired immunodeficiency syndrome. *N. Engl. J. Med.* 313:1493-97.

Hoffman, R. S. 1984. Neuropsychiatric complications of AIDS. *Psychosomatics* 25:393-400.

Holland, J. C. B. 1985. Psychosocial and neuropsychiatric sequelae of AIDS and AIDS-associated disorders: an overview. Paper presented at the International Conference on Acquired Immune Deficiency Syndrome (AIDS), 14-17 April. Atlanta, Georgia.

Holtz, M., J. Dobro, and R. Palinkas. 1983. Psychological impact of AIDS. *J.A.M.A.* 250:167.

Horowitz, M. T. 1973. *Stress response syndromes.* New York: Jason Aranson.

Hunsmann, G., J. Schneider, and H. Bayer. 1985. Seroepidemiology of HTLV-III/LAV in the Federal Republic of Germany. *Klin. Wochenschr.* 63:233-35.

Institute of Medicine. 1986. *Confronting AIDS: directions for public health, health care and research.* Washington, D.C.: National Academy Press.

Jaffe, H. W., J. Bregman, and R. Selik. 1983. AIDS in the United States: the first 1,000 cases. *J. Infect. Dis.* 148:339-45.

Jaffe, H. W., K. Choi, and P. Thomas. 1983. National case-control study of Kaposi's sarcoma and *Pneumocystis carinii* pneumonia in homosexual men. Part 1. Epidemiologic results. *Ann. Intern. Med.* 99:145-51.

Jaffe, H. W., W. Darrow, and D. Echenberg. 1985. The acquired immunodeficiency syndrome in a cohort of homosexual men: a six-year follow-up study. *Ann. Intern. Med.* 103:210-14.

Jett, J. R., J. Kuritsky, and A. Katzmann. 1984. Acquired immunodeficiency syndrome associated with blood-product transfusions. *Ann. Intern. Med.* 99:621-24.

Johnson, B. D. 1973. *Marijuana users and drug subcultures.* New York: John Wiley.

———. 1980. Toward a theory of drug subcultures. In *Theories on drug abuse,* ed. D. J. Lettiere. NIDA Research Monograph 30. Rockville, Maryland: National Institute on Drug Abuse, 110-19.

Johnson, B. D., P. Goldstein, and E. Preble. 1985. *Taking care of business: the economics of crime by heroin abusers.* Lexington, Massachusetts: Lexington Books.

Joncas, J. H., G. Delage, and Z. Chad. 1983. Acquired (or congenital) immunodeficiency syndrome in infants born of Haitian mothers (letter). *N. Engl. J. Med.* 308:842.

Jonsen, A. R., M. Siegler, and W. Winslade. 1982. *Clinical ethics.* New York: Macmillan.

Joseph, J. G., C. Emmons, and R. Kessler. 1985. Changes in sexual behavior of gay men: relationships to perceived stress and psychological symptomatology. Paper presented at the International Conference on the Acquired Immune Deficiency Syndrome (AIDS), 14-17 April, Atlanta, Georgia.

Kaplan, E. L., and P. Meier. 1958. Nonparametric estimation from incomplete observations. *J. Am. Stat. Assoc.* 53:457-81.

Karasu, T. B. 1978. Utilization of a psychiatric consultation service. *Psychosomatics* 19:467-73.

Kathleen v. Robert, 150 Cal.Apped 992, 198 Cal Rptr 273 (1984).

Kemani, E., S. Drob, and M. Alpert. 1984. Organic brain syndromes in three cases of AIDS. *Comp. Psychiat.* 25:292-97.

Kimball, C. P. 1981. *The biopsychosocial approach to the patient.* Baltimore, Maryland: Williams & Wilkins.

Klatzmann, D., F. Barre-Sinoussi, and M. Nugeyre. 1984. Selective tropism of lymphadenopathy associated virus (LAV) for helper inducer T lymphocytes. *Science* 225:59-63.

Klein, R. S., C. Harris, and C. Small. 1984. Oral candidiasis in high-risk patients as the initial manifestation of the acquired immunodeficiency syndrome. *N. Engl. J. Med.* 311:354-58.

Krown, S. E. 1984. Kaposi's sarcoma and AIDS: clinical manifestations and treatment. *J. Psychosocial Oncol.* 2:1-17.

Kubler-Ross, E. 1962. *On death and dying.* New York: MacMillan Publishing Co.

Kuehnle, J., and R. Spitzer. 1981. DSM-III classification of substance use disorders. In *Substance abuse: clinical problems and perspectives*, eds. J. Lowinson and R. Ruiz. Baltimore, Maryland: Williams and Wilkins.

Landesman, S. H., H. Ginzburg, and S. Weiss. 1985. Special report: the AIDS epidemic. *N. Engl. J. Med.* 312:521-25.

Larsen, K. S., M. Reed, and S. Hoffman. 1980. Attitudes of heterosexuals toward homosexuality. *J. Sex Res.* 16:245-49.

Laurence, J., F. Brun-Vezinet, and S. Schutzer. 1984. Lymphadenopathy associated viral antibody in AIDS: immune correlations and definition of a carrier state. *N. Engl. J. Med.* 311:1269-73.

Lawrence, D. N., K. Lui, D. Bregman, T. Peterman, and W. Morgan. 1985. A model-based estimate of the average incubation and latency period for transfusion-associated AIDS. Paper presented at the International Conference on Acquired Immune Deficiency Syndrome (AIDS), 14 April. Atlanta, Georgia.

Levengood, R., P. Lowinger, and K. Schoof. Heroin addiction in the suburbs – An epidemiologic study. *Am. J. Public Health* 63:209-14.

Levy, J. A., A. Hoffman, and S. Kramer. 1984. Isolation of lymphocytopathic retrovirus from San Francisco patients with AIDS. *Science* 225:840-42.

Levy, J. A., L. Kaminsky, and W. Morrow. 1985. Infection by the retrovirus associated with the acquired immunodeficiency syndrome: clinical, biological, and molecular features. *Ann. Intern. Med.* 103:604-9.

Levy, R. M., D. Bredesen, and M. Rosenblum. 1985. Neurological manifestations of the acquired immune deficiency syndrome (AIDS): experience at UCSF and review of the literature. *J. Neurosurg.* 62:475-95.

Lewis, B. F., and R. Galea. 1986. A survey of the perceptions of drug abusers concerning the acquired immunodeficiency syndrome (AIDS). *Health Matrix* 4:14-17.

Lo, B., and R. Steinbrook. 1983. Deciding whether to resuscitate. *Arch. Intern. Med.* 143:1561-63.

Louria, D., T. Hensle, and J. Rose. 1967. The major medical complications of heroin addiction. *Ann. Intern. Med.* 67:1-22.

Lowenstein, R. J., and S. Sharfstein. 1983-84. Neuro-psychiatric aspects of AIDS. *Int. J. Psychiat. Med.* 13:255-61.

Maayan, S., G. Wormser, and D. Hewlett. 1985. Acquired immunodeficiency syndrome (AIDS) in an economically disadvantaged population. *Arch. Intern. Med.* 145:1607-12.

Macdonald, D. I. 1986. Coolfont report: a PHS plan for prevention and control of AIDS and AIDS virus. *Public Health Reports* 101:34-38.

Macek, C. 1982. Acquired immunodeficiency syndrome cause(s) still elusive. *J.A.M.A.* 248:1423-31.

Malebranch, R., J. Guerin, and A. Raroche. 1983. Acquired immunodeficiency syndrome with severe gastrointestinal manifestation in Haiti. *Lancet* 1:873-76.

Malyon, A. K., and A. Pinka. 1983. Acquired immune deficiency syndrome: a challenge to psychology. *Profess. Psychol.* 7:1-10.

Marmor, M., A. Friedman-Kien, and L. Laubenstein. 1982. Risk factors for Kaposi's sarcoma in homosexual men. *Lancet* 1:183-87.

Marmor, M., A. Friedman-Kien, and S. Zolla-Pazner. 1984. Kaposi's sarcoma in homosexual men: a seroepidemiologic case-control study. *Ann. Intern. Med.* 100:809-15.

Marmor, M., D. Des Jarlais, and S. Friedman. 1984. The epidemic of acquired immunodeficiency syndrome (AIDS) and suggestions for its control in drug abusers. *J. Substance Abuse Treatment* 1:237-47.

Martin, J. L. 1986. Sexual behavior patterns, behavior change, and occurrence of antibody to LAV/HTLV-III among New York City gay men. Paper presented at the International Conference on AIDS, 23-26 June. Paris, France.

Massachusetts Department of Public Health. 1987. Radio presentation.

Masur, H., M. Michelis, and J. Greene, 1984. An outbreak of community-acquired *Pneumocystis carinii* pneumonia: initial manifestation of cellular immune dysfunction. *N. Engl. J. Med.* 311:328.

Matter of Application to quash subpoena duces tecum in grand jury proceedings, 56 N.Y.2d 348, 452 N.Y.S.2d 361, 437 N.E.2d 1118 (1981).

McDonough, R. J., J. Madden, and A. Falek. 1980. Aberration of T and null lymphocyte frequencies in the peripheral blood of human opiate addicts: in vivo evidence for opiate receptor sites on T lymphocytes. *J. Immunol.* 125:2539-43.

McKusick, L., W. Hortsman, and T. Coates. 1985. AIDS and sexual behavior reported by gay men in San Francisco. *Am. J. Public Health* 75:493-96.

Melbye, M., R. Biggar, and P. Ebbesen. 1984. Seroepidemiology of HTLV-III antibody in Danish homosexual men: prevalence, transmission, and disease outcome. *Br. Med. J.* 289:573-75.

Miller, J. D. 1983. *National survey on drug abuse: main findings, 1982.* Rockville, Maryland: National Institute on Drug Abuse.

Moll, B., E. Emeson, and C. Small. 1983. Inverted ratio of inducer to suppressor T-lymphocyte subsets in drug abusers with opportunistic infections. *Clin. Immunol. Immunopathol.* 24:417-23.

Monthly AIDS Data. 1984. New Jersey State Department of Health.

Moore, J. 1986. HTLV-III seropositivity in 1971-1972 parenteral drug users: a case of false positives or evidence of viral exposure. *N. Engl. J. Med.* 314:1387-88.

Moos, R., ed. 1977. *Coping with physical illness.* New York: Plenum.

Morgan, W. M., and J. Curran. Acquired immunodeficiency syndrome: current and future trends. *Public Health Reports* 101:459-64.

Morin, S. F., and W. Batchelor. 1984. Responding to the psychological crisis of AIDS. *Public Health Reports* 99:4-9.

Morris, L., A. Distenfeld, and E. Amorosi. 1982. Autoimmune thrombocytopenic purpua in homosexual men. *Ann. Intern. Med.* 96(part 1):714-17.

Moss, A. R. 1984. Mortality associated with mode of presentation in the acquired immune deficiency syndrome. *J. Natl. Cancer Inst.* 73:1281-84.

National Academy of Sciences. 1986. *Mobilizing against AIDS.* Cambridge, Massachusetts: Harvard University Press.

National Hemophilia Foundation Medical and Scientific Advisory Council. 1984. *Recommendations concerning AIDS and therapy of hemophilia.* New York: National Hemophilia Foundation.

National Institute on Drug Abuse. 1982. *Client Oriented Data Acquisition Process (CODAP)*. Annual data 1981, series E, no. 25, Statistical Series. Rockville, Maryland.

National Institute on Drug Abuse. 1982. *National drug and alcoholism treatment utilization survey.* Summary report on drug abuse treatment units, September, Rockville, Maryland.

Navia, B. A., and R. W. Price. 1986. Dementia complicating AIDS. *Psychol. Ann.* 16:158-66.

Needlestick transmission of HTLV-III from a patient infected in Africa. 1984. *Lancet* 1:1376-77.

Newmeyer, J. 1985. Drug abuse in the San Francisco Bay area: June 1985. In *Patterns and trends in drug abuse: a national and international perspective.* Bethesda, Maryland: National Institute on Drug Abuse.

Newsweek Poll on homosexuality. 1983. *Newsweek*, 8 August p. 33.

New York State Office of Substance Abuse Services. 1983. *AIDS Newsletter*, December.

New York City Department of Health, Surveillance Office. 1987. *AIDS Surveillance Update*, 28 January.

Nichols, S. E., Jr. 1983. Psychiatric aspects of AIDS. *Psychosomatics* 24:1083-9.

Nichols, S. E. Psychotherapy and AIDS. In *Avenues to understanding psychotherapy in gay men and lesbians*, eds. T. S. Stein and C. J. Cohen. New York: Plenum Press (in press).

Nichols, S. E. 1984. The social climate when the acquired immune deficiency syndrome developed. In *Psychiatric implications of the acquired immune deficiency syndrome*, eds. S. E. Nichols and D. G. Ostrow. Washington, D.C.: American Psychiatric Press, 85-92.

Nicholson, J. K. A., J. McDougal, and H. Jaffe. 1984. Exposure to human T-lymphotropic virus type III/lymphadenopathy-associated virus and immunologic abnormalities in asymptomatic homosexual men. *Ann. Intern. Med.* 103:37-42.

Novick, D., M. Kreek, and D. Des Jarlais. Antibody to LAV in parenteral drug abusers and methadone maintained patients: therapeutic, historical and ethical aspects. In press.

——. Antibodies to LAV in New York City: historical and ethical considerations. In *Proceedings of the 46th Annual Scientific Meeting, Committee on Problems of Drug Dependence*, ed. L. Harris. Bethesda, Maryland: National Institute on Drug Abuse. In Press.

O'Donnell, J. A. 1976. *Young men and drugs* – A nationwide survey. National Institute on Drug Abuse, Research Monograph Series 5. DHEW Publication No. (ADM) 76-311. Washington, D.C.: U.S. Government Printing Office.

O'Donnell, J. A., and J. Jones. 1968. Diffusion on the intravenous technique among narcotic addicts in the United States. *J. Health Soc. Behav.* 9:120-89.

Ochitill, H., M. Perl, and J. Dilley. 1984-85. Case reports of psychological disturbances in patients with AIDS. *Int. J. Psychiat. Med.* 14:259-63.

Offenstadt, G., P. Pinta, and P. Hericord. 1983. Multiple opportunistic infection due to AIDS in a previously healthy black woman from Zaire (letter). *N. Engl. J. Med.* 308:775.

Oleske, J., A. Minnefor, and R. Cooper. 1983. Immune deficiency syndrome in children. *J.A.M.A.* 249:2345-49.

Osmond, D., A. Moss, P. Bachetti, P. Volberding, F. Barre-Sinoussi, and J. Chermann. 1985. A case-control study of risk factor of AIDS in San Francisco. In *The International Conference on the Acquired Immunodeficiency Syndrome: Abstracts.* Philadelphia, Pennsylvania: American College of Physicians.

Pape, J. W., B. Liautaud, and F. Thomas. 1983. Characteristics of the acquired immunodeficiency syndrome in (AIDS) in Haiti. *N. Engl. J. Med.* 309:945-50.

——. 1985. The acquired immunodeficiency syndrome in Haiti. *Ann. Intern. Med.* 103:674-78.

Parkes, C. M. 1971. Psychosocial transitions; a field for study. *Soc. Sci. Med.* 5:101-15.

Perlin, S., ed. 1975. *A handbook for the study of suicide.* New York: Oxford University Press.

Peterman, T. A., H. Jaffe, and P. Feorino. 1985. Transfusion-associated acquired immunodeficiency syndrome in the United States. *J.A.M.A.* 254:2913-17.

Petito, C. K., B. Navja, E. Cho, B. Jordan, D. George, and R. Prince. 1985. Vacuolar myelopathy pathologically resembling subacute combined degeneration in patients with the acquired immunodeficiency syndrome. *N. Engl. J. Med.* 312:874-78.

Piot, P., H. Tailman, and K. Minlangu. 1984. Acquired immunodeficiency syndrome in a heterosexual population in Zaire. *Lancet* 2:65-69.

Plumb, M. M., and J. Holland. 1977. Comparative studies of psychological function in patients with advanced cancer. *Psychosom. Med.* 39:264-75.

Polk, B. F. 1987. Predictors of the acquired immunodeficiency syndrome developing in a cohort of seropositive homosexual men. *N. Engl. J. Med.* 316:61-66.

Preble, E., and J. H. Casey. 1969. Taking care of business: the heroin user's life on the street. *Int. J. Addictions* 4:1-24.

President's Commission for the Study of Ethical Problems in Medicine and Biomedical Problems in Medicine and Biomedical and Behavioral Research. 1983. *Deciding to forego life-sustaining treatment*, a Report on the Ethical, Medical and Legal Issues in Treatment Decisions. Washington, D.C.: Government Printing Office.

Protection of identity of research subjects, 44 FED. REG. 20382-87, 1979.

Ramsey, R. B., E. Palmer, and J. McDougal. 1984. Antibody to lymphadenopathy associated virus in hemophiliacs with and without AIDS. *Lancet* 2:397-98.

Redfield, R. R., P. Markham, and S. Salahuddin. 1985a. Frequent transmission of HTLV-III among spouses of patients with AIDS-related complex (ARC) and the acquired immunodeficiency syndrome (AIDS): a family study. *J.A.M.A.* 253:1571-73.

——. 1985b. Heterosexually acquired HTLV-III/LAV disease (AIDS-related complex and AIDS), epidemiologic evidence for female-to-female transmission. *J.A.M.A.* 254:2094-6.

Rivin, B. E., J. Monroe, and B. Hubschuman, 1984. AIDS outcome: a first follow-up (letter). *N. Engl. J. Med.* 311:857.

Robertson, J. R., A Bucknall, and P. Welsby. 1986. Epidemic of AIDS related virus (HTLV-III/LAV) infection among intravenous drug abusers. *Br. Med. J.* 292:527-29.

Rodrigo, J. M., M. Serra, E. Aguilar, D. Del Olmo, V. Gimeno, and L. Aparisi. 1985. HTLV-III antibodies in drug addicts in Spain. *Lancet* 2:156-57.

Rogers, C. R. 1974. In retrospect: 46 years. *Am. Psychol.* 29:115-23.

Rosenstock, I. M. 1966. Why people use health services. *Milbank Mem. Fund Quarterly* 44(suppl.):94-124.

Rossi, A. S. 1980. The middle years of parenting. In *Life-span development and behavior*, vol. 3, eds. P. Baltes and O. Brim Jr. New York: Academic Press.

Rubinstein, A., M. Sickick, and A. Gupta. 1983. Acquired immunodeficiency with reverse T4/T8 ratios in infants born to promiscuous and drug-addicted mothers. *J.A.M.A.* 249:2350-56.

Sabbath, J. 1969. The suicidal adolescent: the expendable child. *J. Am. Acad. Child Psychiat.* 8:272-89.

Safai, B., M. Sarngadharan, and J. Groopman. 1984. Seroepidemiological studies of human T-lymphotropic retrovirus type III in acquired immunodeficiency syndrome. *Lancet* 1:1438-40.

San Francisco Department of Public Health. 1986. San Francisco AIDS cases by age, group, race/ethnicity and patient group through 4/30/86, May, San Francisco, California.

San Francisco Department of Public Health. 1987. AIDS in IV drug users, San Francisco. 1979-86. *San Francisco Epidemiol. Bull.* 2:1-2.

Sarngadharan, M. G., M. Popovic, and L. Bruch. 1984. Antibodies reactive with human T-lymphotropic retroviruses (HTLV-III) in the serum of patients with AIDS. *Science* 224:506-8.

Schneidman, E. S. 1981. *Suicide thoughts and reflections, 1960-1980.* New York: Human Sciences Press.

Schupbach, J., O. Haller, and M. Vogt. 1985. Antibodies to HTLV-III in Swiss patients with AIDS and pre-AIDS and in groups at risk for AIDS. *N. Engl. J. Med.* 312:265-70.

Scott, G. B., B. Buck, and J. Letterman. 1984. Acquired immuno-deficiency syndrome in infants. *N. Engl. J. Med.* 310:76-81.

Selik, R. M., H. Haverkos, and J. Curran. 1984. Acquired immune deficiency syndrome (AIDS) trends in the United States, 1978-1982. *Am J. Med.* 76:493-500.

Sells, S. B., ed. 1974. *The effectiveness of drug abuse treatment: evaluation of treatment*, vol. 1. Cambridge, Massachusetts: Ballinger Publishing Co.

Selwyn, P. A., C. Cox, C. Feiner, C. Lipshutz, and R. Cohen. 1985. Knowledge about AIDS and high-risk behavior among intravenous drug abusers in New York City. Paper presented at the Annual Meeting of the American Public Health Association, 18 November, Washington, D.C.

Shaw, G., M. Harper, and B. Hahn. 1985. HTLV-III infection in brains of children and adults with encephalopathy. *Science* 227:177-81.

Sheretz, R. J. 1985. Acquired immunodeficiency syndrome: a perspective for the medical practitioner. *Med. Clin. N. Am.* 69:637-55.

Sherlock, S. 1981. *Diseases of the liver and biliary system.* Oxford, England: Blackwell Scientific Publications.

Shine, D., B. Moll, and E. Emeson. 1985. Serologic, immunologic, and clinical features of I.V. drug abusers without AIDS. In *The International Conference on the Acquired Immunodeficiency Syndrome: Abstracts.* Philadelphia, Pennsylvania: American College of Physicians.

Shortell, S. M., and R. Daniels. 1974. Referral relationships between internists and psychiatrists in fee-for-service practice. *Med. Care* 12:229-40.

Shumaker, S. A., and A. Brownell. 1985. Toward a theory of social support. *Social Forces* 40:11-33.

Siegal, F. P., C. Lopez, and G. Hammer. 1981. Severe acquired immunodeficiency in homosexual males manifested by chronic perianal and herpes simplex lesions. *N. Engl. J. Med.* 305:1439-44.

Siegel, K., and L. Bauman. 1986. Patterns of change in sexual practices among gay men in New York City. Paper presented at the Annual Meetings of the American Sociological Association, August, New York City.

Siegel, R. L., and D. Hoefer. 1981. Bereavement counseling for gay individuals. *Am. J. Psychother.* 35:517-25.

Simpson, D. D., L. Savage, and S. Sells. 1978. *Data book on drug treatment outcomes.* Fort Worth, Texas: Institute of Behavioral Research.

Singer, E., and T. Rogers. 1986. Public opinion and AIDS. *AIDS and Public Policy* 1:8-13.

Small, C. B., R. Klein, and G. Friedland. 1983. Community-acquired opportunistic infections and defective cellular immunity in heterosexual drug abusers and homosexual men. *Am. J. Med.* 74:433-41.

Snider, W. D., D. Simpson, and S. Nielson. 1983. Neurological complications of acquired immune deficiency syndrome: analysis of 50 patients. *Ann. Neurol.* 14:403-18.

Sontag, S. 1977. *Illness as metaphor.* New York: Vintage Books.

Sourcebook of Criminal Justice Statistics, 1984. 1985. Washington, D.C.: General Printing Office, p. 629.

Spira, T. J., D. Des Jarlais, and M. Marmor. 1984. Prevalence of antibody to lymphadenopathy-associated virus among drug-detoxification patients in New York. *N. Engl. J. Med.* 311:467-68.

Spira, T. J., D. Des Jarlais, and D. Bokos. 1985a. HTLV-III/LAV antibodies in intravenous drug (IV) abusers—Comparison of high and low risk areas for AIDS. Paper presented at the International Conference on Acquired Immune Deficiency Syndrome (AIDS), 14-17 April, Atlanta, Georgia.

——. 1985b. HTLV-III/LAV antibodies in intravenous (IV) drug abusers—Comparison of high and low risk areas for AIDS. In

The International Conference on the Acquired Immunodeficiency Syndrome: Abstracts. Philadelphia, Pennsylvania: American College of Physicians.

Stoneburner, R. L., and A. Kristal. 1985a. Increasing tuberculosis incidence and its relationship to acquired immunodeficiency syndrome in New York City. Paper presented at the International Conference on Acquired Immune Deficiency Syndrome (AIDS), 14-17 April, Atlanta, Georgia.

——. 1985b. Increasing tuberculosis incidence and its relationship to acquired immunodeficiency syndrome in New York City. In *The International Conference on the Acquired Immunodeficiency Syndrome: Abstracts.* Philadelphia, Pennsylvania: American College of Physicians.

Thomas, P. A., H. Jaffe, T. Spira, R. Reiss, I. Guerrero, and D. Auerbach. 1985. Unexplained immunodeficiency in children: a surveillance report. *J.A.M.A.* 252:639-44.

Tripp, C. A. 1975. *The homosexual matrix.* New York: McGraw-Hill.

Tross, S., R. Price, and J. Sidtis. 1985. Psychological and neuropsychological function in AIDS spectrum disorder patients. Paper presented at the International Conference on Acquired Immune Deficiency Syndrome (AIDS), 14-17 April, Atlanta, Georgia.

Tucker, J., C. Ludlam, and A. Craig. 1984. HTLV-III infection associated with glandular-fever-like illness in a haemophiliac (letter). *Lancet* 1:585.

Tyhurst, J. S. 1951. Reactions to community disaster: the natural history of psychiatric phenomena. *Am. J. Psychiat.* 107:764-69.

Van de Perre, P., P. Le Page, and P. Kestlyn. 1984. Acquired immunodeficiency syndrome in Rwanda. *Lancet* 2:62-65.

Van de Wijngaart, G. F. 1984. The "Junkie League" promoting the interests of the Dutch hard-drug user. Paper presented at The 14th International Institute of the Prevention and Treatment of Drug Dependence, May, Athens, Greece.

Vieira, J., E. Frank, T. Spira, and S. H. Landesman. 1983. Acquired immune deficiency in Haitians; opportunistic infections in previously healthy Haitian immigrants. *N. Engl. J. Med.* 308:125-29.

Wallace, S. E., and A. Eser, eds. 1981. *Suicide and euthanasia: the rights of personhood.* Knoxville, Tennessee: University of Tennessee Press.

Weinberg, S., and C. Williams. 1984. *Male homosexuals: their problems and adaptations.* New York: Oxford University Press.

Weis, R. S. 1976. Transition states and other stressful situations: their nature and programs for their management. In *Support systems and mutual help*, eds. G. Kaplan and M. Killilea. New York: Grune & Stratton, 213-32.

Weisman, A. D., and J. Worden. 1976-77. The existential plight in cancer: significance of the first 100 days. *Int. J. Psychiat. Med.* 7:1015.

Weiss, S. H., H. Ginzburg, and J. Goedert. 1985. Risk for HTLV-III exposure to AIDS among parenteral drug abusers in New Jersey. Paper presented at the International Conference on Acquired Immune Deficiency Syndrome (AIDS), 14-17 April, Atlanta, Georgia.

——. 1985. Risk for HTLV-III exposure and AIDS among parenteral drug abusers in New Jersey. In *The International Conference on the Acquired Immunodeficiency Syndrome: Abstracts.* Philadelphia, Pennsylvania: American College of Physicians.

Weiss, S. H., J. Goedert, and M. Sarngadharan. 1985. Screening test for HTLV-III (AIDS agent) antibodies: specificity, sensitivity, and applications. *J.A.M.A.* 253:221-25.

Weiss, S. H., W. Saxinger, and D. Rechtman. 1985. HTLV-III infection among health care workers: association with needle-stick injuries. *J.A.M.A.* 254:2089-93.

Weissman, M. W. 1976. Clinical depression among addicts maintained on methadone in the community. *Am. J. Psychiat.* 13:1434-38.

Weppner, R. S., ed. 1977. *Street ethnography.* Beverly Hills, California: Sage.

Wikler, A. 1980. A theory of opioid dependence. In *Theories on drug abuse*, eds. D. J. Lettieri, M. Sayers, and H. W. Pearson. Rockville, Maryland: National Institute on Drug Abuse.

Womser, G. P. 1983. Acquired immunodeficiency syndrome in male prisoners: new insights into an emerging syndrome. *Ann. Intern. Med.* 98:297-303.

Wong-Staal, F., and R. Gallo. 1985. Human T-lymphotropic retroviruses. *Nature* 317:395-403.

Wong-Staal, F., G. Shaw, and B. Hahn. 1985. Genetic diversity of human T-lymphotropic virus type III (HTLV-III). *Science* 229:759-65.

Zagury, D., J. Bernard, and J. Leibowitch. 1984a. HTLV-III in cells cultured from semen of two patients with AIDS. *Science* 226:449-51.

Index